This book belongs to:

_____

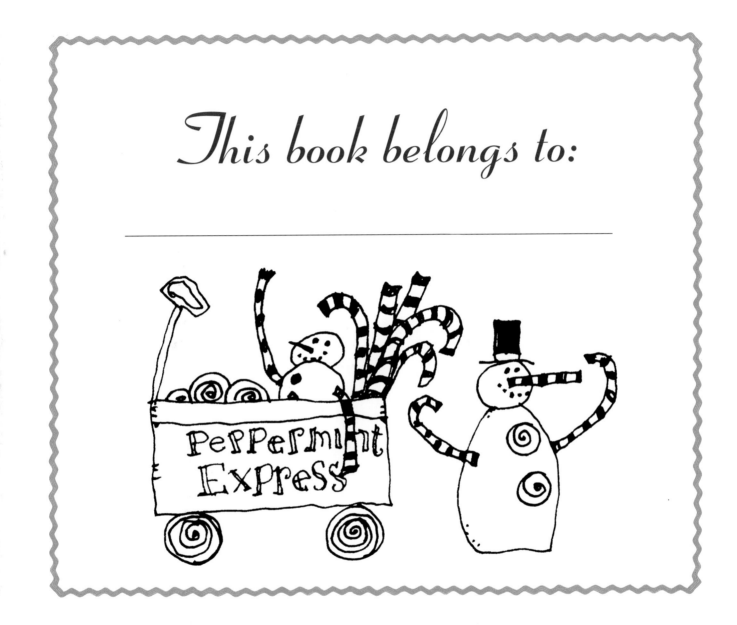

Old-Fashioned Fruitcake
(page 65)

SHAPE

lowfat
& easy

151 fast, delicious, nutritious, low-calorie recipes for weight loss from the editors of SHAPE

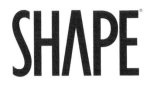

David Pecker **Chairman, President, CEO**
Bonnie Fuller **EVP, Chief Editorial Director**
Barbara Harris **EVP, Editorial Director, Active Lifestyle Group**
Anne M. Russell **Editor in Chief**
Jacqueline C. Moorby **Art Director**

Joe Weider **Founding Chairman**
Ben Weider **President, International Federation of Bodybuilders**

SHAPE
Lowfat & Easy
Jeanine Detz **Editor**
Jennie Brewton **Art Director**
Colm Doherty **Designer**
Monica Gullon **Contributing Editor**
Amy Spitalnick **Copy Editor**
Fiona Maynard **Director, Rights and Permissions**
Renee Thompson **Manufacturing Manager**
Steve Lombardi **Director, Product Development**
James Lombardi **Manager, Product Development**

Recipes by Colleen Dunn Bates, Kathleen Daelmemans, Nancy Fox, Ramin Ganeshram, Elaine Glusac, Rozanne Gold, Monica Gullon, Beth Hensperger, Judith Benn Hurley, Angela Hynes, Robin Vitetta-Miller, M.S., Paul E. Piccuito, Victoria Abbott Riccardi, Nancy Rommelmann, Jenna Schnuer, Elizabeth Somer, M.A., R.D., Evelyn Tribole and Bradley J. Wilcox.

Photography by Mary Ellen Bartley, Leigh Beisch, Beatriz Da Costa, Reed Davis, Gentl & Hyers, Lisa Hubbard, Richard Jung, Catherine Ledner, Rita Maas, Anthony-Masterson, Jonelle P. Miller, Pornchai Mittongtare, Lisa Romerein, David Prince, Maria Robledo, David Roth, Ann Stratton, Lisa Thompson, Luca Trovato, Ondine Vierra and Jonelle Weaver.

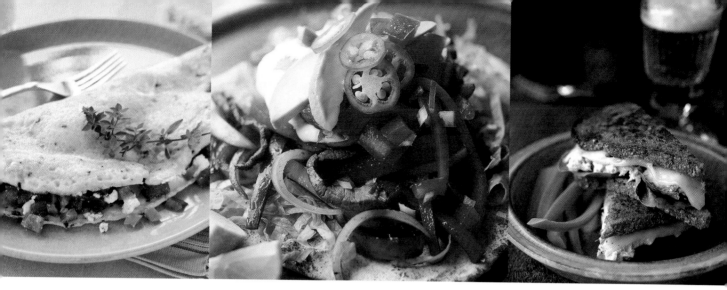

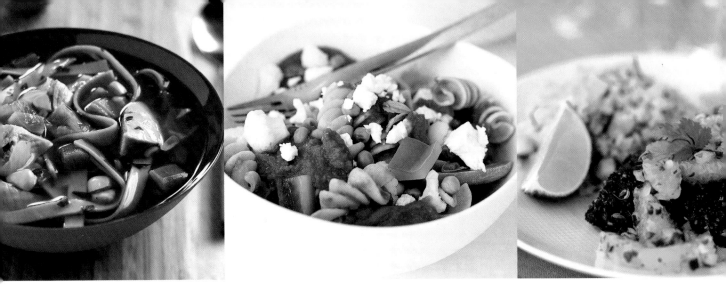

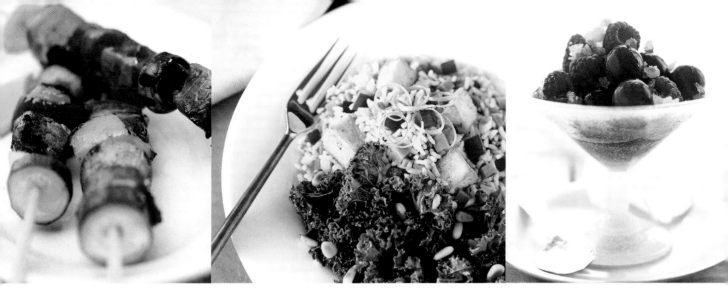

Classic Roast Chicken With Vegetables

Eat Well, Live Well

Do you love delicious food, but still want to look great and live healthfully? You can have your cake and eat it too – with a little help from SHAPE. The right recipes can help you lose weight, fight disease, boost energy levels and make your tastebuds tingle.

We've collected 151 favorites that reflect SHAPE's philosophy: A healthy diet is about celebration, not deprivation. That's why you'll find broccoli *and* chocolate on these pages, as well as dozens of other yummy and good-for-you ingredients. Our dishes offer a kaleidoscope of colors, scents and flavors to delight the senses: from the intense hues of tropical fruits and the earthy aroma of spices to the cool, refreshing taste of fresh herbs. Let them inspire you to embark on a healthier path that includes nurturing your spirit and mind, and strengthening your body through exercise.

Our recipes were created with the SHAPE Food Pyramid in mind. Based on the latest scientific studies regarding health and longevity, the Pyramid combines the best aspects of existing models and adds important new features. Here's a tier by tier look at our Pyramid, from the bottom up, along with a sneak peak at what you'll find in *Lowfat & Easy*.

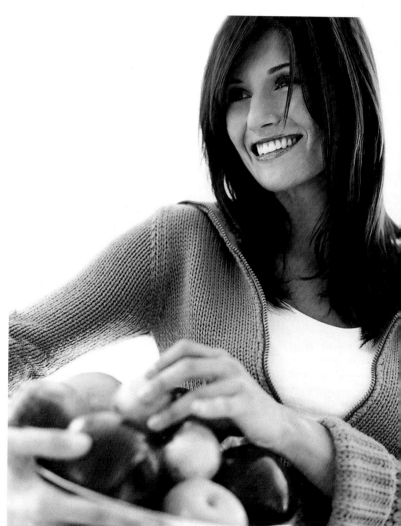

First Tier 8 or more servings a day of vegetables and fruits
Serving size: 1 piece, 1 cup raw, ½ cup canned or cooked, 1 ounce dried, 6 ounces juice

Packed with disease-fighting antioxidants, fruits and veggies are the building blocks of a healthy diet. Enjoy them fresh, frozen, canned or dried in every color of the rainbow. Choose vitamin-rich juices such as orange and tomato and skip sugary, refined ones.

The *Lowfat & Easy* way: Watermelon, Grilled Peach and Blackberry Salad with Honey-Yogurt Dressing; Oranges, Beets and Greens With Goat-Cheese Toast Points; Curried Pumpkin Soup; Broccoli Bake; Veggie Hippie Hero; Warm Rhubarb Compote With Vanilla-Yogurt Timbale

Second Tier 8 or more servings a day of water
Serving size: 1 cup

Elevate water's humble status by serving it in beautiful pitchers and glassware. Perk up ordinary tap water by adding citrus or cucumber slices, bruised fresh herbs (like mint and basil) or frozen berries.

Third Tier 6 or more servings a day of whole grains
Serving size: 1 slice bread; ½ English muffin; ½ hamburger bun; ½ bagel; 1 ounce ready-to-eat cereal; ½ cup cooked pasta, rice or cereal; 1 tortilla

Whole-grain foods take longer to eat, so they're more satisfying. They're also lower in calories. For example, a cup of cooked whole-wheat spaghetti has 6 grams of fiber and 170 calories, while the same amount of enriched spaghetti has only 2 grams of fiber, but 200 calories.

The *Lowfat & Easy* way: Cinnamon-Wheat Pancakes With Hot Boysenberry Compote; Quinoa Salad With Vegetables and Feta; Chicken Barley Soup With Vegetables; Grilled Turkey Club

Fourth Tier 3 servings a day of nonfat milk and dairy products and fortified soy milk
Serving size: 1 cup milk, 1 ounce cheese, 1 cup yogurt, 1 cup soy milk

Nonfat and 1 percent milk products are excellent sources of calcium. Flavored yogurts are high in sugar, so choose plain and serve with fresh berries instead. If you opt for soy milk, make sure it's fortified with vitamin D and calcium.

The *Lowfat & Easy* way: Three-Cheese Vegetable Quesadillas; Eggplant, Roasted Red Peppers and Mozzarella Sandwich; Mac 'n Cheese; Greek Pizza; Vanilla-Pistachio Panna Cotta

Fifth Tier 1-2 servings a day of legumes: beans, chickpeas, lentils, soy beans
Serving size: ¾ cup cooked

Legumes are high in protein and fiber, and packed with disease-protective nutrients. If you don't have the patience for their longer cooking times, buy canned or partially cooked frozen legumes.

The *Lowfat & Easy* way: White-Bean Soup With Mustard Greens; Cuban Black Bean Soup With Cod; Warm Lentil Vegetable Salad With Feta, Dried Currants and Dill; Lebanese-Style Chickpea Salad **3-4 servings a week of fish**
Serving size: 3 ounces

(Mercury Alert: Because mercury pollutants concentrate in larger fish, all women of childbearing age, as well as those who are pregnant or nursing, have been warned to avoid eating shark, swordfish, king mackerel and tilefish. The U.S. Food and Drug Administration and the Environmental Protection Agency also caution that women in these groups should eat no more than 12 ounces of all fish and shellfish per week.)

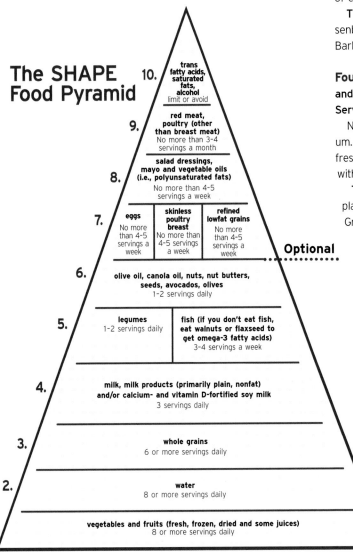

The SHAPE Food Pyramid

10. trans fatty acids, saturated fats, alcohol
limit or avoid

9. red meat, poultry (other than breast meat)
No more than 3-4 servings a month

8. salad dressings, mayo and vegetable oils (i.e., polyunsaturated fats)
No more than 4-5 servings a week

7. eggs — No more than 4-5 servings a week | skinless poultry breast — No more than 4-5 servings a week | refined lowfat grains — No more than 4-5 servings a week

6. olive oil, canola oil, nuts, nut butters, seeds, avocados, olives
1-2 servings daily

Optional

5. legumes — 1-2 servings daily | fish (if you don't eat fish, eat walnuts or flaxseed to get omega-3 fatty acids) — 3-4 servings a week

4. milk, milk products (primarily plain, nonfat) and/or calcium- and vitamin D-fortified soy milk
3 servings daily

3. whole grains
6 or more servings daily

2. water
8 or more servings daily

1. vegetables and fruits (fresh, frozen, dried and some juices)
8 or more servings daily

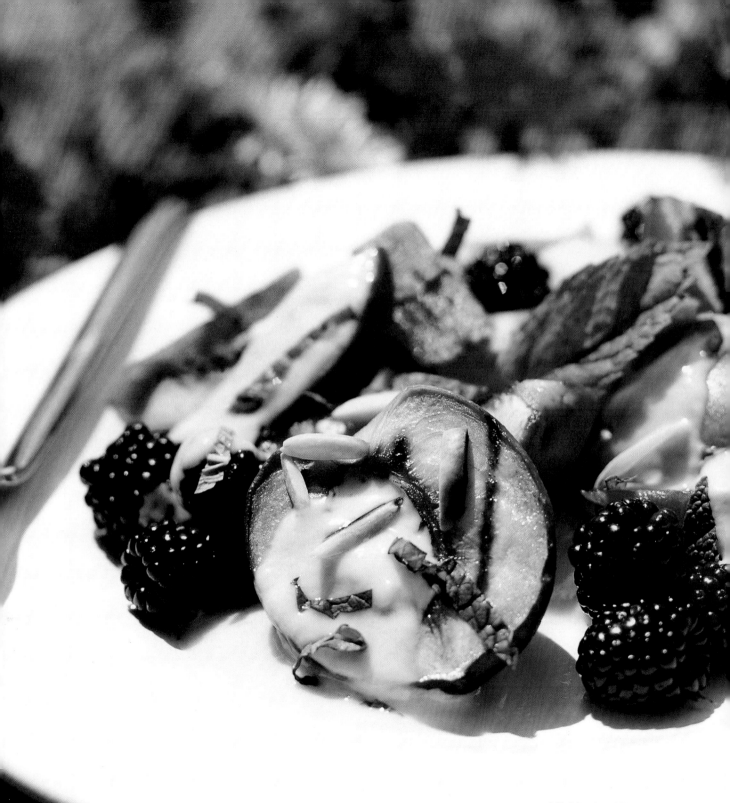

*Grilled Peach and Blackberry Salad
With Honey-Yogurt Dressing*

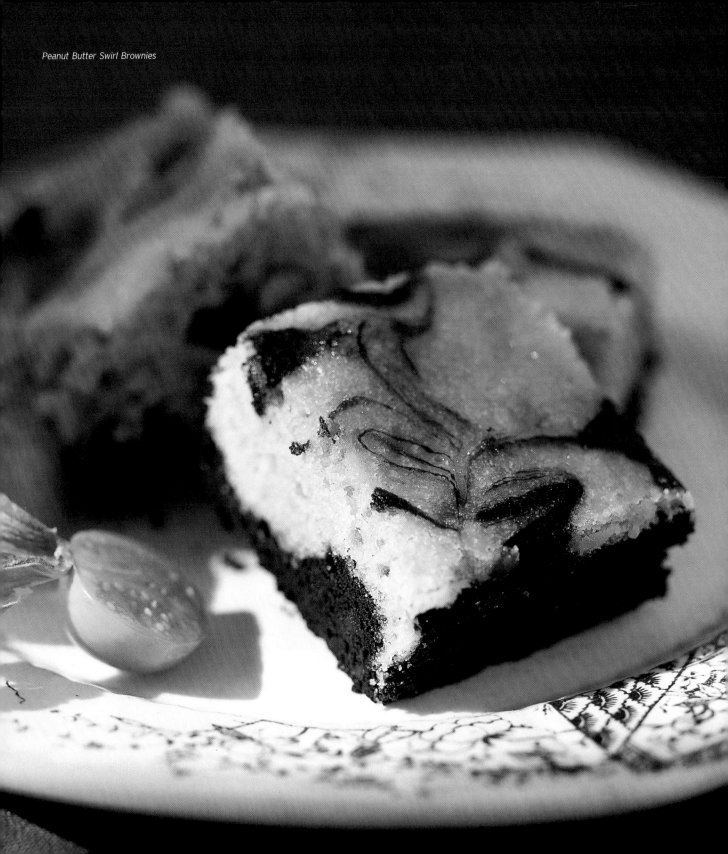

Peanut Butter Swirl Brownies

Fish oils, aka omega-3 fatty acids, may lower your risk for heart disease and help prevent breast cancer. Don't eat fish? Substitute flaxseed or walnuts; they contain linolenic acid, a precursor to omega-3s that offers similar benefits.

The *Lowfat & Easy* way: Romaine-Wrapped Tilapia With Red Onions and Capers; Poached Chilean Sea Bass With Garlicky Bread Crumbs; Pepper-Seared Tuna With Cool Mango Salsa; Trout Enchiladas; Red-Hot Sesame Spinach-Salmon Salad

Sixth Tier 1-2 servings a day of olive or canola oil, nuts, nut butters, seeds, avocados or olives

Serving size: 1 tablespoon of oil or nut butter, $\frac{1}{3}$ ounce of nuts and seeds, $\frac{1}{3}$ avocado, 20 medium olives

While these foods are high in fat, it's monounsaturated – the healthy type that's essential to the body's absorption of vitamins and protects against heart disease. Nuts, seeds, avocado and olives are more nutritious than oils, so give them priority.

The *Lowfat & Easy* way: Avocado Energizer; Chicken Salad With Raspberries and Walnuts; Fried Rice With Carrots, Tomato and Pine Nuts; Peanut Butter Swirl Brownies

Seventh Tier (Optional) 4-5 servings or less a week of each: eggs, skinless poultry breast, refined grains

Serving size: 1 egg, 3 ounces skinless poultry breast, 1 slice bread, $\frac{1}{2}$ English muffin, $\frac{1}{2}$ hamburger bun, $\frac{1}{2}$ bagel, $\frac{1}{2}$ cup cooked cereal or pasta

Eggs offer protein and minerals. Skinless poultry breast meat is low in saturated fat and is an excellent source of protein and iron. Refined grains are lower in vitamins and fiber than whole grains, but they still give you carbs.

The *Lowfat & Easy* way: Greek Omelet With Tomatoes and Feta Cheese; Eggs Florentine With Lowfat Hollandaise; Grilled Lime Chicken Sandwiches With Spicy Slaw; Moroccan Chicken and Arugula Salad With Olives and Figs; Pasta Salad With Almonds and Grapes

Eighth Tier (Optional) No more than 4-5 servings a week of polyunsaturated fats (salad dressings, mayonnaise, vegetable oils other than canola and olive)

Serving size: 1 tablespoon

Polyunsaturated fats don't raise heart disease risk, but they may increase risk of breast, colon and pancreatic cancers.

Ninth Tier (Optional) No more than 3-4 servings a month of red meat or poultry other than breast meat

Serving size: 3 ounces

Red meat is a rich source of iron and zinc, but it's also high in saturated fat. Eating more than 12-16 ounces a month increases your risk of colon cancer and heart disease.

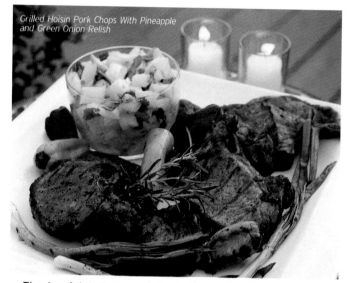

Grilled Hoisin Pork Chops With Pineapple and Green Onion Relish

The *Lowfat & Easy* way: Curried Lamb Patties With Chutney; Broiled Flank Steak With Orange-Glazed Carrots and Sweet Potatoes; Shepherd's Pie With Root Vegetables; Saigon Beef With Noodles; Grilled Hoisin Pork Chops With Pineapple and Green Onion Relish

Tenth Tier (Optional) Limit or avoid trans fatty acids (fried, fast and baked foods, convenience and snack foods, margarine), saturated fats (butter, fatty dairy products) and alcohol

Saturated fats and trans fatty acids have no nutritional value and are major culprits in the development of heart disease. Although alcohol may reduce risk for heart disease, more than one small drink a day increases a woman's risk for breast cancer.

Now that you know the optimal way to eat, it's time to get cooking! This book is conveniently divided into categories based on the casual way we dine: *Breakfast*, *Salads*, *Sandwiches*, *Soups*, *Pizzas and Pastas*, *Seafood*, *Meat and Poultry*, *Sides*, and, yes, *Desserts*. Each recipe includes prep and cook times, as well as nutrition information. Throughout the book you'll find hints, tips and techniques to inform, inspire and motivate you in your quest to stay in shape. Just look for the following icons: sauce pan (food-prep or cooking tip), apple (nutrition tip) and scale (weight-loss tip).

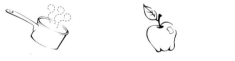

We know you'll love making these *Lowfat & Easy* dishes. Enjoy them mindfully, setting a beautiful table and taking the time to savor every bite. Eating well and losing weight really can be satisfying and simple. Turn the page and start today.

–*Anne M. Russell, Editor in Chief*, SHAPE magazine

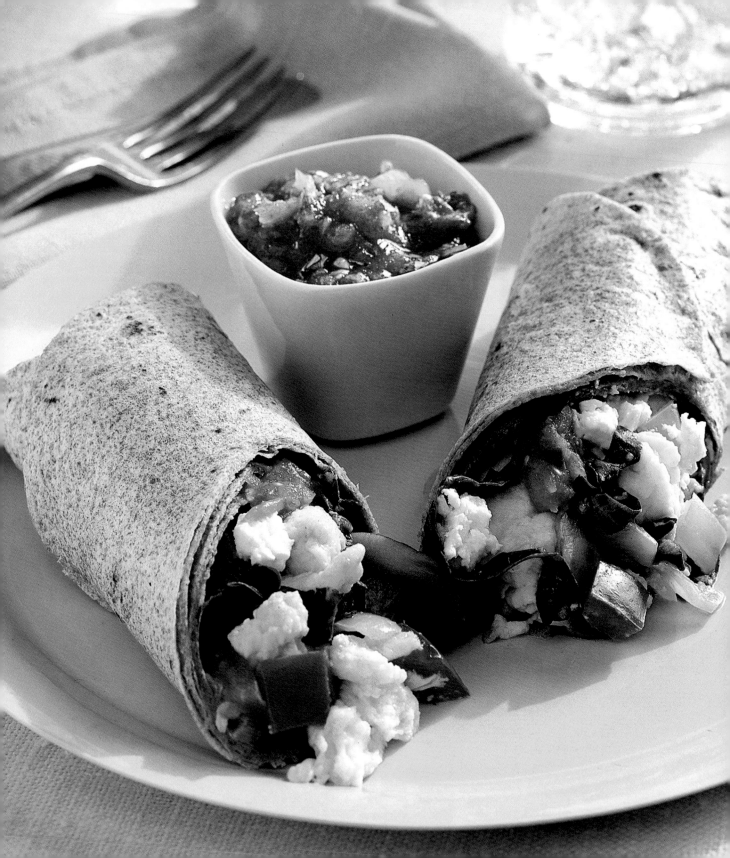

breakfast

No matter what your schedule is, it's possible to start the day off with a healthy breakfast. Pressed for time? Zap yourself a Micro Monte Cristo Breakfast Sandwich, whip up a Berry Blast smoothie or grab a Ginger Date Muffin that you've baked the night before. On leisurely weekend mornings, try Apple Crepes or savor Cinnamon-Wheat Pancakes With Hot Boysenberry Compote.

recipes

Greek Omelet With Tomatoes and Feta Cheese

Serves 2
Prep time: 10 minutes
Cook time: 4-6 minutes

Olive-oil cooking spray
6 large egg whites
½ teaspoon dried oregano
½ cup diced fresh tomatoes
½ cup diced green bell peppers
2 tablespoons crumbled feta cheese
Salt and ground black pepper to taste

Spray a large nonstick skillet with cooking spray and set pan over medium-high heat.

Whisk together egg whites and oregano. Add egg mixture to pan and cook 3-5 minutes, until egg whites are cooked through to the top, frequently lifting the sides of egg whites with a spatula to allow uncooked portions to slide underneath (tilt the pan to help them do this).

Top one side of egg mixture with tomatoes, bell pepper and feta cheese. Using the spatula, fold over untopped side. Cook omelet 1 more minute, until feta melts. Season with salt and black pepper and cut omelet in half to serve.

NUTRITION SCORE
Per serving (½ omelet): 109 **calories**
30% **fat** (3.6 g; 2 g saturated)
20% **carbs** (5 g), 1 g **fiber**
50% **protein** (14 g)

No time to heat up an omelet pan? Try one of these 5-minute breakfasts: 1 slice whole-grain toast, 2 tablespoons natural peanut butter and ½ grapefruit; or 1 cup vanilla yogurt, 2 tablespoons wheat germ, 1 tablespoon ground flaxseed and 1 banana.

Blueberry-Apricot Muffins With Almond Streusel Topping

Makes 12 muffins
Prep time: 10 minutes
Cook time: 20-25 minutes

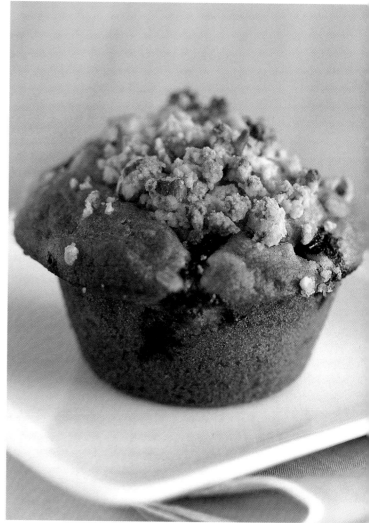

Cooking spray
2 cups all-purpose flour, divided
¾ cup whole-wheat flour
1 cup quick-cooking oats
1 cup granulated sugar
1 tablespoon baking powder
1 teaspoon baking soda
¼ teaspoon salt
¾ cup nonfat milk
¾ cup apricot nectar
½ cup lowfat vanilla yogurt
1 egg
3 tablespoons light margarine, melted and divided
2 teaspoons vanilla extract
1½ cups blueberries, fresh or frozen (keep frozen until ready to use)
¼ cup chopped almonds
1 tablespoon light brown sugar

Preheat oven to 400° F. Coat a 12-cup muffin pan with cooking spray. In a large bowl, combine 1¾ cups of the all-purpose flour with the next 6 ingredients. Mix thoroughly with a fork, make a well in the center and set aside.

In a large bowl, whisk together milk, apricot nectar, yogurt, egg, 2 tablespoons of the margarine, and vanilla. Fold mixture into dry ingredients until just blended. Fold in blueberries. Spoon batter into prepared muffin pan, filling each cup (batter will be heaping in the cup). To make the streusel topping, in a small bowl combine remaining ¼ cup flour, almonds, brown sugar and remaining 1 tablespoon margarine. Sprinkle mixture over muffins.

Bake 20-25 minutes, until a wooden pick comes out clean. Cool muffins in pan, on a wire rack, 10 minutes before removing from pan.

NUTRITION SCORE
Per serving (1 muffin): 274 **calories**
14% **fat** (4 g; 1 g saturated)
76% **carbs** (52 g), 3 g **fiber**
10% **protein** (7 g)

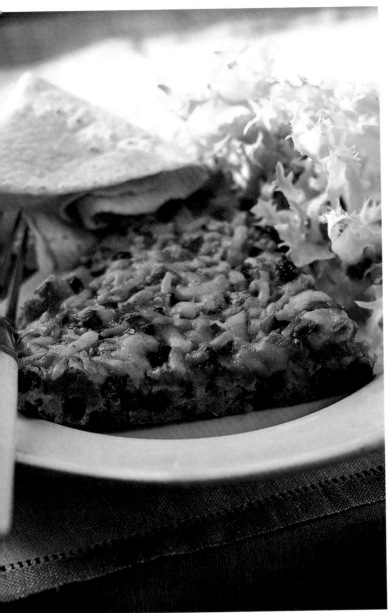

Egg Strata

Serves 4
Prep time: 10 minutes
Cook time: 6-10 minutes

Cooking spray
8 slices whole-grain pumpernickel bread, cut into ½-inch cubes
1 14.5-ounce can diced tomatoes with basil, garlic and oregano
1 cup shredded reduced-fat Cheddar cheese
1 cup nonfat milk
4 large eggs
2 teaspoons Dijon mustard
¼ teaspoon ground black pepper
2 tablespoons grated Parmesan cheese

Preheat broiler. Coat a microwave-safe, shallow baking dish (about 7 by 11 inches) with cooking spray. Arrange pumpernickel cubes in the bottom of dish. Spoon tomatoes over bread, then sprinkle Cheddar cheese over tomatoes. Set aside.

In a small bowl, whisk together milk, eggs, Dijon mustard and black pepper. Pour mixture over tomato-and-cheese-topped bread. Sprinkle with Parmesan. Cover dish with fitted lid or paper towel.

Microwave on high 6-10 minutes (it's best to undercook and keep checking), until eggs are set, rotating dish once during cooking. Place dish under broiler for 1 minute, until top is golden brown. Let stand 2 minutes before slicing into 4 equal portions.

NUTRITION SCORE
Per serving (¼ of strata): 373 **calories**
31% **fat** (13 g; 6 g saturated)
42% **carbs** (39 g), 6 g **fiber**
27% **protein** (25 g)

Eggs Florentine With Lowfat Hollandaise

Serves 4
Prep time: 5 minutes
Cook time: 5 minutes

Eggs Florentine

 4 oat-bran English muffins, split
16 fresh baby spinach leaves (or 8 regular spinach leaves)
 1 tablespoon white vinegar
 4 large eggs

Lowfat Hollandaise

 1 egg yolk
⅔ cup nonfat milk
 1 tablespoon all-purpose flour
 1 tablespoon fresh lemon juice
Salt and ground black pepper to taste

Toast English muffins. Top 4 halves with 4 baby spinach leaves each (or 2 leaves if using regular spinach). Cover with foil to keep warm; set aside.

To poach eggs, fill a large saucepan or high-sided skillet with 2 inches of water. Add vinegar and set pan over medium-high heat. Bring to a simmer. Crack eggs, one at a time, into a small bowl and slide each egg carefully into simmering water (this prevents yolk from breaking). Simmer 3-5 minutes, until whites are cooked and yolk is as desired. Using a slotted spoon or spatula, remove eggs from water and place on top of spinach. Cover with foil to keep warm.

Meanwhile, to prepare hollandaise, combine egg yolk, milk and flour in a small saucepan. Whisk until blended and set pan over medium heat. Simmer 2 minutes, until mixture thickens, stirring constantly with a wire whisk. Remove from heat and whisk in lemon juice. Season with salt and pepper.

Spoon hollandaise sauce over eggs and serve alongside remaining English muffin half.

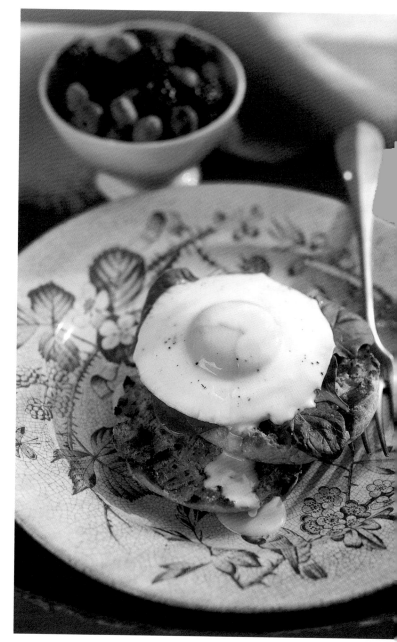

NUTRITION SCORE
Per serving (1 egg, 1 English muffin): 235 **calories**
28% **fat** (7.4 g; 2.5 g saturated)
51% **carbs** (30 g), 2 g fiber
21% **protein** (12.4 g)

Breakfast Burrito With Roasted Salsa Mexicana

Serves 6
Prep time: 20 minutes
Cook time: 15 minutes

Salsa

- 2 tomatoes, quartered
- ½ red onion, coarsely chopped
- 2 tomatillos, papery skin removed and halved
- 1 jalapeño chili pepper, halved lengthwise and seeded
- 1 clove garlic, peeled and halved
- ½ teaspoon olive oil
- Salt and ground black pepper to taste
- Juice of ½ lime
- 1 tablespoon chopped fresh cilantro

Burrito

- 2 teaspoons olive oil, divided
- 2 tablespoons finely diced red onion
- ½ cup sliced white or cremini mushrooms
- 2 tablespoons seeded, finely diced Anaheim chile peppers
- 2 tablespoons seeded, finely diced tomatoes
- 1 cup trimmed, thinly sliced spinach leaves
- Salt to taste
- 6 eggs
- 6 egg whites
- ¼ cup crumbled feta cheese
- 6 8-inch whole-wheat tortillas
- Fresh, chopped cilantro

To prepare the salsa, preheat oven to 400° F. In a small bowl, combine tomatoes, onion, tomatillos, jalapeño and garlic. Add olive oil, salt and black pepper; toss to coat. Place mixture on baking sheet and roast 15 minutes, until softened and lightly browned. Transfer to a blender and process to a coarse consistency. Place mixture in a bowl and stir in lime juice and cilantro. (Can be kept in the refrigerator, covered, for up to 5 days, and frozen for up to 3 months.)

To make the burrito, brush a large skillet with 1 teaspoon of the olive oil and set pan over medium-high heat. Add onion and cook 2–3 minutes, until softened, stirring frequently. Add mushrooms and peppers and cook until mushroom liquid is almost evaporated. Add tomatoes and spinach and cook 2–3 minutes, until spinach begins to wilt, stirring frequently. Season with salt. Set mixture aside in a bowl.

In a medium bowl, whisk together eggs and egg whites until blended. Brush the same skillet with remaining olive oil and set pan over medium heat. Add beaten eggs and cook 1–1½ minutes, until eggs are scrambled but still wet, stirring constantly. Stir in cooked vegetable mixture. Sprinkle feta cheese over top and season with salt, if desired. Transfer mixture to a bowl and set aside.

Preheat the same skillet over medium heat. Place tortillas in skillet and cook 20 seconds per side, until hot. Put tortillas on a flat surface and spoon ½ cup of cooked egg mixture onto center of each tortilla. Drizzle 2 tablespoons salsa over each serving and roll tortillas into 1½-inch cylinders. Serve immediately, or cover with a clean kitchen towel and place on a baking pan in a 200° F oven for up to 20 minutes. (You can refrigerate the egg mixture for up to 3 days; freezing is not recommended.)

To serve, slice each rolled tortilla in half diagonally and garnish with dollops of salsa and chopped cilantro.

NUTRITION SCORE
Per serving (1 burrito, 3 tablespoons salsa): 224 **calories**
38% **fat** (9 g; 3 g saturated)
35% **carbs** (20 g), 11 g **fiber**
27% **protein** (15 g)

The tomatillo is a small green fruit, similar to a tomato, with a paperlike husk. A traditional ingredient in Mexican cooking, it contains the antioxidant lutein, which may prevent diseases of the eye.

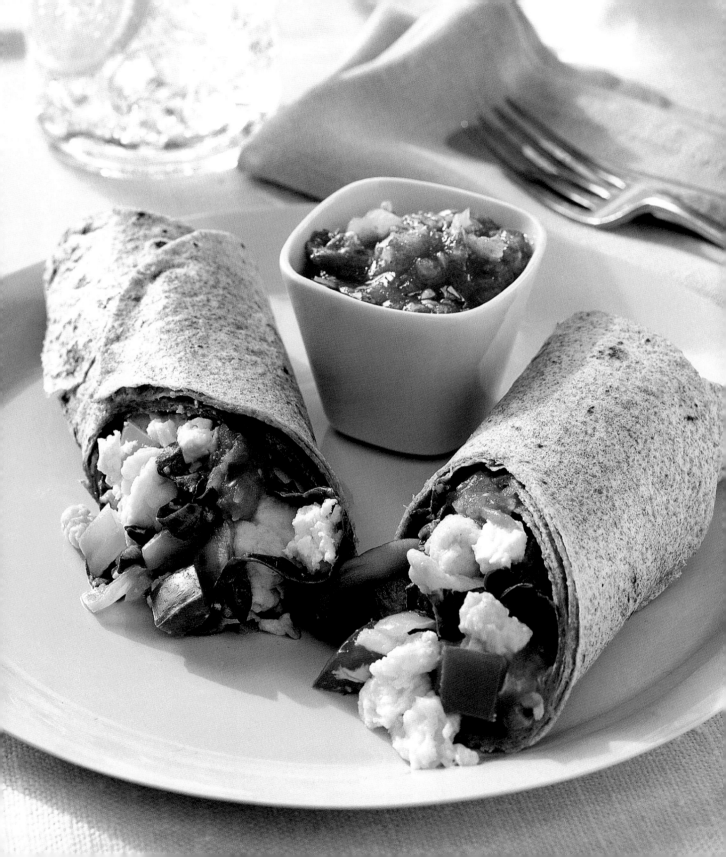

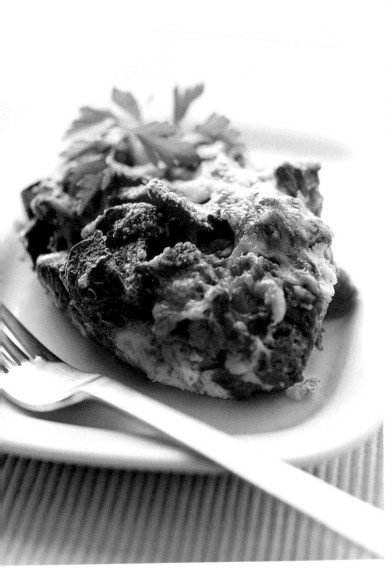

Mexican Frittata With Black Beans and Rice

Serves 4
Prep time: 8 minutes
Cook time: 5-9 minutes

- 4 large eggs
- ½ cup nonfat milk
- 1 15-ounce can black beans, rinsed and drained
- 1 14-ounce can diced tomatoes with green pepper and onion
- ½ cup instant brown rice
- 1 4.5-ounce can diced green chilies
- 2 teaspoons ground cumin
- ¼ teaspoon ground black pepper
- 2 teaspoons olive oil
- ¼ cup reduced-fat shredded Mexican four-cheese blend

In a large bowl, whisk together eggs and milk. Add the next 6 ingredients and mix well. Let mixture stand 5 minutes.

Preheat broiler. Heat oil in a large oven-safe skillet over medium heat. Add egg mixture and cook 3-5 minutes, until almost cooked through to the surface, frequently smoothing the top with the back of a large spoon.

Place skillet under broiler; cook 1-2 minutes, until top is done. Sprinkle with shredded cheese and return skillet to broiler. Broil 1-2 minutes, until cheese is golden. Slice into 4 equal wedges and serve warm or at room temperature.

NUTRITION SCORE
Per serving (1 wedge): 448 **calories**
21% **fat** (10.5 g; 3.5 g saturated)
60% **carbs** (67 g), 17 g **fiber**
19% **protein** (21 g)

Southwestern Potato Hash With Black Beans and Tofu

Serves 4
Prep time: 3-4 minutes
Cook time: 11 minutes

- 1 14.5-ounce can whole new potatoes, drained and diced
- 1 14.5-ounce can diced tomatoes with green pepper and onion
- 1 15-ounce can black beans, rinsed and drained
- ½ cup diced firm tofu
- 1 teaspoon dried oregano
- ½ cup reduced-fat shredded Mexican four-cheese blend

Preheat broiler. Place potatoes, tomatoes, beans, tofu and oregano in a medium pan over medium-high heat. Simmer 5 minutes, until liquid is absorbed and potatoes are tender.

Sprinkle cheese on top of potato mixture. Place pan under broiler for 1 minute, until cheese melts.

NUTRITION SCORE
Per serving (1½ cups): 308 **calories**
16% **fat** (5.5 g; 2 g saturated)
60% **carbs** (46 g), 12 g **fiber**
24% **protein** (18.5 g)

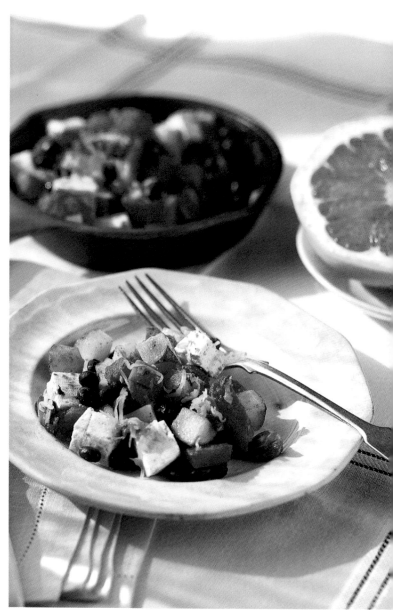

According to a survey of more than 2,600 students at Michigan State University in East Lansing, women who eat breakfast may be more likely to consume less fat throughout the day than breakfast skippers.

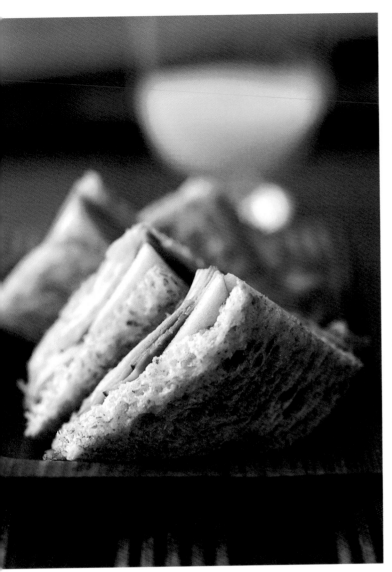

Micro Monte Cristo Breakfast Sandwich

Serves 4
Prep time: 10 minutes
Cook time: 3-5 minutes

- 8 slices whole-grain bread
- 8 teaspoons honey mustard
- 2 Granny Smith apples, thinly sliced
- 4 ounces lean baked ham
- 4 ounces Swiss cheese
- 4 egg whites
- 1 cup nonfat milk
- ⅛ teaspoon ground nutmeg

Spread 4 slices of bread with mustard. Top each slice with apples, ham and cheese. Cover with other bread slice.

In a microwave-safe pan, whisk egg whites, milk and nutmeg. Add sandwiches and coat both sides. Cover with plastic wrap and microwave on high 3-5 minutes.

NUTRITION SCORE
Per serving (1 sandwich): 393 **calories**
17% **fat** (9 g; 5 g saturated)
61% **carbs** (44 g), 5.4 g **fiber**
22% **protein** (26 g)

Whole-grain bread is rich in fiber and B vitamins; apples offer cholesterol-lowering soluble fiber; Swiss cheese and nonfat milk are great sources of calcium; egg whites are an excellent source of high-quality protein.

Cinnamon-Wheat Pancakes With Hot Boysenberry Compote

Serves 4
Prep time: 10 minutes
Cook time: 5 minutes for sauce, 7 minutes for pancakes

Compote
- 2 cups frozen boysenberries
- ⅓ cup apple juice
- 1 tablespoon sugar
- 1 tablespoon cornstarch

Pancakes
- 1 teaspoon baking soda
- 1½ cups buttermilk
- 1 cup whole-wheat flour
- 1 tablespoon cinnamon
- 1 tablespoon sugar
- 2 egg whites
- 1 teaspoon vanilla
- Cooking spray

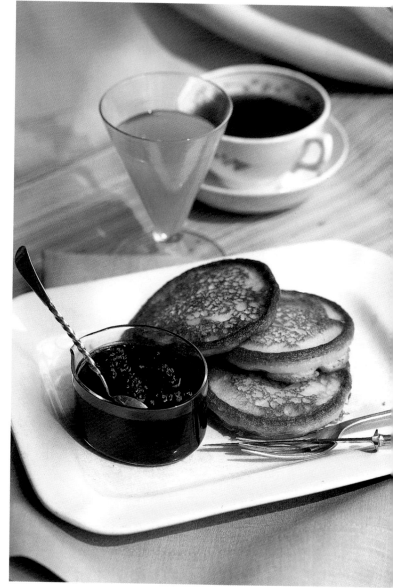

To make compote, combine boysenberries and apple juice in a small saucepan; simmer for 5 minutes. In a separate bowl, combine sugar and cornstarch and add to berry mixture, gently stirring until contents of pan boils. Remove from heat and let compote cool slightly until it thickens.

To make pancakes, dissolve baking soda in buttermilk in a small bowl; set aside. In a larger bowl, combine flour, cinnamon and sugar. Add buttermilk mixture, egg whites and vanilla, and blend. Spray griddle with vegetable-oil cooking spray. Ladle pancake mixture onto griddle and cook until pancakes are light brown on both sides. Serve with boysenberry compote.

NUTRITION SCORE
Per serving (2 pancakes, 2 tablespoons compote): 228 **calories**
6% **fat** (2 g; 0.6 g saturated)
77% **carbs** (46 g), 7 g fiber
17% **protein** (10 g)

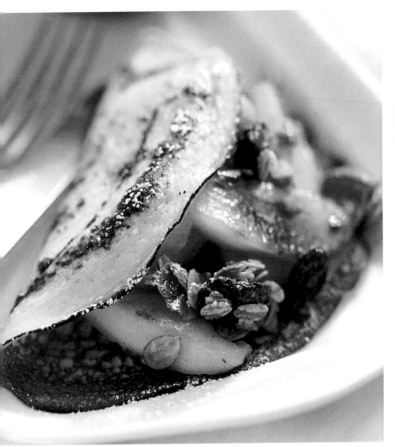

Apple Crepes

Batter

Makes 8 crepes
Prep time: 3 minutes
Cook time: 8-10 minutes

   1 cup nonfat milk
   ⅓ cup water
   4 large egg whites
   1 teaspoon vanilla extract
   1 cup all-purpose flour
   2 tablespoons granulated sugar
   1 teaspoon canola oil

In a large bowl, whisk together milk, water, egg whites and vanilla. Whisk in flour and sugar. Then follow "Crepe Making 101" below.

Serves 4
Prep time: 5-10 minutes
Cook time: 5 minutes

   4 Granny Smith apples, peeled, cored and diced
   ¾ cup raisins
   ⅓ cup packed brown sugar
   ¼ cup water
   1 lemon, zest and juice
   ½ teaspoon cinnamon
   8 crepes (see recipe for batter above)
   1 cup lowfat granola

Combine first 6 ingredients in a medium saucepan. Simmer over medium heat 5 minutes, until apples are tender and liquid is reduced. Arrange crepes on a flat surface. Top with apple mixture and granola. Roll up and serve.

NUTRITION SCORE
Per serving (2 filled crepes): 356 **calories**
5% **fat** (2 g; 0 g saturated)
90% **carbs** (80 g), 5 g **fiber**
5% **protein** (5 g)

CREPE MAKING 101

Fear of making crepes does have some basis in reality. You can ruin them (pretty easily) with two common mistakes. The first is pan temperature: You need to pre-heat your pan to medium-high heat, so that a drop of water bounces on the surface. If the pan is too hot, the water will quickly evaporate, and the crepe will burn. If the pan isn't hot enough, the water will lie flat, and the crepe will not cook properly. The second common mistake is batter quantity: Add just enough to coat the surface of the pan so it's almost see-through. Too much makes a pancake. Chef Michael Kalajian offers these tips:

1. Always use a shallow nonstick skillet (or a crepe pan). Set it over medium-high heat and let it get hot before coating with nonstick spray.

2. Use just 3-4 tablespoons of batter for each crepe and pour it from a small pitcher or glass measuring cup; then tilt pan to coat the bottom evenly.

3. Cook 1-2 minutes on the first side, until bottom sets and starts to bubble. Then run a thin knife or spatula under edges, lift crepe and flip over. Cook 30 seconds, until bottom is speckled with golden dots.

Berry Orange-Oat Muffins

Serves 12
Prep time: 15 minutes
Cook time: 15 minutes

Cooking spray
½ cup rolled oats
½ cup lowfat buttermilk
1½ cups whole-wheat flour
1 teaspoon baking powder
½ teaspoon baking soda
½ teaspoon ground cinnamon
¼ teaspoon salt
1 medium orange
½ cup granulated sugar
¼ cup canola oil
1 whole egg
1 cup blueberries (fresh or frozen)
½ cup dried cranberries

Preheat oven to 400° F. Lightly coat 12 muffin cups with cooking spray. Stir together oats and buttermilk in a small bowl and set aside for 5 minutes.

Whisk flour, baking powder, baking soda, cinnamon and salt together in a medium bowl. Grate rind from orange and add to a large bowl; squeeze ½ cup orange juice and add to rind. Whisk in sugar, oil and egg until mixture is smooth. Blend in oatmeal mixture, followed by flour mixture. Stir until ingredients are just combined; then gently fold in berries.

Spoon batter into prepared muffin tins and bake for 15 minutes, or until a toothpick inserted in center of muffin comes out clean.

NUTRITION SCORE
Per serving (1 muffin): 180 **calories**
25% **fat** (5 g; 0.5 g saturated)
67% **carbs** (30 g), 1 g **fiber**
8% **protein** (3 g)

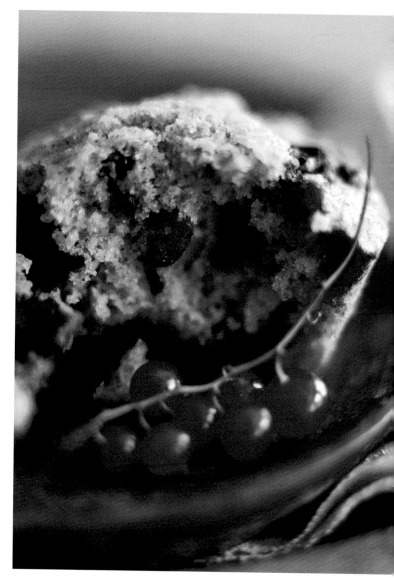

The anthocyanins that give fruits like blueberries and strawberries their distinctive colors may help ward off heart disease by preventing clot formation. Fiber-rich oats, blueberries, cranberries and oranges (including the peel) abound with phytochemicals.

Apple-Blueberry Coffee Cake

Serves 12
Prep time: 15 minutes
Cook time: 30-35 minutes

Cooking spray
2 cups whole-wheat flour
¾ cup granulated sugar
2 teaspoons baking powder
½ teaspoon salt
1 cup cinnamon applesauce
½ cup nonfat milk
2 tablespoons butter or margarine, melted
1 egg
1 teaspoon vanilla extract
1 cup frozen blueberries or cranberries (do not thaw)

Streusel topping
½ cup sliced almonds
2 tablespoons light brown sugar
2 tablespoons whole-wheat flour
1 egg white
½ teaspoon ground cinnamon

Preheat oven to 350° F. Coat an 11-by-7-inch baking pan with cooking spray and set aside.

In a large bowl, combine flour, sugar, baking powder and salt. Make a well in the center and set aside. Whisk together applesauce, milk, butter, egg and vanilla. Fold into dry ingredients until just blended; then fold in berries. Pour into prepared pan.

Combine topping ingredients in a small bowl. Mix well; spread over batter. Bake 30-35 minutes, until a wooden pick inserted in the center comes out clean. Cool in pan on wire rack for 10 minutes. Cut into 12 pieces.

Apples offer a terrific source of dietary fiber to help curb your appetite, and they contain pectin, a type of fiber known to lower LDL cholesterol.

NUTRITION SCORE
Per serving (1 slice): 216 **calories**
24% **fat** (5.8 g; 1.7 g saturated)
67% **carbs** (36 g), 4 g **fiber**
9% **protein** (5 g)

Ginger Date Muffins

Makes 12 muffins
Prep time: 10 minutes
Cook time: 15-17 minutes

Cooking spray
- 1 cup all-purpose flour
- ¼ cup whole-wheat flour
- ⅓ cup brown sugar
- 1¼ teaspoons ground ginger
- ½ teaspoon baking powder
- ¼ teaspoon baking soda
- ¼ teaspoon cinnamon
- ¼ teaspoon nutmeg
- ⅛ teaspoon salt
- ½ cup applesauce
- ⅓ cup molasses
- 3 tablespoons lowfat buttermilk
- 2 egg whites
- 1½ cups chopped dates

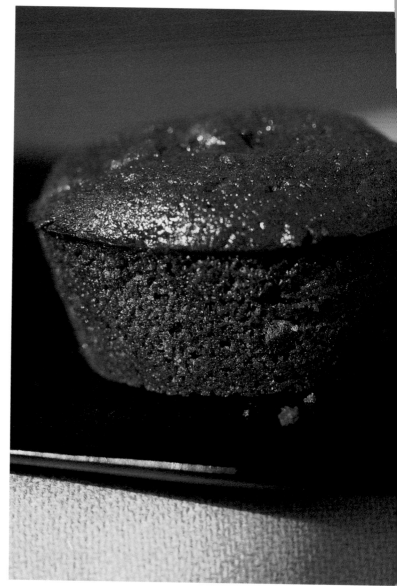

Preheat oven to 400° F. Lightly coat a 12-cup muffin pan with cooking spray.

In a large bowl, combine flours, sugar, ginger, baking powder, baking soda, cinnamon, nutmeg and salt.

In a small bowl, combine applesauce, molasses, buttermilk and egg whites. Add the applesauce mixture to the flour mixture. Stir just until combined. Fold in dates.

Divide batter among muffin cups. Bake 15-17 minutes or until golden and muffins are pulling away from the pan.

NUTRITION SCORE
Per serving (1 muffin): 154 **calories**
2% **fat** (0.3 g)
92% **carbs** (37.3 g), 2g **fiber**
6% **protein** (2.6 g)

It takes 3,500 calories to gain or lose a pound. If you want to shed a pound a week, carve 500 calories off your day by thinking through your food choices and increasing your exercise.

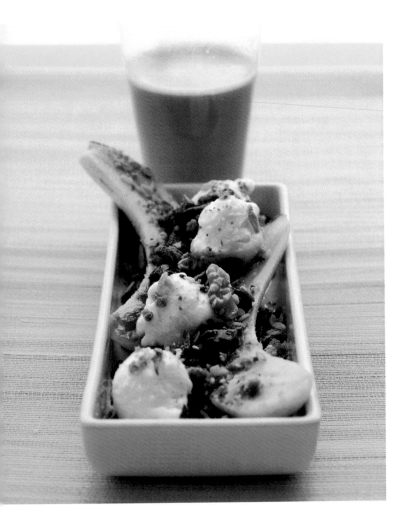

Breakfast Banana Split

Serves 1
Prep time: 5 minutes

- 1 small banana
- ⅓ cup nonfat vanilla frozen yogurt
- ¼ cup lowfat granola
- 1 tablespoon all-fruit preserves
- 2 tablespoons chopped walnuts

Halve the banana lengthwise. Top with 4 melon-ball-size scoops of nonfat vanilla frozen yogurt, the lowfat granola, all-fruit preserves and chopped walnuts.

NUTRITION SCORE
Per serving: 414 **calories**
23% **fat** (11 g; 1.3 g saturated)
69% **carbs** (71 g), 5 g **fiber**
8% **protein** (8 g)

There is a reason that bananas are the snack of choice at triathlons and 10ks: A medium banana supplies 26 grams of carbohydrates as well as healthy doses of the minerals potassium and magnesium, which are important in regulating muscle contractions.

Piña Colada Pick-Me-Up

Serves 2
Prep time: 5 minutes

- ½ cup lowfat silken tofu
- ¾ cup frozen pineapple chunks
- ½ cup lowfat coconut or piña colada flavor yogurt
- 1 tablespoon flaxseed oil
- ¼ teaspoon coconut extract
- ⅓ cup water

In a blender, mix tofu and pineapple chunks on whip setting for about 20 seconds, until well incorporated. Next, add yogurt, flaxseed oil, coconut extract and water. Continue to whip for 15 seconds. Freeze leftovers. (To reuse, defrost for about 10 minutes; then blend for about 40 seconds or until smooth.)

NUTRITION SCORE
Per serving (7 ounces): 132 **calories**
45% **fat** (7 g; 0.65 g saturated)
49% **carbs** (16 g), 0.6 g **fiber**
6% **protein** (2 g)

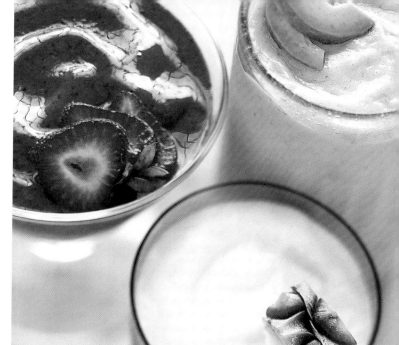

Avocado Energizer

Serves 2
Prep time: 5 minutes

- ¼ cup fresh mashed avocado
- ½ cup lowfat milk
- 1 teaspoon honey
- 1 banana, frozen, then broken into 3 pieces
- ½ cup frozen mango pieces
- ⅓ cup peach nectar

In a blender, whip together avocado and milk. Add honey, banana and mango. Whip another 10 seconds or until smooth. Add peach nectar and mix 5 seconds. Freeze leftover smoothie. (To reuse, defrost for about 10 minutes; then place in blender for 40 seconds.)

NUTRITION SCORE
Per serving (7 ounces): 207 **calories**
27% **fat** (7 g; 1.6 g saturated)
67% **carbs** (68 grams), 3.9 g **fiber**
6% **protein** (4 grams)

Berry Blast

Serves 2
Prep time: 10 minutes

- ½ cup frozen sliced or whole strawberries
- ½ cup lowfat silken tofu
- ½ cup frozen blueberries
- ½ cup frozen raspberries
- ¼ cup low-cal cranberry juice
- ¼ teaspoon vanilla extract
- 2 tablespoons wheat germ
- 1 tablespoon sugar

Allow frozen strawberries to defrost slightly (about 7 minutes on the countertop or 20 seconds in microwave on defrost mode).

Meanwhile, in a blender, mix tofu, blueberries and raspberries on whip for 10 seconds. Add strawberries. Mix 5 seconds. Add remaining ingredients and mix 5 seconds. Freeze leftovers. (To reuse, defrost for about 10 minutes; then blend for about 40 seconds or until smooth.)

NUTRITION SCORE
Per serving (8 ounces): 141 **calories**
9% **fat** (1 g; 0.07 g saturated)
72% **carbs** (26 g), 6 g **fiber**
19% **protein** (7 g)

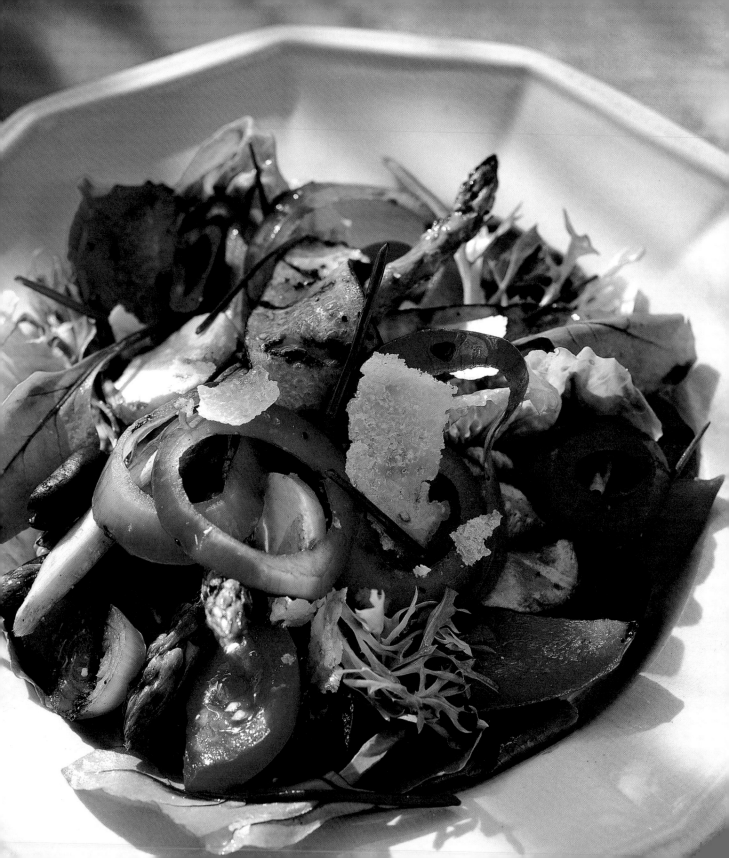

salads

Research indicates that starting lunch or dinner with a salad can reduce the total number of calories consumed at that meal. Besides helping regulate calorie intake, salads offer a delicious opportunity to load up on a variety of fiber-packed, nutrient-dense fruits and veggies: from spinach, beets and fennel to green mangoes, persimmons and jicama. When a light meal is what you crave, choose a protein-packed dish like Beef Fajita Salad or Warm Lentil Vegetable Salad With Feta, Dried Currants and Dill.

recipes

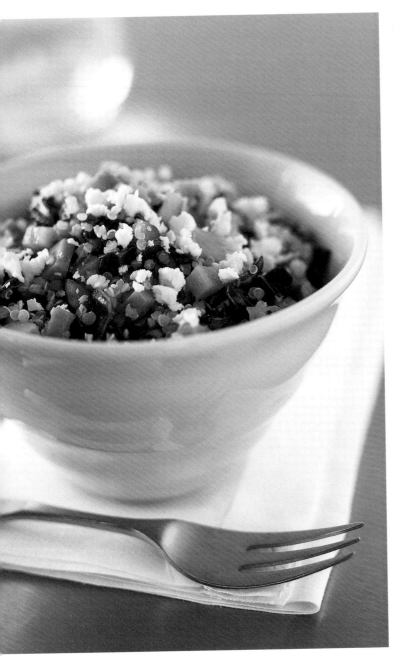

Quinoa Salad With Vegetables and Feta

Serves 2
Prep time: 10 minutes
Cook time: 10 minutes

- ½ cup quinoa
- 1 cup water
- 1 green bell pepper, seeded and diced
- 1½ cups chopped carrots
- 1 cup diced red cabbage
- ½ cup minced red onion
- ¼ cup minced sun-dried tomatoes (from oil-packed jar), drained
- 1 tablespoon red wine vinegar
- 2 teaspoons Dijon mustard
- 1 teaspoon olive oil
- Salt and ground black pepper to taste
- 2 tablespoons feta cheese

Rinse quinoa under cold water and drain. Combine quinoa and 1 cup water in a medium saucepan. Bring water to a boil, reduce heat, cover and cook 10 minutes, until liquid is absorbed. Transfer quinoa to a large bowl and add green pepper, carrots, cabbage, onion and sun-dried tomatoes.

In a small bowl, whisk together vinegar, mustard and oil. Pour mixture over quinoa mixture and toss to combine. Season with salt and pepper. Spoon mixture onto individual plates, and top each serving with 1 tablespoon feta cheese.

NUTRITION SCORE
Per serving (2 cups salad, 1 tablespoon feta cheese): 325 **calories**
29% **fat** (10 g; 3 g saturated)
58% **carbs** (47 g), 8 g fiber
13% **protein** (11 g)

Quinoa contains more high-quality protein than any other grain because it's a complete protein, supplying all the essential amino acids. You can find this low-carb grain in health-food stores and some supermarkets.

Asian Peanut Noodle Salad With Veggies, Tofu and Macadamia Nuts

Serves 8
Prep time: 15 minutes
Cook time: 15 minutes

Peanut sauce

  4 tablespoons creamy peanut butter
  4 tablespoons lite coconut milk
  1 teaspoon toasted sesame oil
  1 tablespoon freshly grated ginger
  1 teaspoon chopped garlic
  Juice of 2 limes
2-3 tablespoons reduced-sodium soy sauce (to taste)
1-3 teaspoons Tabasco sauce (to taste)
  ½ cup hot water

Noodle salad

1¼ cup extra-firm tofu, diced into ½-inch pieces
  2 teaspoons toasted sesame oil, divided
  2 cups broccoli florets
  1 cup snow peas, ends trimmed and cut into thirds
  1 cup carrots, cut into matchstick
  1 pound whole-wheat cooked linguine, rinsed in cool water
  2 tablespoons chopped macadamia nuts

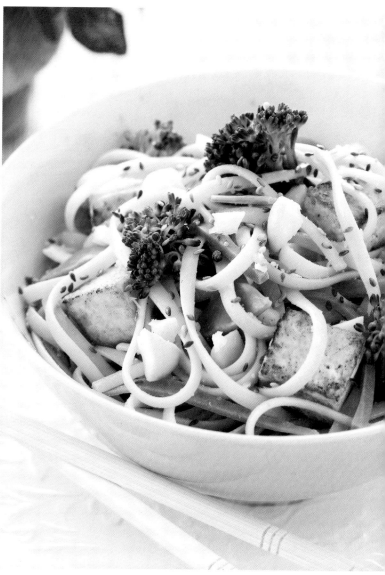

To make the peanut sauce, purée ingredients in a blender until smooth. Place in a covered container and refrigerate to thicken while you prepare the salad. To make the noodle salad, in a large nonstick pan, stir-fry diced tofu in 1 teaspoon of the sesame oil until golden on all sides, about 3-4 minutes. Remove tofu and set aside.

Pour the other teaspoon of sesame oil in pan and add broccoli, stir-frying for 3-4 minutes. Then add the snow peas and carrots and stir-fry an additional 3-4 minutes. Vegetables should still be crunchy.

In a large bowl, toss cooked linguine, tofu and veggies with peanut sauce until all are well-coated. Transfer to a serving platter and garnish with macadamia nuts.

NUTRITION SCORE
Per serving (1¼ cups): 362 **calories**
28% **fat** (11 g; 2 g saturated)
53% **carbs** (48 g), 8 g **fiber**
19% **protein** (17 g)

Lebanese-Style Chickpea Salad

Serves 6
Prep time: 10 minutes

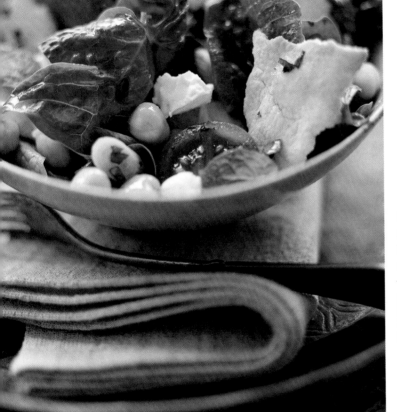

½ cup lemon juice

Salt to taste

½ teaspoon ground cumin

2 tablespoons olive oil

4 thinly sliced scallions (white part only)

2 cups sliced cucumber

1 pint cherry tomatoes, halved

2 cups cooked chickpeas

½ cup chopped flat-leaf parsley

½ cup chopped mint

1 bag pre-washed spinach

2 6-inch toasted pitas, broken into bite-size pieces

Salt and pepper to taste

In a large bowl, whisk together lemon juice, salt, cumin and oil. Add scallions, cucumber, cherry tomatoes, chickpeas, parsley and mint. Toss to combine. Add spinach and pita chips. Toss again; season with salt and pepper. Serve immediately.

NUTRITION SCORE
Per serving (1 cup): 230 **calories**
23% **fat** (6 g; <1 g saturated)
63% **carbs** (36 g), 8 g **fiber**
14% **protein** (8 g)

A quarter-cup of lemon juice contains half the RDA for vitamin C, an antioxidant that may protect cell membranes and DNA from damage that can lead to cancerous changes.

Beef Fajita Salad

Serves 4
Prep time: 5-7 minutes
Cook time: 8 minutes

Olive-oil cooking spray
8   6-inch whole-wheat tortillas
1   teaspoon ground cumin, divided
2   tablespoons reduced-sodium soy sauce
1   teaspoon liquid smoke seasoning
1   16-ounce package frozen pepper stir-fry mix
    (green, red, yellow bell peppers and onion),
    thawed
¾   pound lean roast beef, sliced into thin strips
4   cups chopped romaine lettuce (or 1 bag of any
    pre-washed romaine salad mix)
1   Haas avocado, peeled, pitted and diced

Preheat oven to 400° F. Coat a baking sheet with olive-oil spray.
Place four tortillas on baking sheet and sprinkle with ½ teaspoon
cumin. Bake 8 minutes, until golden. Remove from oven; transfer
to individual plates. Set aside.

Meanwhile, in a large skillet, combine remaining cumin, soy
sauce and liquid smoke. Set pan over medium-high heat and bring
mixture to a simmer. Add vegetable mix and cook 3 minutes, until
tender. Using tongs or a slotted spoon, remove vegetables from
pan; set aside. To the same pan, add roast beef and simmer
2 minutes, until hot.

Top toasted tortillas with lettuce, then vegetables and roast
beef. Arrange avocado on top. Serve with additional tortillas on
the side.

NUTRITION SCORE
Per serving (1 cup lettuce, 1 cup vegetable mixture, 3 ounces beef,
¼ avocado, 2 tortillas): 340 **calories**
26% **fat** (9.8 g; 2.7 g saturated)
45% **carbs** (38 g), 23 g **fiber**
29% **protein** (25 g)

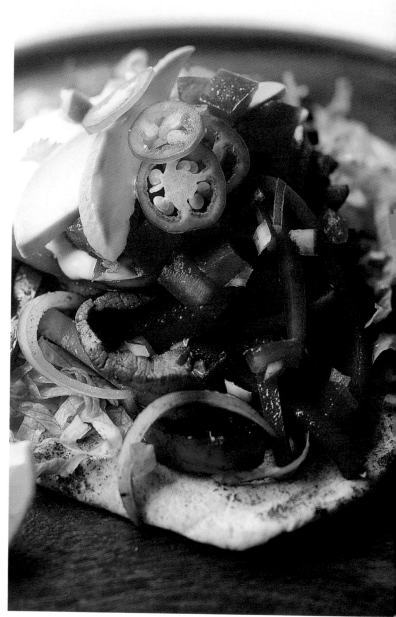

Gazpacho-Shrimp Salad

Serves 4
Prep time: 10 minutes
Cook time: 2 minutes

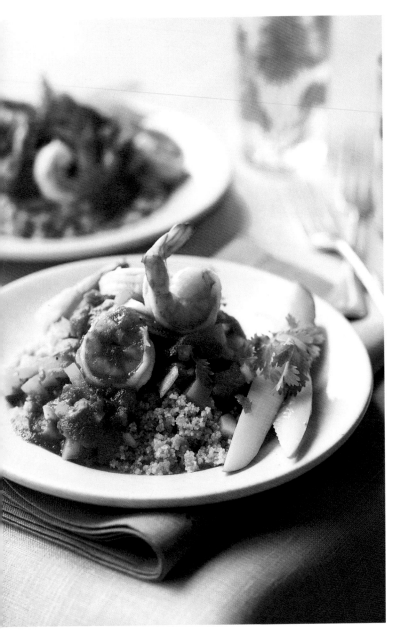

1   cup uncooked whole-wheat couscous
1   pound medium shrimp, peeled and deveined
2   14.5-ounce cans diced tomatoes with green
     pepper and onion
1   small cucumber, diced
1   yellow bell pepper, seeded and diced
2   tablespoons chopped fresh cilantro
½   teaspoon ground coriander
Salt and ground black pepper to taste

Prepare couscous according to package directions. Meanwhile, in a large saucepan over medium-high heat, combine shrimp and enough water to cover. Bring to a boil. Once water boils (shrimp will be bright pink and cooked through; about 2–3 minutes), drain and plunge shrimp into ice water.

In a large bowl, combine tomatoes, cucumber, bell pepper, cilantro and coriander. Mix well. Add shrimp and toss to combine. Season with salt and pepper.

Transfer couscous to 4 plates and top with shrimp mixture.

NUTRITION SCORE
Per serving (2 cups vegetables with shrimp, ¾ cup couscous):
348 **calories**
5% **fat** (2 g; 0 g saturated)
64% **carbs** (56 g), 11 g **fiber**
31% **protein** (27 g)

Getting enough protein, carbs and fat after a workout can help speed the muscle-building process. A light meal such as this one is the perfect way to revive yourself post-gym.

Red-Hot Sesame Spinach-Salmon Salad

Serves 6
Prep time: 30 minutes
Cook time: 20 minutes

Dressing

- ¼ cup scallions, thinly sliced (about 2 medium)
- ¼ cup soy sauce
- ¼ cup rice vinegar
- 2 tablespoons water
- 2 cloves garlic, minced
- 2 teaspoons toasted sesame seeds
- 2 teaspoons toasted sesame oil
- 1 teaspoon chili paste

Salad

- 2 teaspoons toasted sesame oil
- 6 scallions, trimmed and sliced into 1-inch batons (white and green parts)
- ¾ pound shiitake mushroom caps, sliced
- 3 cups corn
- 6 4-ounce salmon fillets, about 1½ inches thick
- Cooking spray
- 18 cups cleaned spinach leaves
- 3 cups bean sprouts
- 2 sweet red peppers, cored, seeded and thinly sliced

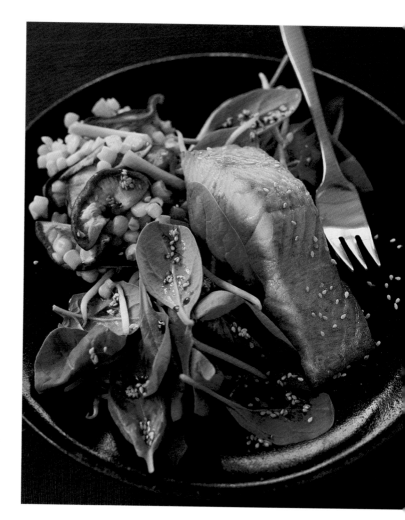

Preheat broiler. Whisk together dressing ingredients in a small bowl. Set aside.

To make salad, heat oil in a large nonstick skillet over medium-high heat. Add scallions and mushrooms. Sauté for 6 minutes. Stir in corn, cover and set aside.

Spray each salmon fillet with cooking spray. Place on a foil-lined baking sheet. Broil 8 minutes or until salmon is juicy and just cooked through.

Divide spinach, bean sprouts and peppers among 6 plates. Top with an equal portion of warm mushroom mixture. Slide a spatula under each piece of salmon (skin may stick to foil) and place atop mushroom mixture. Top with dressing and serve immediately.

NUTRITION SCORE
Per serving (3 cups salad, 4 ounces salmon): 351 **calories**
31% **fat** (12 g; 2 g saturated)
30% **carbs** (35 g), 10 g **fiber**
39% **protein** (34 g)

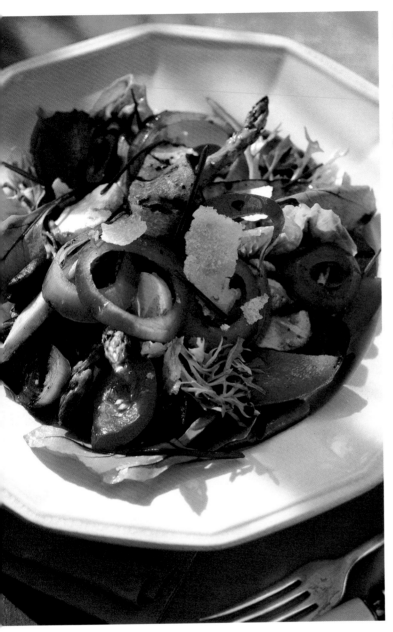

Grilled Vegetable Salad

Serves 6
Prep time: 20 minutes
Cook time: 15 minutes

3   tablespoons olive oil
1   tablespoon balsamic vinegar
1   medium red onion, cut into ½-inch-thick rounds
1   bunch asparagus
3   small zucchini, each cut lengthwise into 4 slices
2   large bell peppers, cut into 2-inch-wide strips
1   teaspoon salt
10 cups (1-2 bags) mixed baby greens
4   medium tomatoes, chopped
⅓   cup grated Parmesan cheese
¼   cup chopped fresh basil
¼   cup fresh chives
12 large brine-cured kalamata olives, halved (plus
    2 tablespoons of brine)
½   of a 3.5-ounce package chilled goat cheese, cut
    horizontally into 6 slices

Heat barbecue to medium-high. Whisk together oil and vinegar in a small bowl. Place onion, asparagus, zucchini and peppers on grill. Brush with half of the oil mixture and sprinkle with salt. Grill asparagus and onion about 6 minutes per side; zucchini and peppers, 4 minutes per side. (Or roast them on a baking sheet in a 400° F oven for 4-6 minutes.)

In a large bowl, combine greens, tomatoes, Parmesan cheese, basil and chives. Whisk the olives and brine into the remaining oil mixture and drizzle over the greens. Toss to coat. Divide greens among 6 plates. Top with grilled vegetables, one slice of goat cheese, and olives. Serve immediately.

NUTRITION SCORE
Per serving (2 cups of greens, 1 cup vegetables): 222 **calories**
55% **fat** (13.6 g; 3.8 g saturated)
30% **carbs** (18 g), 5.4 g **fiber**
15% **protein** (10 g)

Watermelon, Grilled Peach and Blackberry Salad With Honey-Yogurt Dressing

Serves 8
Prep time: 15 minutes
Cook time: 10-12 minutes

Honey-Yogurt Dressing

- 1 cup lowfat vanilla yogurt
- 2 tablespoons honey
- 1 tablespoon fresh lemon juice

Fruit Mixture

- ½ ripe watermelon, peeled, seeded and cut into 2-inch wedges (about 8 cups)
- 1 pint blackberries, rinsed
- ¼ cup chopped fresh mint
- ½ cup slivered almonds, lightly toasted
- 4 ripe peaches, pitted and halved
- 1 teaspoon vegetable oil

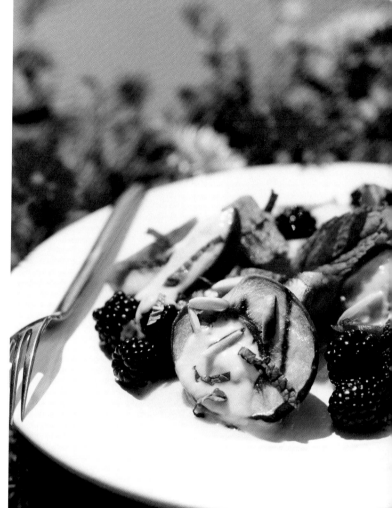

Preheat oven to 300° F. To make the dressing, whisk together the yogurt, honey and lemon juice in a small bowl.

In another bowl, combine the watermelon, blackberries and mint. Refrigerate until ready to use. To toast almonds, spread them out on a baking sheet and place in oven for 5 minutes. Allow them to cool completely.

Brush both sides of the peaches with oil. Place, cut side down, on the barbeque and grill 3-4 minutes, until golden brown. Flip and cook another 1-2 minutes. Remove from barbeque and cut each peach half into 2 pieces. Transfer to a large bowl, add watermelon wedges, blackberries and mint, and toss to combine. Divide peach mixture evenly among 8 plates, drizzle dressing over top and garnish with toasted almonds.

 Unhappy people are more likely to fast, binge, skip meals and eat too few vegetables. They also tend to consume more than 100 extra calories daily. Instead of reaching for food when you feel depressed, call a friend. If the feelings persist, seek professional psychological help.

NUTRITION SCORE
Per serving (1½ cups salad with 2 tablespoons dressing):
187 **calories**
29% **fat** (6 g fat; 1 g saturated)
62% **carbs** (29 g), 5 g **fiber**
9% **protein** (4 g)

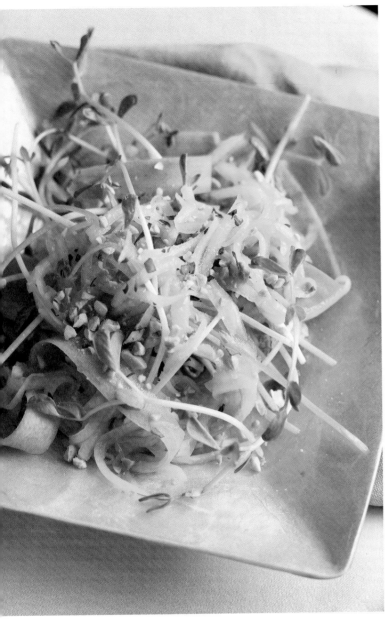

Green Mango Salad and Cilantro Vinaigrette

Serves 4
Prep time: 15 minutes

- ¼ cup toasted cashews
- 1 pound fresh green mango (about 1 large mango)
- 1 cup loosely packed bean sprouts
- ½ carrot, peeled and grated
- 3 tablespoons lemon juice
- 1 tablespoon light soy sauce
- 1 tablespoon bottled fish sauce (available in the Asian foods aisle of your supermarket)
- 1 clove garlic
- 1 teaspoon sugar
- 1 tablespoon chopped fresh cilantro

In a food processor, grind cashews finely. Set aside.

Peel, seed and grate mango. In a medium bowl, combine mango, bean sprouts and carrot. In a small bowl, mix lemon juice with soy and fish sauces.

Using the flat blade of a large knife, crush garlic with sugar to release the oils. Finely mince garlic and add to liquids. Combine with mango mixture. Mound on a platter for serving. Sprinkle with ground cashews and cilantro.

NUTRITION SCORE
Per serving (¾ cup): 143 **calories**
26% **fat** (4.2 g; 0.7 g saturated)
9% **carbs** (27 g), 3 g **fiber**
65% **protein** (3.3 g)

Green mangoes are a staple of Indian, Malaysian and Thai cuisines. For this recipe, choose mangoes with a green skin and hard flesh.

Fennel Salad With Blood Oranges and Fuji Persimmons

Serves 6
Prep time: 20 minutes

- 2 fennel bulbs
- 2 Fuji persimmons (available in winter)
- 2 blood oranges
- 3 tablespoons lemon juice
- Salt and pepper to taste
- ¼ cup extra-virgin olive oil
- 1 bunch watercress tops
- Pinch fennel seeds

Using a mandoline slicer (available at houseware stores), slice fennel bulbs crosswise and as thin as possible. Peel and cut persimmons into small wedges. Using a knife, peel oranges, sectioning and removing all membranes over a bowl to catch juice. Reserve juice that remains.

In a salad bowl, add lemon and orange juices, salt and pepper. Mix until salt dissolves. Slowly add olive oil. Add fennel, persimmons, orange sections and watercress tops. Sprinkle with fennel seeds. Toss and serve.

NUTRITION SCORE
Per serving (1 cup): 188 **calories**
45% **fat** (1.2 g saturated)
49% **carbs** (27 g), 3.1 g **fiber**
6% **protein** (3 g)

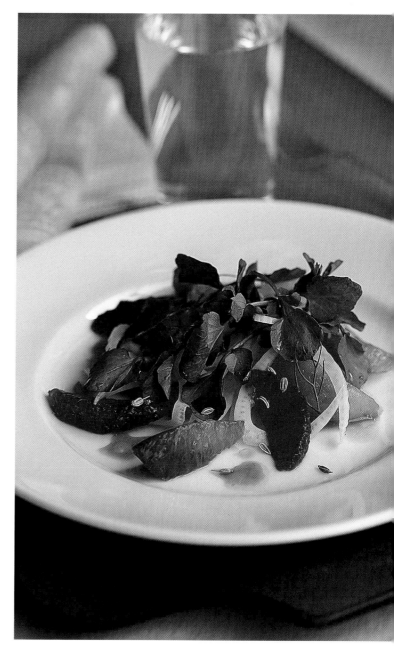

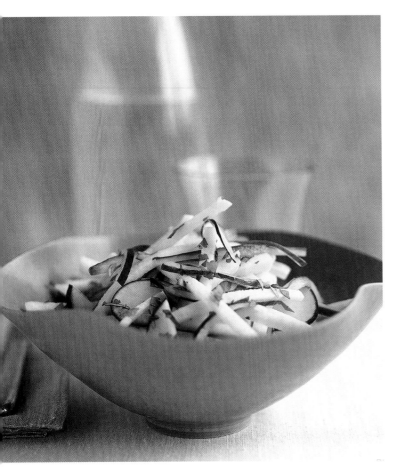

Jicama, Cucumber and Citrus Salad

Serves 4
Prep time: 15 minutes

1 medium jicama (about 1 pound), peeled and cut into 1/4-inch-thick matchsticks (makes about 3 cups)

½ English (seedless) cucumber, cut into 1/4-inch-thick matchsticks

6 radishes, thinly sliced

⅓ cup thinly sliced red onion

¼ cup chopped fresh cilantro

3 tablespoons orange juice

1 tablespoon fresh lime juice

2 teaspoons olive oil

¼ teaspoon salt

In a large bowl, combine jicama, cucumber, radishes, onion and cilantro. Toss to combine. In a small bowl, whisk together orange juice, lime juice, olive oil and salt. Pour over jicama mixture and toss. Serve immediately or cover with plastic and refrigerate up to 2 days.

NUTRITION SCORE
Per serving (1 ½ cups): 79 **calories**
27% **fat** (2 g; 0 g saturated)
67% **carbs** (13 g), 6 g **fiber**
6% **protein** (1 g)

Consuming plenty of fruits and vegetables shows promise in managing diabetes, one of the fastest-growing diseases in the country. This is because the soluble fibers in produce can delay blood glucose absorption from the small intestine.

Crab Salad in Zucchini Bowls With Whole-Grain Rolls and Zesty Olive Oil

Serves 4
Prep time: 15 minutes

- ¼ cup fat-free mayonnaise
- 1 tablespoon chopped fresh cilantro
- 1 teaspoon curry powder
- ½ teaspoon salt
- ¼ teaspoon ground black pepper
- 1 pound fresh lump crabmeat or 2 (6-ounce) cans, drained
- 1 green bell pepper, seeded and diced
- 2 medium zucchini, halved lengthwise and seeds removed with a spoon
- 8 teaspoons olive oil
- ½ teaspoon crushed red pepper flakes
- 4 4-ounce whole-grain rolls

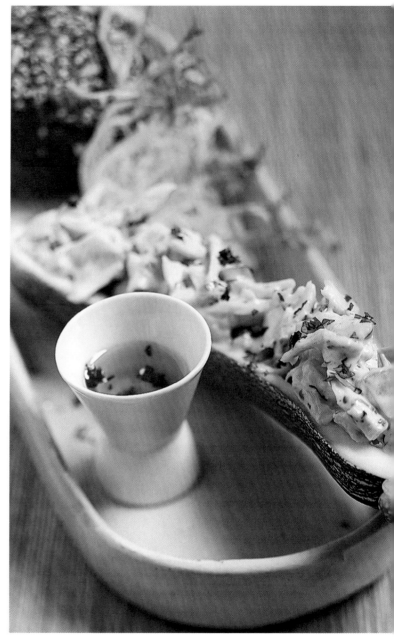

In a medium bowl, combine mayonnaise, cilantro, curry powder, salt and black pepper. Add crabmeat and green pepper and mix gently to combine. Spoon mixture into carved-out zucchini halves.

In a small bowl, combine olive oil and red pepper flakes. Serve crab-stuffed zucchini with rolls and olive-oil mixture on the side as a dip for the bread.

NUTRITION SCORE
Per serving (½ cup crab mixture, ½ zucchini, 1 roll, 2 teaspoons olive oil): 404 **calories**
23% **fat** (10 g; 1 g saturated)
49% **carbs** (49 g), 11 g **fiber**
28% **protein** (28 g)

Warm Lentil Vegetable Salad With Feta, Dried Currants and Dill

Serves 6
Prep time: 30 minutes
Cook time: 20 minutes

- 3 cups water
- 1 cup brown lentils, picked over (to remove pebbles) and rinsed
- 2 large carrots, peeled and diced
- 2 large parsnips, peeled and diced
- ½ cup minced red onion, divided
- ½ cup dried currants
- 2 large beets, peeled and diced
- 1 cup rice wine vinegar
- ⅓ cup chopped fresh dill
- 3 tablespoons sugar
- 2 cloves garlic, minced
- 2 teaspoons olive oil
- Salt and freshly ground black pepper to taste
- 12 cups cleaned mesclun lettuce
- 4 ounces feta cheese, crumbled (about ½ cup)

Combine water, lentils, carrots, parsnips and ¼ cup onion in a large saucepan. Bring to a boil. Reduce heat to low and partially cover; simmer 15 minutes, or until lentils and vegetables are tender. Drain; transfer to salad bowl. Toss with remaining onion and currants.

Steam beets for 10 minutes. Let cool. Combine vinegar, dill, sugar and garlic in a small bowl. Whisk until sugar is dissolved. Whisk in oil. Pour ⅔ of dressing over lentil mixture and toss to combine. Add salt and pepper.

Divide mesclun among 6 large plates. Drizzle with an equal portion of remaining dressing. Top with an equal portion of warm lentil mixture, beets and feta cheese.

NUTRITION SCORE
Per serving (2 cups greens, ⅔ cup lentils): 311 **calories**
17% **fat** (6 g; 3 g saturated)
64% **carbs** (53 g), 16 g **fiber**
19% **protein** (15 g)

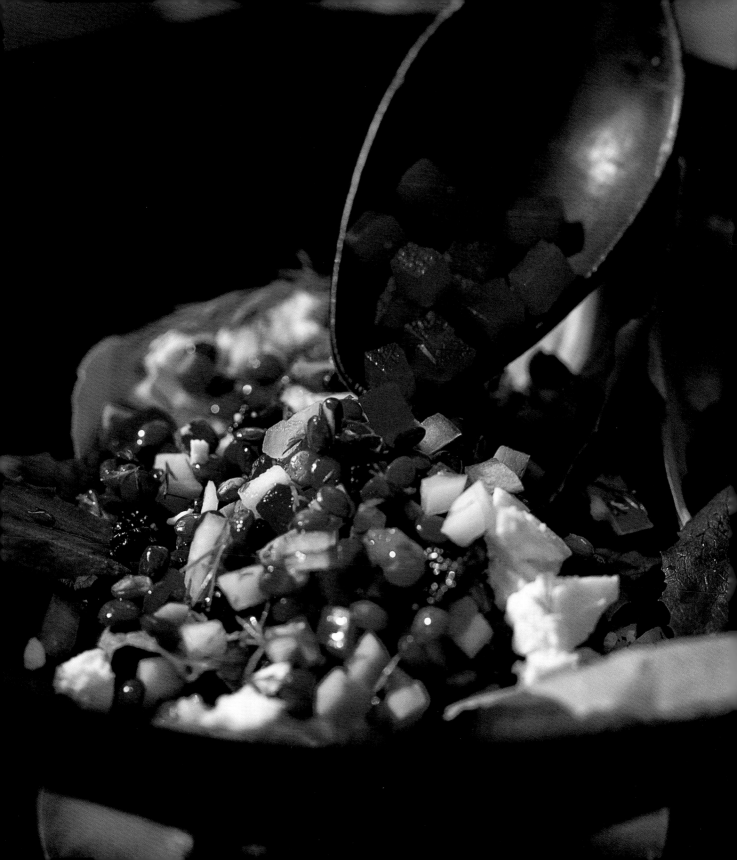

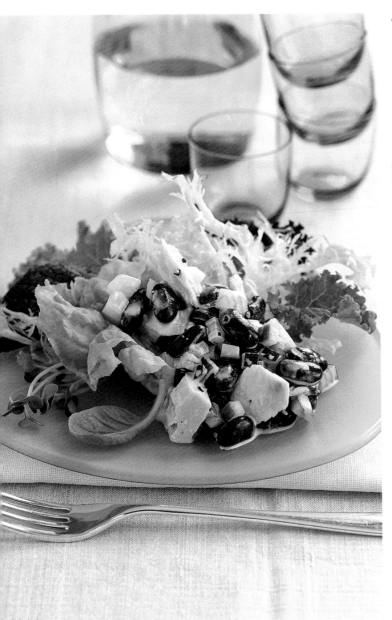

Tuna Salad With Kidney Beans and Red Onion

Serves 4
Prep time: 12 minutes

¼ cup chopped red onion
3 tablespoons cider vinegar
3 tablespoons lowfat mayonnaise
1 tablespoon lemon juice
¼ teaspoon ground black pepper
1 6-ounce can water-packed tuna
½ cup diced seedless cucumber
1 15-ounce can kidney beans, rinsed and drained
8 slices whole-grain bread, toasted

Combine onion and cider vinegar in a small dish. Let stand for at least 5 minutes.

Meanwhile, mix together mayonnaise, lemon juice and pepper in a medium bowl. Break up tuna and add to mayo mixture, along with cucumber and kidney beans. Drain onions in colander and rinse well. Add to tuna and stir to combine. Serve with mixed greens and bread on the side.

NUTRITION SCORE
Per serving (½ cup tuna-bean salad with 2 slices toast):
273 **calories**
11% **fat** (3 g; 0.6 g saturated)
60% **carbs** (40 g), 5 g **fiber**
29% **protein** (20 g)

Grilled Chicken Caesar Salad

Serves 4
Prep time: 8-10 minutes
Cook time: 7 minutes

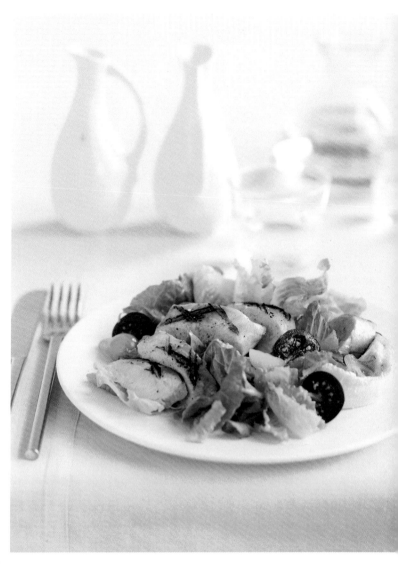

  4 4-ounce skinless, boneless chicken breast halves
Salt and ground black pepper to taste
  1 tablespoon grated Parmesan cheese
  2 teaspoons Dijon mustard
  2 teaspoons olive oil
  1 teaspoon Worcestershire sauce
  1 clove garlic, minced
  ½ cup reduced-sodium, nonfat chicken broth, divided
  2 teaspoons anchovy paste (optional)
  6 cups romaine lettuce leaves (in 2-inch pieces), rinsed, patted dry
16 cherry tomatoes

Preheat grill, broiler or grill pan. Season both sides of chicken with salt and pepper. Cook 5 minutes a side, or until done.

Meanwhile, purée cheese, mustard, oil, Worcestershire sauce, garlic and ¼ cup broth in a blender until smooth. Add remaining broth (and ½ teaspoon anchovy paste, if desired); purée.

In a large bowl, toss romaine with dressing. Divide among 4 plates. Thinly slice grilled chicken crosswise; arrange with tomatoes on romaine.

NUTRITION SCORE
Per serving (1 chicken breast, sliced; 1½ cups lettuce; 2 tablespoons dressing; 4 cherry tomatoes): 200 **calories**
27% **fat** (6 g; 1 g saturated)
14% **carbs** (6.5 g), 2 g **fiber**
59% **protein** (29.5 g)

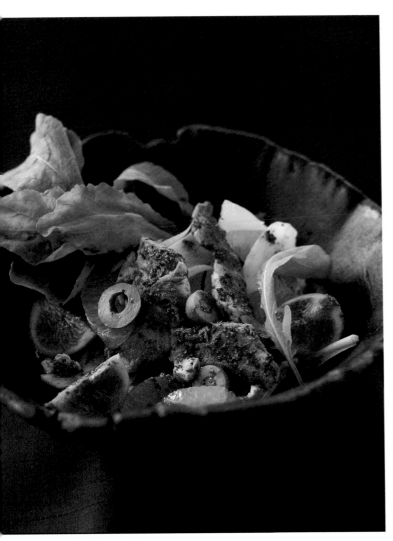

Moroccan Chicken and Arugula Salad With Olives and Figs

Serves 6
Prep time: 35 minutes
Cook time: 10 minutes

3½ teaspoons olive oil, divided
4 boneless, skinless chicken breast halves, cut into bite-size chunks
1 clove garlic, minced
1 teaspoon ground cumin
6 tablespoons orange juice
¼ cup balsamic vinegar
2 tablespoons Dijon mustard
Salt and freshly ground black pepper to taste
18 cups cleaned, trimmed arugula leaves
3 cups thinly sliced fennel
3 oranges, peeled, sectioned and sliced into chunks
12 dried figs, chopped
6 pitted green olives, thinly sliced
2 ounces goat cheese, crumbled (about ¼ cup)

Warm 2 teaspoons of oil in a large nonstick skillet over medium-high heat. Sauté chicken for 2 minutes. Add garlic and cumin; sauté 2 minutes more. Reduce heat to low. Stir in orange juice, vinegar and mustard. Slowly stir in remaining oil to make a warm dressing. Add salt and pepper.

Divide arugula among 6 plates. Sprinkle with fennel and oranges. Spoon warm chicken mixture over salad and top with figs, olives and goat cheese.

NUTRITION SCORE
Per serving (4 cups): 268 **calories**
27% **fat** (8 g; 2 g saturated)
37% **carbs** (26 g), 8 g **fiber**
36% **protein** (24 g)

Pasta Salad With Almonds and Grapes

Serves 4
Prep time: 5 minutes
Cook time: 8-10 minutes

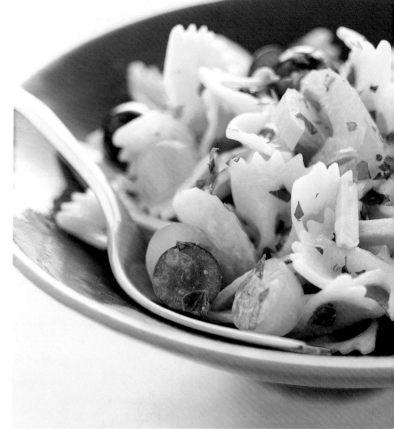

  12 ounces uncooked bow-tie (farfalle) pasta
   4 tablespoons slivered almonds
   1 cup nonfat sour cream
   2 tablespoons nonfat mayonnaise
   1 tablespoon sherry vinegar
   1 cup green grapes, halved
   1 cup red grapes, halved
   2 stalks celery, chopped
   1 tablespoon chopped fresh mint
  Salt and ground black pepper to taste

Cook pasta in a large pot of boiling water for 8-10 minutes, until just tender. Drain and place in a large bowl.

While pasta cooks, place almonds in a small skillet and set pan over low heat. Cook 3-5 minutes, until nuts are golden, shaking the pan frequently to prevent burning. Set aside.

Add sour cream, mayonnaise and vinegar to the pasta and toss to coat noodles. Fold in grapes, celery and mint. Add salt and ground black pepper.

Spoon mixture onto individual plates and top with toasted almonds.

NUTRITION SCORE
Per serving (2 cups): 470 **calories**
11% **fat** (6 g; <1 g saturated)
74% **carbs** (87 g), 3 g **fiber**
15% **protein** (18 g)

 Domestically grown grapes show up in grocery stores from May through January. (Chile provides the bulk of imports the rest of the year.) Try adding grapes to savory salads, toss them into stir-fries or drop them into the roasting pan when you're cooking chicken, turkey or pork.

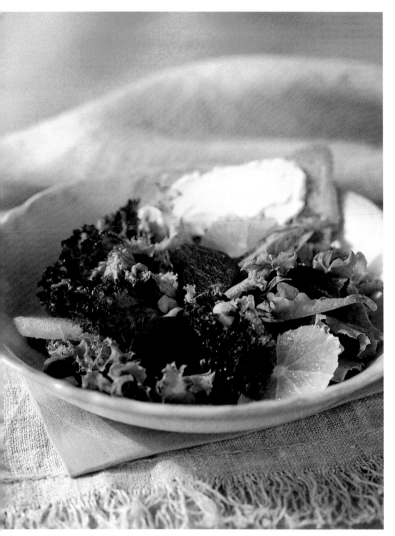

Oranges, Beets and Greens With Goat-Cheese Toast Points

Serves 10
Prep time: 25 minutes

- 1 ounce goat cheese
- 1 ounce lowfat cream cheese
- 2 cups canned beets, drained
- 2 tablespoons sherry vinegar
- 8-10 navel or Valencia oranges
- 1 pound mixed salad greens
- Salt to taste
- 8-10 Melba toasts
- ⅓ cup toasted walnuts, roughly chopped

Vinaigrette

- ¼ cup plus 2 tablespoons orange juice
- 2 tablespoons sherry vinegar
- 4 tablespoons balsamic vinegar
- 2 tablespoons extra-virgin olive oil
- Coarse-grained salt to taste
- Cracked black pepper to taste

In a small nonmetal bowl, whisk together vinaigrette ingredients. Set aside. In another small bowl, whisk together cheeses; refrigerate, covered. In a bowl, toss beets with sherry vinegar. Set aside.

Using a sharp paring knife, trim off the top and bottom of the oranges; then slice away all peel and pith, beginning at the top and paring downward. Slice oranges crosswise into ¼-inch-thick rounds. Set aside.

Place greens in a nonmetal bowl and toss with just enough vinaigrette to coat. Season with salt. Transfer to a platter. Top with orange slices and beets. Just before serving, spread 1 teaspoon of cheese mixture on each toast point and set atop salad. Garnish with toasted walnuts.

NUTRITION SCORE
Per serving (1 cup): 180 **calories**
36% **fat** (7.2 g; 1.4 g saturated)
53% **carbs** (27 g), 5.4 g **fiber**
11% **protein** (4.9 g)

Oriental Salad

Serves 8
Prep time: 10 minutes
Chill time: 60 minutes

2	3-ounce packages lowfat beef ramen noodle soup
1	16-ounce package cabbage slaw or shredded cabbage
¼	cup salted sunflower seeds
⅓	cup slivered almonds, toasted
1½	cups chopped chives
2	tablespoons hot water
½	cup pineapple juice
5	teaspoons dark sesame oil
½	cup white wine vinegar
3	tablespoons sugar

To make the salad, crumble ramen noodles. (Be sure to save one of the flavor packets for the dressing.) In a large bowl, toss together the noodles, cabbage, sunflower seeds, almonds and chives.

To make the dressing, dissolve one beef flavor packet in hot water. Whisk together pineapple juice, oil, vinegar, sugar and dissolved beef flavor mixture. Pour over salad. Cover and chill at least 1 hour, stirring occasionally.

NUTRITION SCORE
Per serving (1 ½ cups): 247 **calories**
34.7% **fat** (9.8 g; <1 g saturated)
53.6% **carbs** (34 g); 6.4 g **fiber**
11.7% **protein** (7.4 g)

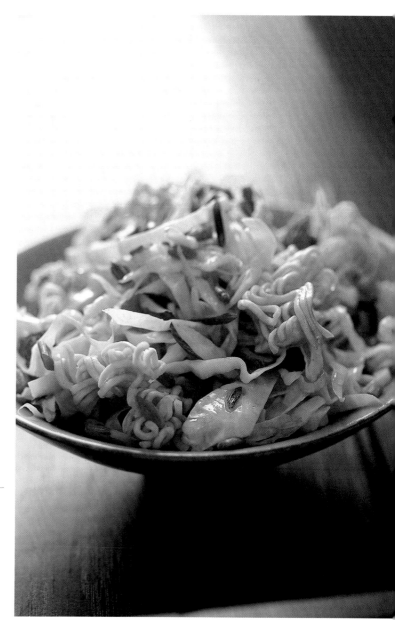

Cabbage contains indoles, a substance (also found in brussels sprouts and broccoli) that helps prevent breast cancer.

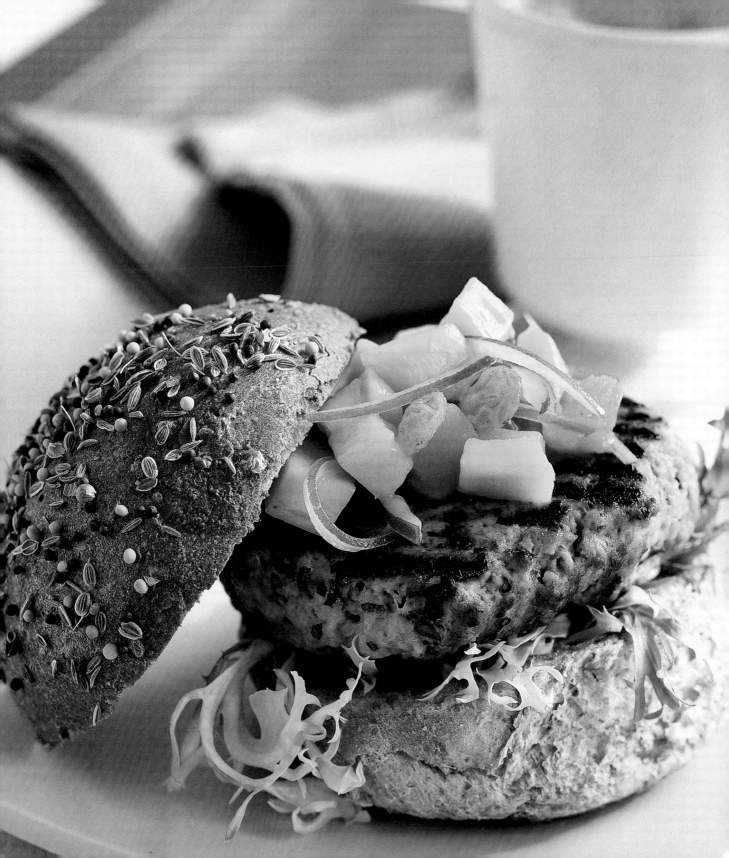

sandwiches

You don't need to give up your lunch favorites in order to eat well. Here we show just how easy it is to assemble healthful versions of the burger, tuna melt, Reuben and club. And lunch at work doesn't have to mean greasy fast-food takeout. You can easily brown-bag it the healthy way with Faux Egg Salad Sandwich or Chicken Salad With Raspberries and Walnuts.

recipes

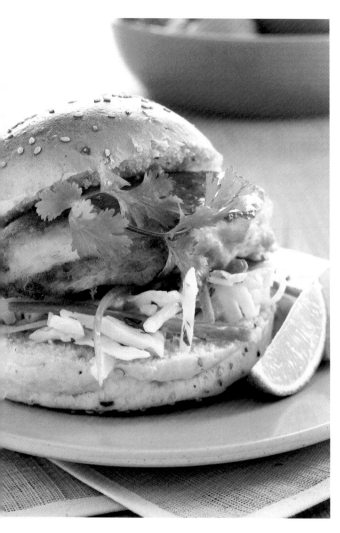

Grilled Lime Chicken Sandwiches With Spicy Slaw

Serves 4
Prep time: 30 minutes
Cook time: 10 minutes

Grilled chicken

  4 skinless, boneless chicken breast fillets, all fat removed
  ½ cup reduced-sodium soy sauce
Juice of 3 limes

Dressing

  ½ cup plain nonfat yogurt
  2 tablespoons mayonnaise
  ⅓ cup apple-cider vinegar
  ¼ teaspoon sugar
  3 tablespoons chopped cilantro
1-2 teaspoons Tabasco sauce (or to taste)
Salt to taste

Slaw

  4 cups shredded raw cabbage
  1 cup shredded raw carrots
  ⅓ cup finely sliced green onions, green parts only
Cooking spray
  4 large whole-grain hamburger buns

NUTRITION SCORE
Per serving (1 sandwich): 363 **calories**
28% **fat** (11 g; 2 g saturated)
34% **carbs** (31 g), 5 g **fiber**
38% **protein** (34 g)

Preheat broiler or grill. Place chicken breasts, soy sauce and lime juice in a medium-size glass or ceramic bowl; cover with plastic wrap and allow to marinate in the refrigerator for at least 30 minutes (and up to 3 hours).

Meanwhile, place dressing ingredients in a small bowl and whisk until well incorporated. In a large bowl, toss dressing with cabbage, carrots and green onions and set aside.

Once chicken has marinated for 30 minutes, lightly coat fillets with cooking spray and grill or broil until chicken is firm and cooked through. (Cook for 4-5 minutes on each side, depending on thickness.) To assemble sandwich, place ½ cup slaw on a whole-grain bun bottom, place chicken breast on top and add 2-3 tablespoons of slaw over chicken. Cover with bun top and serve immediately.

Veggie Hippie Hero

Serves 1
Prep time: 5 minutes

Dressing

- 1 medium carrot, grated (½ cup)
- 2 tablespoons mirin (Japanese rice wine)
- 2 tablespoons seasoned rice wine vinegar
- 1 teaspoon chili oil
- 1 teaspoon grated ginger root
- 1 16-ounce package silken tofu
- 1 small clove of garlic

Sandwich

- 1 2-ounce soft whole-wheat roll
- 3-4 romaine lettuce leaves
- ¼ cup shredded carrots
- 4 ounces reduced-fat Cheddar cheese
- 4-5 ripe tomato slices
- 7-8 cucumber slices
- 7-8 radish slices
- Red onion slices to taste
- 3-4 avocado slices (⅛ of an avocado)
- ⅓ cup alfalfa sprouts

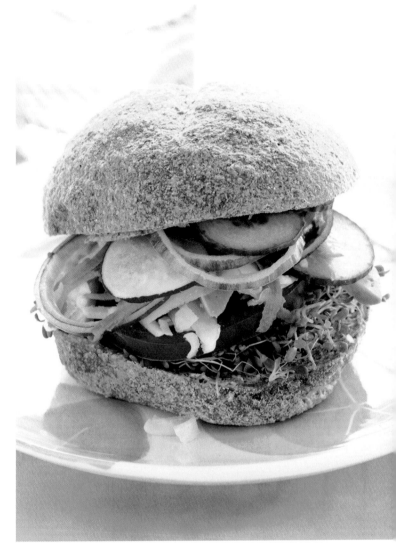

Combine all the dressing ingredients in a blender and blend until smooth. Set aside.

Hollow out the roll, and layer 3-4 romaine lettuce leaves, shredded carrots, shredded Cheddar cheese, tomato slices, cucumber slices, radish slices, red onion slices and avocado slices. Top with alfalfa sprouts and drizzle generously with 2 tablespoons dressing. Cover with the hollowed-out top of the roll.

NUTRITION SCORE
Per serving (1 veggie hero): 452 **calories**
18% **fat** (9 g; 1 g saturated)
41% **carbs** (46 g), 7 g **fiber**
41% **protein** (46 g)

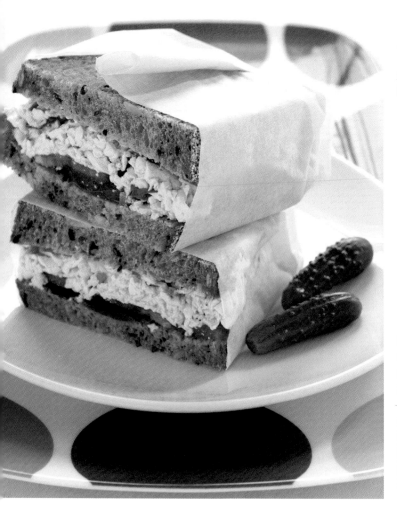

Faux Egg Salad Sandwich

Serves 4
Prep time: 5 minutes

- 1　16-ounce package extra-firm silken tofu
- 2　tablespoons diced celery (1 small rib)
- 3　tablespoons thinly sliced scallion (green parts only)
- 2　tablespoons light mayonnaise
- 1　teaspoon plain whole-milk yogurt
- ½　teaspoon Dijon mustard
- Pinch of turmeric
- Salt and cracked pepper to taste
- 8　slices multigrain bread
- 1　tomato, sliced

Pat tofu dry with paper towels; then grate it. Place grated tofu in a medium-size bowl and add celery, scallion, mayonnaise, yogurt, mustard, turmeric, salt and pepper. Stir until all ingredients are combined. Serve on multigrain bread with sliced tomato.

NUTRITION SCORE
Per serving (½ cup "egg" salad spread on 2 slices multigrain bread):
250 **calories**
20% **fat** (6 g)
53% **carbs** (33 g), 8 g **fiber**
27% **protein** (17 g)

Silken tofu stands in for the eggs in this recipe. Grating the tofu with a large-hole grater (just as you would Cheddar cheese) helps get the texture right.

Tuna Melt

Serves 4
Prep time: 5 minutes
Cook time: 2 minutes

- 2 6-ounce cans chunk white tuna in water, drained
- ⅓ cup fat-free mayonnaise
- ¼ cup diced, water-packed roasted red peppers
- 2 teaspoons Dijon mustard
- ¼ teaspoon ground black pepper
- 1 cup baby spinach leaves, stems trimmed
- 4 slices whole-grain bread
- 4 1-ounce slices reduced-fat Swiss cheese

Preheat broiler. Mix together tuna, mayonnaise, red peppers, mustard and black pepper. Arrange spinach leaves on bread slices. Top spinach with tuna mixture and then cheese slices. Transfer sandwiches to a baking sheet and broil 1–2 minutes, until cheese melts.

NUTRITION SCORE
Per serving (½ sandwich): 251 **calories**
21% **fat** (5.8 g; 2.6 g saturated)
35% **carbs** (22 g), 4 g **fiber**
44% **protein** (27.6 g)

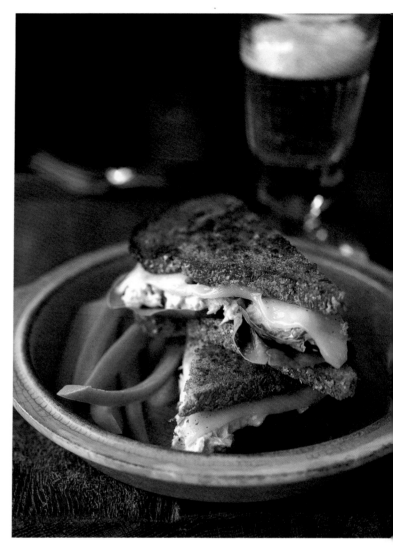

Stick to a 1:3 ratio to eat a 30 percent fat diet without counting fat grams. Balance each high-fat food you eat with three lowfat foods. Follow each high-fat meal with three lowfat ones.

Chicken Salad With Raspberries and Walnuts

Serves 4
Prep time: 10 minutes
Cook time: 2-3 minutes

- ¼ cup chopped walnuts
- 4 cooked skinless chicken breast halves, cut into 1-inch cubes
- 1 cup fresh raspberries or a combination of raspberries and blackberries
- 2 green onions, chopped
- 1 tablespoon raspberry white wine vinegar
- 1 tablespoon olive oil
- 2 teaspoons Dijon mustard
- Salt and ground black pepper to taste
- 4 Boston lettuce leaves, rinsed well and patted dry
- 4 whole-wheat pita pockets, halved

Place walnuts in a small skillet and set pan over medium-high heat. Cook 2-3 minutes, until nuts are golden brown, shaking the pan frequently. Set aside.

In a large bowl, combine chicken, berries, green onions and walnuts. Toss gently to combine.

In a small bowl, whisk together vinegar, oil and mustard. Add to chicken mixture and toss to coat. Season with salt and pepper.

Stuff lettuce leaves into pita pockets. Spoon chicken salad into pita and serve.

NUTRITION SCORE
Per serving (1 pita, 1 cup chicken salad, 1 lettuce leaf): 410 **calories**
29% **fat** (13 g; 2 g saturated)
38% **carbs** (39.25 g), 7 g **fiber**
33% **protein** (34 g)

Be savvy at the salad bar: To avoid going overboard with fatty dressings, load up on juicy ingredients like tomatoes and beets.

Grilled Turkey Club

Serves 2
Prep time: 5 minutes
Cook time: 6-8 minutes

- 4 slices turkey bacon, cooked
- 4 slices 100 percent whole-wheat bread
- 1 tablespoon mustard
- 6 teaspoons light margarine
- 4 ounces sliced turkey breast
- 4 slices fresh tomato
- 2 ounces (½ cup) reduced-fat Cheddar cheese, shredded

Put bacon atop 2 paper towels on a microwave-safe plate; lay another towel on top. Microwave until crisp, about 2 minutes. (The paper towels will absorb much of the fat.) Crumble.

Spread one side of each bread slice with mustard and the other side with 1 teaspoon of margarine.

Top 2 slices of bread each with half of the turkey, tomato, bacon and cheese. Top each stack with a slice of bread, mustard side in.

In a nonstick pan, melt remaining margarine over medium heat. Grill sandwiches until golden, 3-4 minutes per side. Cut in half; serve.

NUTRITION SCORE
Per serving (1 sandwich): 378 **calories**
26% **fat** (10.9 g; 0.5 g saturated)
40% **carbs** (40 g), 6.9 g **fiber**
34% **protein** (33 g)

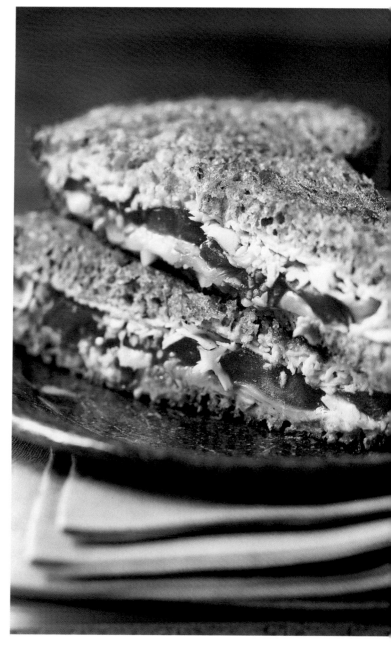

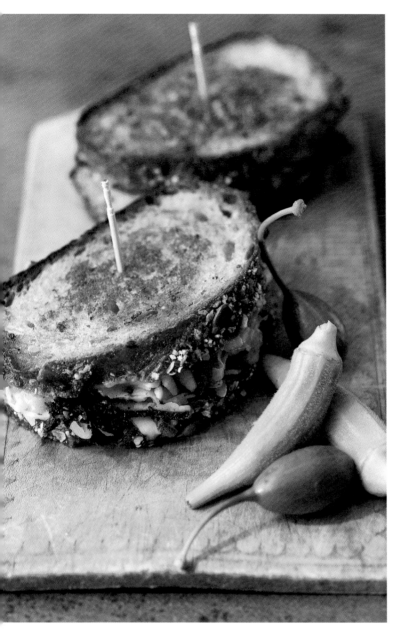

Reuben

Serves 2
Prep time: 4-5 minutes
Cook time: 8 minutes

- 4 slices rye bread
- 6 teaspoons light margarine
- 4 ounces turkey pastrami, sliced
- ½ cup sauerkraut, drained
- 2 ounces reduced-fat mozzarella cheese, shredded

Thousand Island Dressing

- 1 tablespoon reduced-fat mayonnaise
- 1 teaspoon sweet relish
- 1 teaspoon ketchup

Combine dressing ingredients. Spread on one side of each slice of bread; spread 1 teaspoon of margarine on the other side. Pile half of pastrami, sauerkraut and cheese onto the dressing side of two slices of bread. Top with remaining bread, dressing side in.

In a nonstick pan, melt the 2 remaining teaspoons of margarine over medium heat. Grill the sandwiches in the pan until golden (approximately 4 minutes per side). Cut in half and serve immediately.

NUTRITION SCORE
Per serving (1 sandwich): 327 **calories**
33% **fat** (12 g; 0.5 g saturated)
36% **carbs** (29 g), 3.5 g **fiber**
31% **protein** (26 g)

No time for a sandwich? Healthy snacks such as turkey jerkey; energy bars; an apple with peanut butter; and Asian trail mix with rice crackers, peanuts and dried peas will provide energy until your next meal.

Blackened Shrimp Po' Boy

Serves 4
Prep time: 5 minutes, (plus 30 minutes to marinate)
Cook time: 10 minutes

- 1 pound large raw fresh shrimp, peeled and deveined
- 1 tablespoon Cajun blackened seasoning for seafood
- ¼ cup plus 2 tablespoons lowfat mayonnaise
- 2 tablespoons Dijon mustard
- 2 tablespoons lime juice
- 4 6-inch whole-wheat submarine rolls
- 1 tablespoon plus 1 teaspoon butter or margarine, divided
- 2 medium green or red bell peppers, thinly sliced
- 2 cloves garlic, minced

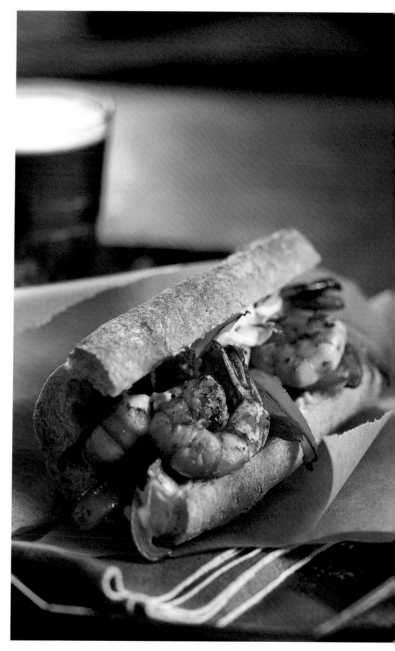

Toss shrimp and Cajun seasoning in a small bowl. Cover with plastic wrap and refrigerate 30 minutes to 1 hour.

Combine mayonnaise, mustard and lime juice; mix well. Set aside. Split submarine rolls. Pull out centers of roll halves, leaving 1-inch shell at edges and ½ inch at bottoms. (The roll centers can be reserved for later use, such as for making bread crumbs.) Set rolls aside.

Melt 1 tablespoon butter in a large nonstick skillet over medium-high heat. Add shrimp and sauté 4-5 minutes or until shrimp are opaque. Remove shrimp from skillet and set aside. Reduce heat to medium. Add remaining butter to skillet. Add peppers and sauté 5 minutes. Add garlic and sauté another 5 minutes or until peppers are tender.

Spread 2 teaspoons of mayonnaise mixture in each roll bottom. Spoon pepper-garlic mixture evenly into roll bottoms. Spoon shrimp evenly over pepper-garlic mixture.

Drizzle remaining mayonnaise mixture evenly over shrimp, and cover with roll tops. Serve immediately.

NUTRITION SCORE
Per serving (1 sandwich): 430 **calories**
29% **fat** (14 g; 4 g saturated)
47% **carbs** (52 g), 5 g **fiber**
24% **protein** (26 g)

Tuna Burgers With Horseradish Mayo

Serves 4
Prep time: 10 minutes
Cook time: 14 minutes

Burgers

- 3 6-ounce cans chunk light tuna in water, drained
- ¼ cup Italian-style dry bread crumbs
- 2 tablespoons fat-free mayonnaise
- 1 tablespoon Dijon mustard
- ¼ teaspoon salt
- ¼ teaspoon ground black pepper
- Cooking spray
- 8 slices whole-wheat bread or 4 whole-wheat hamburger buns, split

Horseradish Mayo

- ½ cup fat-free mayonnaise
- 1 tablespoon chopped fresh parsley
- 1 tablespoon prepared horseradish

Preheat grill or broiler. In a large bowl, combine tuna, bread crumbs, mayonnaise, mustard, salt and pepper. Mix well to combine. Shape mixture into 4 equal patties and transfer to a baking sheet coated with cooking spray.

Broil burgers 5 minutes per side, until light brown on both sides. Transfer burgers to hot grill and grill 2 minutes per side, until grill marks appear.

Meanwhile, to make Horseradish Mayo, combine all ingredients in a small bowl and mix well.

Arrange tuna burgers on bread and top each burger with horseradish mayo.

NUTRITION SCORE
Per serving (1 burger): 294 **calories**
15% **fat** (4.9 g; 1.4 g saturated)
42% **carbs** (31 g), 2 g **fiber**
43% **protein** (31.6 g)

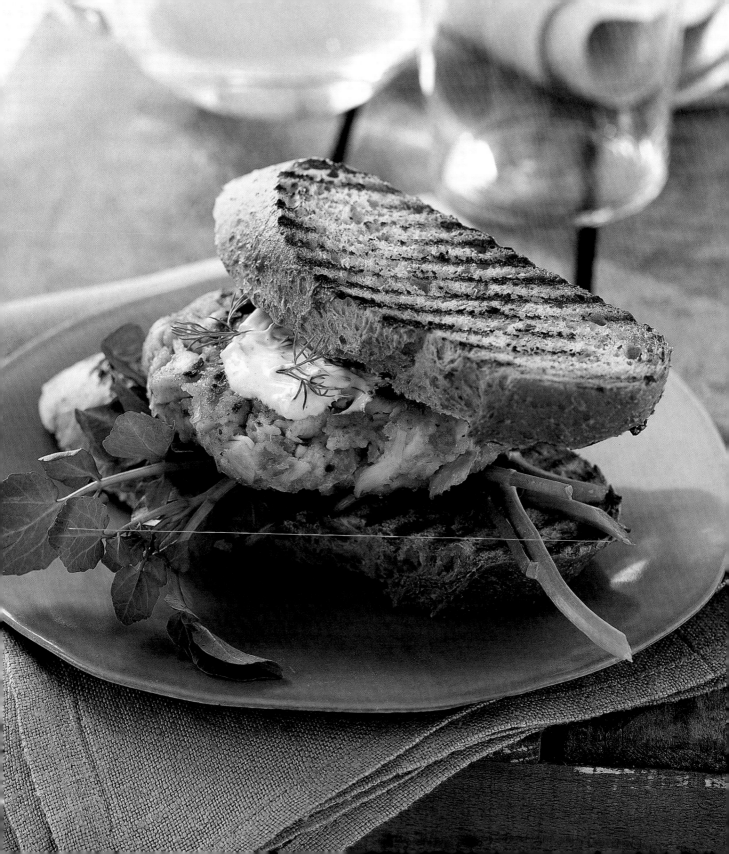

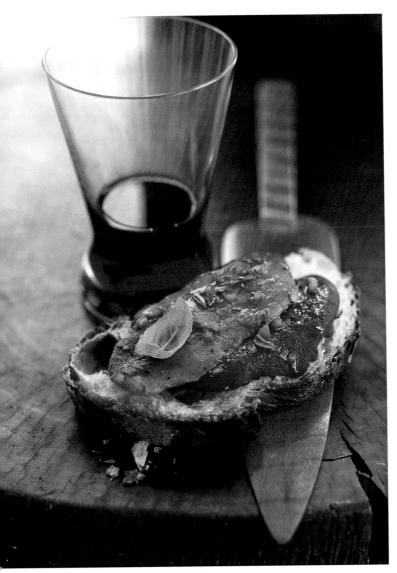

Roasted Pepper Panini With Chili and Basil

Serves 4
Prep time: 15 minutes
Cook time: 5 minutes

4 large bell peppers, sliced and roasted
Olive oil
2 tablespoons minced fresh basil
2 teaspoons balsamic vinegar
1 fresh hot pepper, seeded and minced (use gloves)
4 slices Italian bread, warmed in oven
Pinch sea salt

To blacken peppers, cut in half, rub with olive oil and place on a sheet pan. Broil for about 5 minutes, until skin has blackened. Remove peppers from broiler and wrap tightly in plastic to loosen skin. When cool enough to handle, remove plastic and rub off skin.

Place peppers and remaining ingredients except bread in a medium bowl. Toss well to combine. Spoon over bread.

NUTRITION SCORE
Per serving (1 slice): 124 **calories**
9% **fat** (1.3 g; 0.2 g saturated)
75% **carbs** (24 g), 5.2 g **fiber**
16% **protein** (5.1 g)

From sweet bell to three-alarm-hot, peppers are an incredible source of immunity-boosting vitamin C. One serving provides 235 percent of your RDA for vitamin C plus 53 percent of your daily beta carotene needs.

Hummus and Tzatziki Wrap

Serves 2
Prep time: 10 minutes

- 2 cucumbers, peeled and chopped into bite-size pieces
- 2 cloves garlic, peeled and minced
- 2 cups plain nonfat yogurt
- 4 pita wraps or large whole-wheat tortillas
- 1 15-ounce can garbanzo beans (chickpeas), drained
- 2 teaspoons ground coriander
- 1 teaspoon dried oregano
- 1 teaspoon dried cumin
- Juice of 1 lemon

Stir cucumbers and garlic into yogurt and set aside in refrigerator.

Lay pita wraps or tortillas on a solid, flat surface. Spread garbanzo beans on wraps, leaving 1-inch margin. Smash garbanzos lightly with a fork, being careful not to pierce or tear the wraps. Evenly sprinkle coriander, oregano and cumin over garbanzos. Spread yogurt mixture over the top, maintaining the 1-inch margin. Drizzle fresh lemon juice over yogurt mixture.

Fold left and right margins of the wraps in, and roll them up from the bottom. Secure with a toothpick.

NUTRITION SCORE
Per serving (2 wraps): 468 **calories**
8% **fat** (4 g; 0.4 g saturated)
67% **carbs** (78.8 g), 29 g **fiber**
25% **protein** (29.1 g)

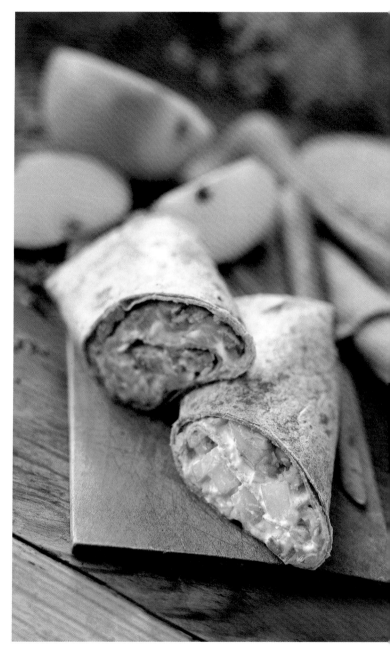

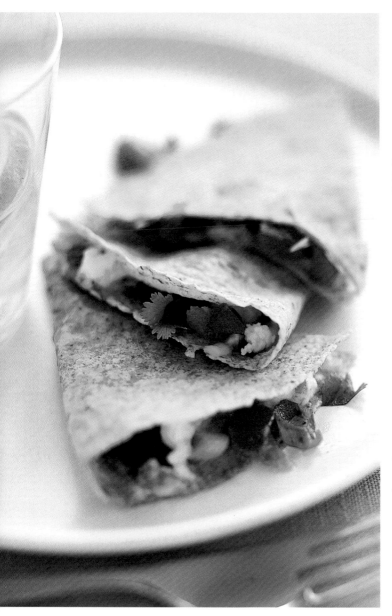

Three-Cheese Vegetable Quesadillas

Serves 4
Prep time: 5 minutes
Cook time: 8 minutes

- ½ cup grated part-skim mozzarella cheese
- ½ cup crumbled feta cheese
- 2 teaspoons crumbled blue cheese
- 1 teaspoon olive oil
- 2 medium tomatoes, diced
- 6 scallions, diced
- 1 jalapeño pepper, seeded and diced
- 2 cloves garlic, minced
- 1 teaspoon chopped fresh oregano or
  ½ teaspoon dried
- 3 tablespoons chopped fresh cilantro
- 8 8-inch flour or whole-wheat tortillas

Combine cheeses in a bowl; set aside.

Heat oil in a large nonstick skillet over medium heat. Add tomatoes, scallions, jalapeño, garlic and oregano and cook 2 minutes, until fragrant, stirring frequently. Stir in cilantro. Remove vegetables from pan; set aside.

Return skillet to heat and add 1 tortilla. Top ½ of tortilla with 2 tablespoons each of cheese mixture and vegetable mixture. Fold over untopped side and cook 1 minute per side, until cheese melts. Remove from pan and cover with foil to keep warm. Cut each quesadilla into 3 wedges and serve warm.

NUTRITION SCORE
Per serving (2 quesadillas/6 wedges): 261 **calories**
29% **fat** (8.5 g; 5 g saturated)
50% **carbs** (33 g), 13 g **fiber**
21% **protein** (14 g)

Veggie Burgers

Serves 4
Prep time: 10 minutes
Cook time: 6 minutes

> 2 cups bulgur-portobello pilaf (see recipe on
>   page 152)
> Cooking spray
> 4 whole-wheat hamburger buns, split
> 1 small onion, sliced
> 1 tomato, sliced
> 4 lettuce leaves

Mash together bulgur pilaf in a mixing bowl, making sure all chickpeas are smashed. Form into 4 patties.

Lightly coat a 10-inch nonstick pan with cooking spray and place on medium heat. When pan is hot, cook burgers 2-3 minutes per side.

Serve on whole-wheat buns with onion, tomato and lettuce.

NUTRITION SCORE
Per serving (1 veggie burger, onion, lettuce, tomato and bun):
181 **calories**
15% **fat** (3 g; 0.4 g saturated)
72% **carbs** (32.5 g), 6 g **fiber**
13% **protein** (6 g)

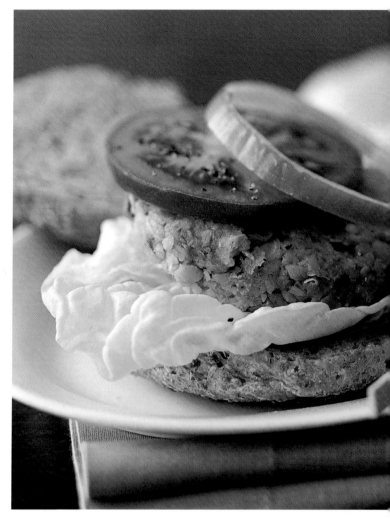

Bored of ketchup? Top your burger with honey mustard ($1/3$ cup honey, 2 tablespoons mustard, 1 tablespoon lightly toasted mustard seeds) or try chili cream ($1/2$ cup nonfat sour cream, 2 teaspoons each chili powder and ground cumin).

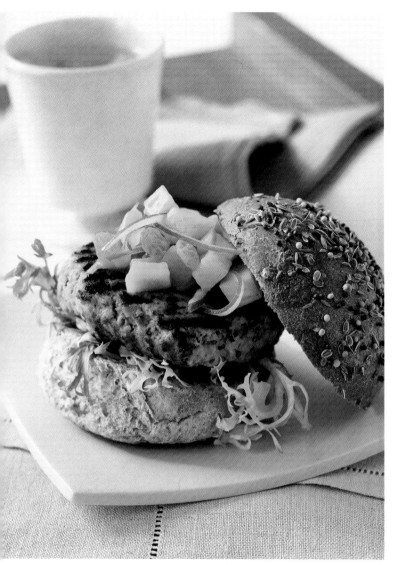

Curried Pork Burgers With Mango Chutney

Serves 4
Prep time: 20 minutes
Cook time: 10 minutes

Mango Chutney
- 2 cups diced fresh mango (about 2 ripe mangoes)
- ¼ cup raisins
- 3 tablespoons minced red onion
- 2 tablespoons balsamic vinegar
- 2 tablespoons water

Burgers
- 1 pound lean ground pork
- 2 tablespoons chopped fresh parsley
- 2½ teaspoons curry powder
- ½ teaspoon salt
- ¼ teaspoon ground black pepper
- 4 whole-wheat hamburger buns, split

To make the chutney, in a small saucepan combine mango, raisins, onion, vinegar and water. Set pan over medium heat and simmer 10 minutes, until mango just starts to break down. Remove from heat and set aside.

Preheat grill or broiler.

To make the burgers, in a large bowl combine pork, parsley, curry powder salt and pepper. Mix well to combine. Shape mixture into 4 equal patties.

Grill or broil burgers (on a baking sheet when broiling) 5 minutes per side, until browned on the outside and cooked through.

Arrange burgers on buns and spoon mango chutney over top.

NUTRITION SCORE
Per serving (1 burger on a bun): 364 **calories**
17% **fat** (6.9 g; 2 g saturated)
51% **carbs** (46.4 g), 4 g **fiber**
32% **protein** (29 g)

Eggplant, Roasted Red Peppers and Mozzarella Sandwich

Serves 4
Prep time: 10 minutes
Cook time: 4-6 minutes

- 2 cups sliced baby eggplant (⅛-inch-thick slices)
- Olive-oil cooking spray
- Salt and ground black pepper to taste
- 1 16-ounce whole-grain baguette, halved lengthwise and cut into 4 equal pieces
- 1 cup fresh watercress leaves
- 2 teaspoons olive oil
- 2 roasted red peppers (from water-packed jar), thinly sliced
- 8 ounces part-skim mozzarella cheese, thinly sliced

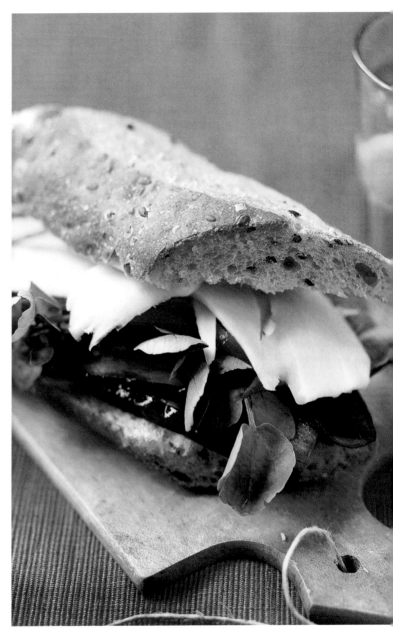

Preheat broiler. Spray both sides of eggplant with cooking spray and season with salt and black pepper. Place eggplant slices on a baking sheet and broil 2-3 minutes per side, until golden brown. Place slices on half of baguette.

Toss watercress leaves with olive oil and place leaves on top of eggplant slices. Layer with roasted red peppers and mozzarella cheese. Top with second half of baguette.

NUTRITION SCORE
Per serving (1 sandwich): 400 **calories**
25% **fat** (11 g; 6 g saturated)
49% **carbs** (49 g), 12 g **fiber**
26% **protein** (26 g)

For a different taste, and a more filling meal, you can add 2 ounces of sliced turkey breast to each sandwich. (This adds 77 calories, 17 grams of protein, 0 carbs and 0.4 gram of fat per serving.)

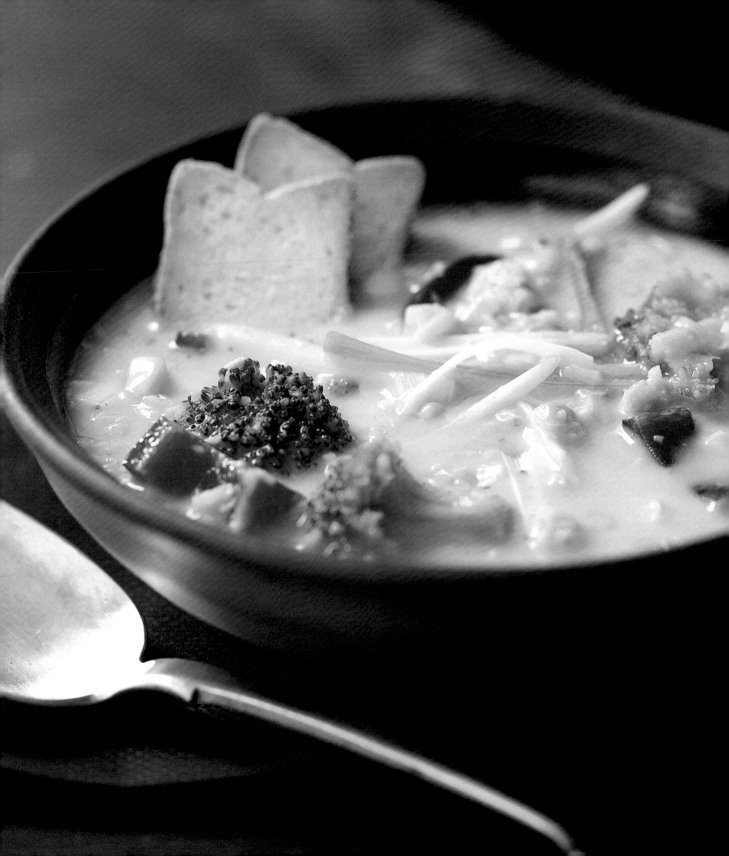

soups

Homemade soup. These words conjure an image of a stockpot filled with delicious ingredients simmering on the stove for hours. But these days, few of us have the luxury of time. So we've created soups that fill your home with a rich, mouthwatering scent in a jiffy, thanks to bold spices, fresh herbs and quick-cooking ingredients. When the weather turns blistering, cool off with no-cook versions like Cucumber Gazpacho and Golden Summer Soup.

recipes

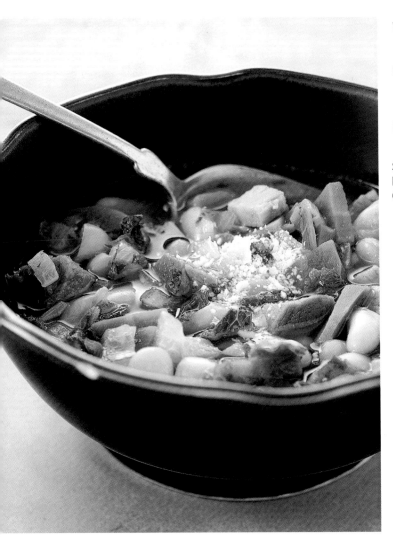

White Bean Soup With Mustard Greens

Serves 4
Prep time: 10 minutes
Cook time: 20 minutes

- 2 teaspoons olive oil
- 1 cup onion, diced
- 1 carrot, diced
- 2 cloves garlic, minced
- 8 ounces baked ham, diced
- 1 teaspoon dried thyme
- 2 bay leaves
- 2 19-ounce cans white beans, rinsed and drained
- 2 14.5-ounce cans reduced-sodium chicken broth
- 2 cups chopped fresh mustard greens
- Salt and ground black pepper to taste
- 4 tablespoons grated Parmesan cheese

Heat oil in a large saucepan over medium heat. Add onion, carrot and garlic and sauté 3 minutes, until soft. Add ham and cook 2 minutes. Stir in thyme and bay leaves; then add beans and broth and bring mixture to a boil. Reduce heat, partially cover and simmer 20 minutes. Remove and discard bay leaves.

Add mustard greens and simmer 1 minute, until greens wilt. Remove from heat and season with salt and black pepper.

Ladle soup into bowls and top with Parmesan cheese.

NUTRITION SCORE
Per serving (1½ cups soup, 1 tablespoon cheese): 441 **calories**
12% **fat** (6 g; 2 g saturated)
56% **carbs** (62 g), 15 g **fiber**
32% **protein** (35 g)

Your refrigerator may chill the flavor right out of onions and garlic. Store these pungent bulbs at room temperature in a dark, well-ventilated place. They should stay flavorful for up to eight weeks.

Chicken and Spinach-Noodle Soup

Serves 4
Prep time: 10 minutes
Cook time: 10 minutes

   1 pound skinless, boneless chicken breast, cut into
     1-inch pieces
   ½ cup chopped onion
   2 medium carrots, chopped, approximately 2 cups
   2 cloves garlic, minced
   1 teaspoon dried thyme
   2 bay leaves
   3 14.5-ounce cans reduced-sodium chicken broth
   4 ounces uncooked spinach fettuccine
     (or macaroni), broken into 2-inch pieces
   ½ cup frozen corn, thawed
   2 tablespoons chopped fresh parsley
   Salt and ground black pepper to taste

In a large stockpot, combine chicken, onion, carrots, garlic, thyme and bay leaves. Pour chicken broth into pot and set pot over high heat. Bring to a boil.

Reduce heat to medium-high. Add spinach pasta, partially cover and cook 3–5 minutes, until noodles are tender. Remove from heat, discard bay leaves and stir in corn and parsley. Season with salt and black pepper; ladle soup into bowls and serve.

NUTRITION SCORE
Per serving (2 cups): 307 **calories**
11% **fat** (4 g; <1 g saturated)
43% **carbs** (33 g), 3 g **fiber**
46% **protein** (35 g)

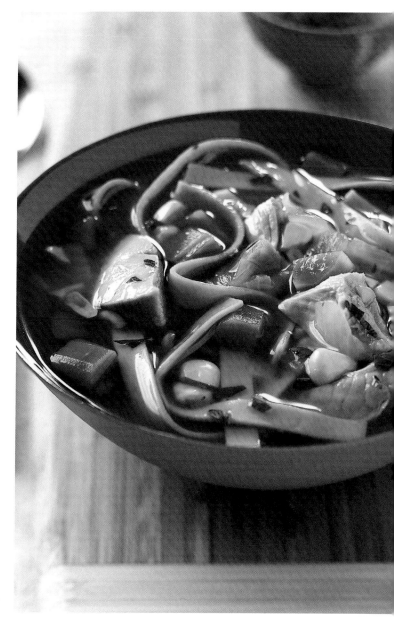

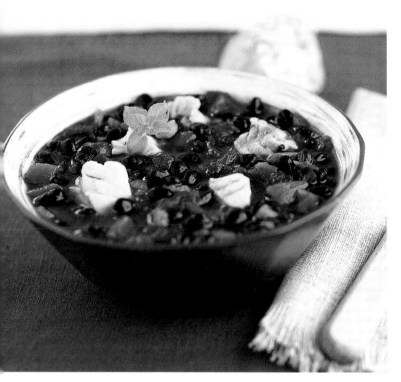

Cuban Black Bean Soup With Cod

Serves 4
Prep time: 20 minutes
Slow-cook time: 8-10 hours

1 pound dry black beans, rinsed and drained
2 14.5-ounce cans reduced-sodium chicken broth
1 14.5-ounce can diced tomatoes
1 14-ounce can diced green chilies
1 8-ounce cod steak, cut into 1-inch cubes
½ cup onion, minced
2 cloves garlic, minced
2 tablespoons red-wine vinegar
1 teaspoon dried oregano
2 teaspoons dried thyme
2 teaspoons ground cumin
½ teaspoon ground black pepper
Salt to taste
4 whole-grain rolls

Place beans in a slow cooker (6-quart size or larger) and add enough water to cover by 4-5 inches. Bring to a boil and cook 10 minutes. Drain water. Add remaining ingredients, mix well, cover and cook on low for 8-10 hours. Ladle soup into bowls, season with salt and serve rolls on the side.

NUTRITION SCORE
Per serving (2 cups soup, 1 roll): 511 **calories**
5% **fat** (3 g; <1 g saturated)
66% **carbs** (84 g), 28 g **fiber**
29% **protein** (37 g)

Your body gets hungry every three to five hours, so you need to eat five to six healthful, lowfat mini meals daily to stay full and to curb cravings.

Creamy Asparagus Soup

Serves 4
Prep time: 10 minutes
Cook time: 12-15 minutes

- 1 pound fresh asparagus, tough ends removed and stalks cut into 1-inch pieces
- ½ cup chopped onion
- 2 14.5-ounce cans reduced-sodium chicken or vegetable broth
- 2 bay leaves
- 1 cup nonfat milk
- 3 tablespoons cornstarch
- ½ cup nonfat sour cream
- 1 teaspoon fresh lemon juice
- ½ teaspoon salt
- ¼ teaspoon ground black pepper

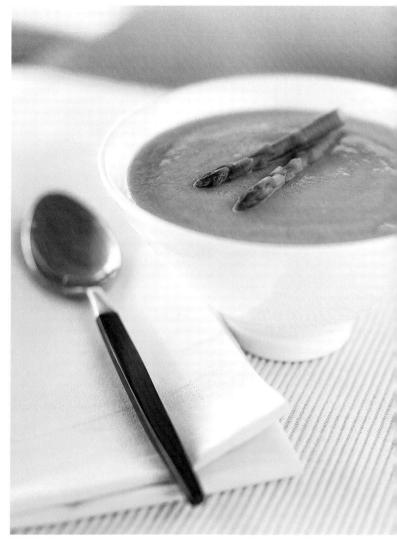

In a large saucepan, combine asparagus, onion and 1 can of broth. Set pan over high heat and bring to a boil. Reduce heat, partially cover and simmer 8-10 minutes, until asparagus is tender. Cut off asparagus tips and set aside.

In a blender, purée remaining asparagus mixture until smooth. Return purée to pan, add remaining broth and bay leaves and bring to a simmer. Whisk together milk and cornstarch. Add milk mixture to pan and simmer 2 minutes, until mixture thickens, stirring constantly.

Place sour cream in a small bowl. Add a spoonful of asparagus mixture and stir to heat sour cream. Add sour-cream mixture to saucepan along with lemon juice, salt and pepper. Simmer 1 minute, to heat through. Remove bay leaves and discard. Ladle soup into bowls and top with reserved asparagus tips.

NUTRITION SCORE
Per serving (1½ cups): 123 **calories**
6% **fat** (<1 g; 0 g saturated)
62% **carbs** (19 g), 2 g **fiber**
32% **protein** (10 g)

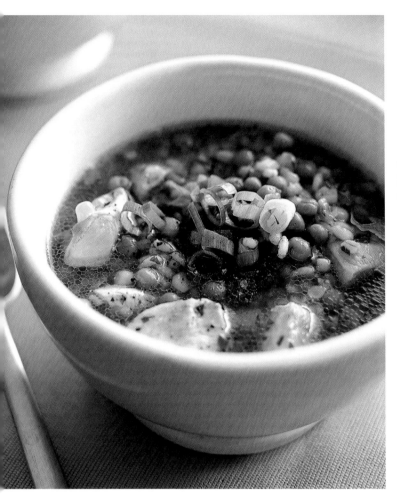

Chicken Barley Soup With Vegetables

Serves 4
Prep time: 5 minutes
Cook time: 15 minutes

  2 teaspoons olive oil
  4 green onions chopped, with white and green
     parts divided
  1 pound skinless, boneless chicken breasts, cut
     into ½-inch pieces
  1 teaspoon dried thyme
  2 bay leaves
  3 14.5-ounce cans reduced-sodium chicken broth
  ⅔ cup quick-cooking barley
  ½ cup frozen corn
  ½ cup frozen peas
  1 tablespoon chopped fresh parsley
     Salt and ground black pepper to taste

Barley (a great vegetable-based protein source) is rich in fiber and B vitamins. Since it's a whole grain, it will keep you feeling satisfied longer.

Heat oil in a large saucepan over medium-high heat. Add white part of the onion and cook 1 minute. Add chicken and cook 3 minutes, until browned on all sides, stirring frequently. Toss in thyme and bay leaves and stir to coat chicken and onion.

Add broth and barley and bring to a boil. Reduce heat to low; cover and simmer 10 minutes, until tender. Stir in corn and peas and simmer 1 minute longer. Remove from heat and stir in parsley.

Season with salt and black pepper. Remove bay leaves and serve topped with green onion.

NUTRITION SCORE
Per serving (1½ cups): 296 **calories**
18% **fat** (6 g; 1 g saturated)
36% **carbs** (27 g), 4 g **fiber**
46% **protein** (34 g)

Minestrone With Pesto Soup

Serves 4
Prep time: 10 minutes
Cook time: 35 minutes

- ½ cup chopped onion
- ½ head savoy cabbage (the loose-leaf cabbage that's milder than common green cabbage), chopped, approximately 3 cups
- 2 cups peeled, seeded and cubed butternut squash, cut into 1-inch pieces
- 2 small red potatoes, cut into 1-inch cubes (unpeeled)
- 2 tablespoons tomato paste
- 1 teaspoon dried thyme
- 4 14.5-ounce cans reduced-sodium vegetable or chicken broth
- 2 cups four-color veggie radiatore or tri-color pasta spirals
- Salt and ground black pepper to taste
- 8 teaspoons prepared basil pesto

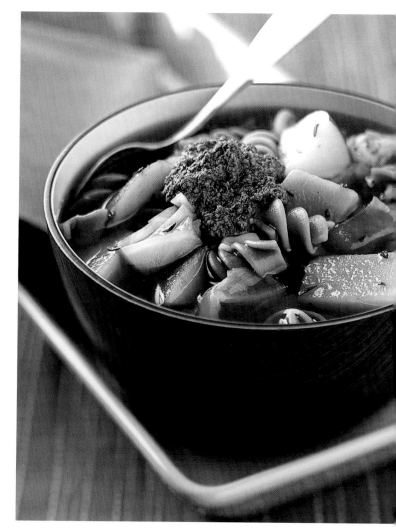

In a large stockpot, combine vegetables, tomato paste and thyme. Pour in the broth and set the pot over high heat. Bring mixture to a boil.

Reduce heat to medium-high. Add pasta, partially cover and cook until tender (about 30 minutes). Season with salt and black pepper. Ladle soup into bowls and top each with pesto.

Eat half a butternut squash and you'll get half the Recommended Dietary Allowance (RDA) for vitamin C and a healthy dose of iron, calcium and fiber.

NUTRITION SCORE
Per serving (2 cups with 2 teaspoons pesto): 208 **calories**
16% **fat** (4 g; <1 g saturated)
67% **carbs** (35 g), 5 g **fiber**
17% **protein** (9 g)

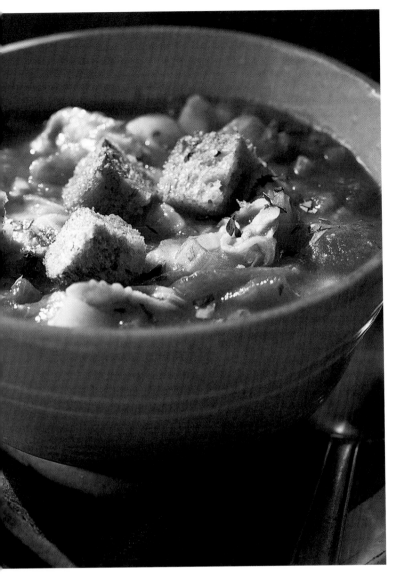

Manhattan Clam Chowder With Whole-Grain Croutons

Serves 4
Prep time: 5 minutes
Cook time: 8 minutes

4 slices whole-grain bread, cut into 1-inch cubes
Olive-oil cooking spray
2 teaspoons Old Bay seasoning, divided
2 celery stalks, chopped
2 10-ounce cans whole baby clams, drained
2 cups fat-free chicken broth
2 14.5-ounce cans diced tomatoes with green pepper and onion
2 Idaho potatoes, peeled and cut into ½-inch cubes

Preheat oven to 400° F. Spread bread cubes out on a large baking sheet. Spray bread with cooking spray; sprinkle with 1 teaspoon Old Bay. Bake 8 minutes, until lightly toasted; set aside.

Meanwhile, coat a large saucepan with cooking spray and set pan over medium-high heat. Sauté celery and clams for 2 minutes. Add remaining Old Bay and stir to coat. Add broth, tomatoes and potatoes and bring to a boil. Reduce heat to medium-low, partially cover and simmer 8 minutes, until potatoes are fork-tender.

Ladle soup into bowls and top with croutons. Serve.

Cooking tomatoes actually boosts their levels of the antioxidant lycopene.

NUTRITION SCORE
Per serving (1½ cups soup, ½ cup croutons): 251 **calories**
9% **fat** (2.5 g; 0.7 g saturated)
63% **carbs** (39.5 g), 8 g **fiber**
28% **protein** (17.5 g)

Quick Corn Chowder

Serves 4
Prep time: 3 minutes
Cook time: 12 minutes

- ⅔ cup lowfat milk
- 1½ tablespoons cornstarch
- 1 16-ounce bag frozen combination broccoli, corn and red peppers (cut up any large pieces)
- 1 15-ounce can cream-style corn
- ½ cup thinly sliced scallions
- 1 cup canned chicken broth
- ½ teaspoon cumin
- ¾ teaspoon pepper (or to taste)

In a large saucepan, dissolve cornstarch in milk. Add all vegetables, broth and cumin. Bring to boil, stirring often. Reduce heat to medium-low. Simmer until vegetables are tender, approximately 10 minutes. Add pepper; serve.

NUTRITION SCORE
Per serving (1¼ cups): 179 **calories**
8% **fat** (1.5 g; 0.3 g saturated)
78% **carbs** (39 g), 4.1 g **fiber**
14% **protein** (6.6 g)

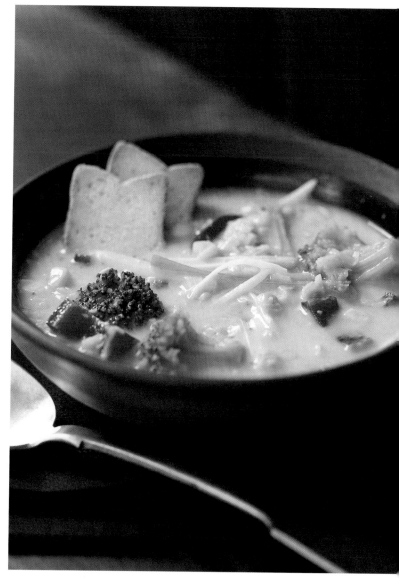

Frozen produce is just as healthy as its fresh counterpart. What's more, it's ready-to-use, which makes food prep a cinch.

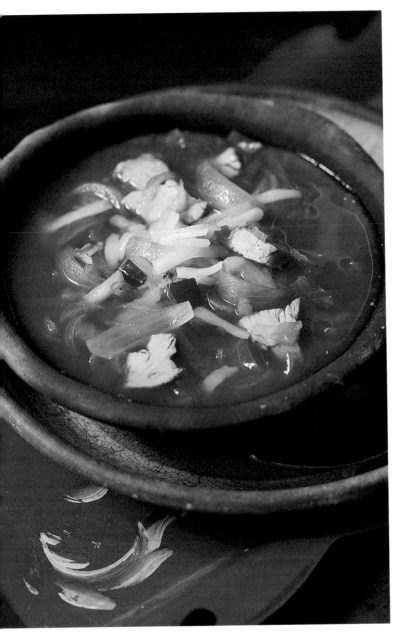

Tortilla Soup

Serves 4
Prep time: 3 minutes
Cook time: 10 minutes

  1 14.5-ounce can chicken broth
  1 cup cooked skinless chicken breast, diced
  1 medium onion, chopped
  2 ounces (½ of a 4-ounce can) diced green chilies
1½ teaspoons chili powder
  1 cup baked corn tortilla chip pieces
  ½ cup reduced-fat Cheddar cheese, shredded
  1 small tomato, chopped

In a medium saucepan, combine chicken broth, chicken breast, onion, green chilies and chili powder. Bring to a boil.

Reduce heat; simmer uncovered 10 minutes, until onion is tender.

Ladle into bowls, add ¼ cup chips to each, and sprinkle each with cheese and tomato. Serve.

NUTRITION SCORE
Per serving (1 cup): 155 **calories**
19% **fat** (3.3 g; 0.3 g saturated)
41% **carbs** (16 g), 1.9 g **fiber**
40% **protein** (16 g)

Eat at home more often. Women who ate in restaurants more than five times a week consumed almost 300 more calories a day than did those who dined out less, a University of Memphis study found.

Egg Drop Soup

Serves 4
Prep time: 5 minutes
Cook time: 10-12 minutes

- 6 cups reduced-sodium, nonfat chicken broth
- 1 ounce dried black or shiitake mushrooms
- 1 tablespoon reduced-sodium soy sauce
- 1 tablespoon sherry wine
- ¾ cup frozen petite green peas
- 2 large eggs, lightly beaten with a wire whisk
- 2 tablespoons chopped fresh cilantro
- 2 green onions, chopped
- 4 whole-grain rolls

In a medium saucepan over high heat, combine chicken broth and dried mushrooms. Bring to a boil, reduce heat to medium and simmer 5 minutes.

Strain liquid through a paper-towel-lined sieve (or coffee filter), reserving liquid. Rinse mushrooms under cold water to remove grit, and slice into thin strips (remove any tough stems if necessary).

Return strained liquid and sliced mushrooms to saucepan and set pan over high heat. Add soy sauce and sherry and bring mixture to a boil. Stir in peas. Gradually add eggs in a thin, slow stream, and stir gently with a wooden spoon for 30 seconds. Remove from heat and stir in cilantro and green onions. Serve rolls on the side.

NUTRITION SCORE
Per serving (1 cup soup, 1 roll): 241 **calories**
21% **fat** (5.6 g; 1 g saturated)
48% **carbs** (29 g), 3 g **fiber**
31% **protein** (18.5 g)

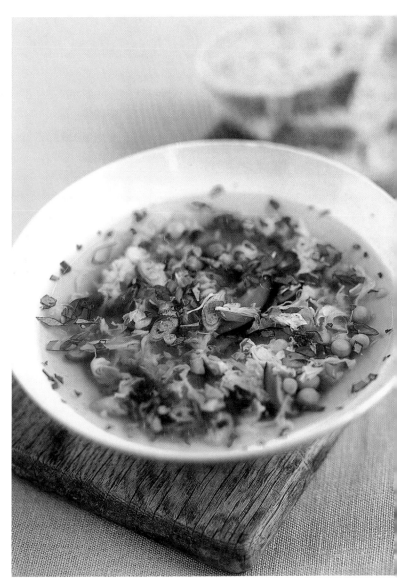

Spicy Carrot Soup

Serves 6
Prep time: 15 minutes
Cook time: 30 minutes

- 2 pounds carrots, peeled and cut into 1-inch pieces (about 6 cups)
- 5 cups low-sodium chicken broth, canned or homemade
- 1 dried hot chile pepper, any type (optional)
- 4 teaspoons minced fresh ginger
- 3 cloves garlic, peeled
- 1 teaspoon curry powder
- 1 teaspoon ground cumin
- ½ teaspoon freshly ground black pepper
- 3 tablespoons chopped fresh cilantro leaves

In a 5-quart saucepan, combine all ingredients except cilantro. Bring mixture to a boil; then reduce heat to low and simmer 30 minutes or until carrots are tender.

Transfer mixture to a food processor in batches, 2-3 cups at a time. Purée until smooth. Return the purée to saucepan and reheat. Stir in chopped cilantro. Serve promptly.

NUTRITION SCORE
Per serving (1 cup): 85 **calories**
6% **fat** (0.6 g; 0.1 g saturated)
76% **carbs** (17 g), 6 g **fiber**
18% **protein** (4 g)

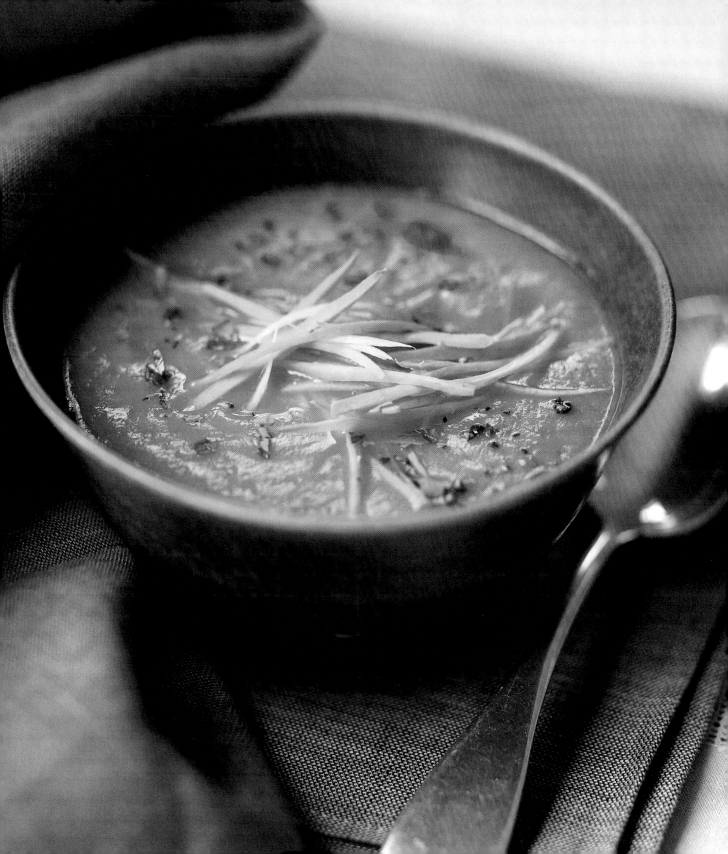

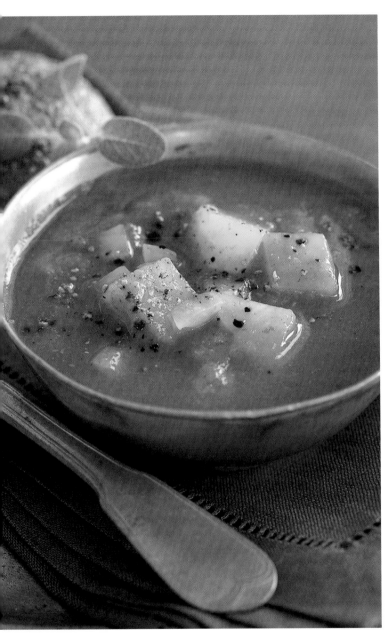

Curried Pumpkin Soup

Serves 4
Prep time: 5 minutes
Cook time: 10-12 minutes

¾ cup chopped Spanish onion

2 teaspoons olive oil

2½ teaspoons curry powder

4 cups reduced-sodium, nonfat chicken or
  vegetable broth

1 15-ounce can pumpkin

2 Idaho potatoes, peeled and cut into 1-inch cubes

¼ cup chopped fresh cilantro

Salt and pepper to taste

4 whole-grain rolls

In a large saucepan, sauté onion in oil 2 minutes. Add curry powder, cilantro, salt and pepper; stir to coat. Add broth, pumpkin and potatoes and bring to a boil. Reduce heat to medium, partially cover and cook 8-10 minutes, until potatoes are tender.

Remove from heat and stir in cilantro. Serve with rolls.

NUTRITION SCORE
Per serving (2 cups soup, 1 roll): 238 **calories**
17% **fat** (4.5 g; 1 g saturated)
67% **carbs** (40 g), 6 g **fiber**
16% **protein** (9.5 g)

Cup for cup, pumpkins have almost twice the beta carotene of spinach. Beta carotene is converted in the body to vitamin A, which is necessary for healthy eyes and skin.

Tomato-Basil Alphabet Soup

Serves 4
Prep time: 10 minutes
Cook time: 10 minutes

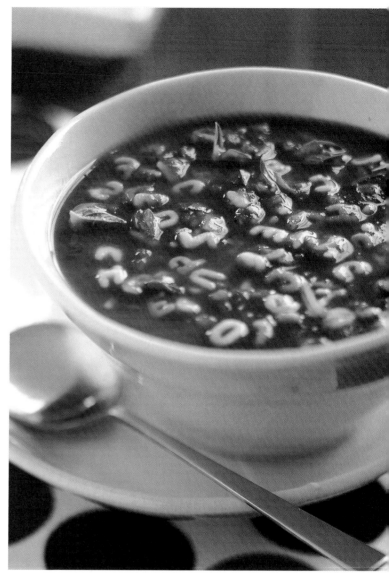

- 2 teaspoons olive oil
- 1 leek, rinsed well and chopped (white parts only), approximately 1 ½ cups
- 2 celery stalks, chopped
- 1 tablespoon sugar
- 1 teaspoon dried thyme
- ⅛ teaspoon cayenne pepper
- 1 28-ounce can diced tomatoes
- 3 14.5-ounce cans reduced-sodium vegetable or chicken broth
- 1 cup durum-wheat vegetable alphabet pasta with beet, spinach and carrot powders or any small whole-wheat pasta
- ¼ cup chopped fresh basil
- Salt and ground black pepper to taste

Heat oil in a large stockpot over medium-high heat. Add leek, celery and sugar and cook 3 minutes, until tender. Add thyme and cayenne pepper and stir to coat.

Transfer mixture to a blender or food processor and add diced tomatoes. Purée until smooth; return purée to stockpot. Place the pot over high heat, add broth and bring mixture to a boil. Stir in pasta and cook 3 minutes, until pasta is tender.

Remove from heat and stir in basil. Season with salt and black pepper; ladle soup into bowls and serve.

NUTRITION SCORE
Per serving (2 cups): 212 **calories**
12% **fat** (3 g; <1 g saturated)
71% **carbs** (38 g), 5 g **fiber**
17% **protein** (9 g)

Cauliflower Vichyssoise With Chive Cream

Serves 8
Prep time: 10 minutes
Cook time: 30 minutes
Chill time: 1 hour

1 large head cauliflower (about 2 ½ pounds)
5 cups water
½ teaspoon coarse salt
1 large bunch chives (with chive flowers attached, if possible)
1 cup half-and-half
Salt and pepper to taste

Trim base of cauliflower; remove leaves and any dark spots. Break into florets. Put in a medium pot. Add water and coarse salt (water won't cover cauliflower). Cut enough chives into ¼-inch lengths to fill ⅔-cup. Add ⅓-cup chives to cauliflower. Set the rest aside.

Bring cauliflower mixture to a boil. Lower heat, cover pot, and cook for 25 minutes, or until cauliflower is very soft. Transfer half of cauliflower and cooking liquid to a food processor or blender. Add ⅓-cup half-and-half and whip until ultrasmooth. Transfer to a bowl and repeat with remaining cauliflower and cooking liquid and another ⅓-cup of half-and-half. Season soup with salt and pepper. Let cool. Cover and refrigerate until cold.

In a small saucepan, bring to a boil remaining half-and-half and chives, 2 tablespoons water and a pinch of salt. Lower heat; simmer for 1 minute. Transfer to a blender. Purée until very smooth. Let cool. Cover and refrigerate until cold.

To serve, season with salt and pepper, ladle into chilled bowls and drizzle with chive cream. Garnish with broken-up chive flowers or minced chives.

NUTRITION SCORE
Per serving (1 cup soup plus 2¼ teaspoons chive cream):
73 **calories**
49% **fat** (4 g; 2 g saturated)
30% **carbs** (6 g), 2 g **fiber**
21% **protein** (4 g)

Cold Corn and Pepper Soup

Serves 6
Prep time: 15 minutes
Cook time: 30 minutes
Chill time: 1 hour

4 cups fresh corn kernels
2 yellow peppers, cored, seeded and chopped
2 14.5-ounce cans reduced-sodium chicken broth
1 cup water
2 cloves garlic
 Salt and pepper to taste
2 tablespoons fresh dill, chopped, for garnish

In a large saucepan, bring first 5 ingredients to a boil. Reduce heat to low; simmer 25 minutes. Transfer soup (in batches) to blender and whip until velvety. Pour through sieve into a bowl, pushing on sieve with back of spoon to drain off solids. Season with salt and pepper; chill. Ladle into bowls; garnish with fresh chopped dill.

NUTRITION SCORE
Per serving (1 cup): 150 **calories**
12% **fat** (2 g; 0.3 g saturated)
73% **carbs** (27.5 g), 2.5 g **fiber**
15% **protein**

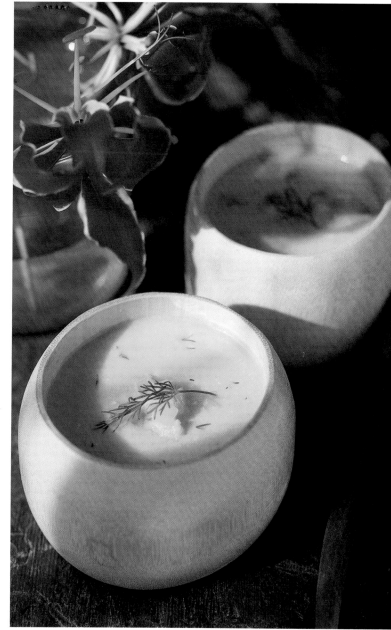

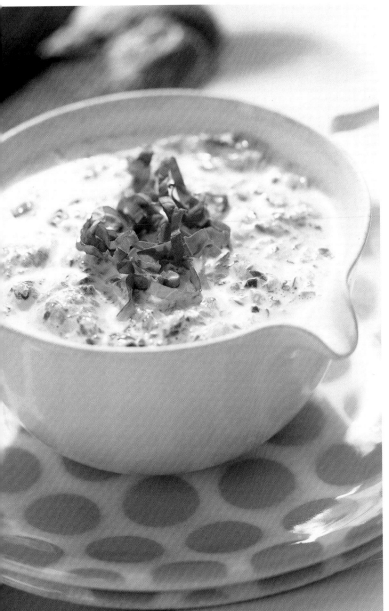

Cucumber Gazpacho

Serves 4
Prep time: 5 minutes
Chill time: 1 hour

 3 cups cucumbers, seeded and chopped
1 ½ cups spinach leaves
 1 cup nonfat plain yogurt
 1 cup fat-free chicken broth
 1 garlic clove

Place all ingredients in a food processor or blender and blend until chunky, not puréed. Chill for at least 1 hour and serve.

Note: Leftover soup will keep for 2 days in the fridge. It can't be frozen.

NUTRITION SCORE
Per serving (1 cup soup): 50 **calories**
5% **fat** (<1 g; 0 g saturated)
57% **carbs** (7 g), 1 g **fiber**
38% **protein** (5 g)

When the weather's hot, cut calories the cool way. Instead of sugary sodas or lemonade, drink mint moon tea. Toss 2 handfuls of fresh mint in a quart of water. Cover and steep overnight (or at least six hours). Discard leaves and pour over ice. It's a delicious, refreshing no-cal drink.

Golden Summer Soup

Serves 4
Prep time: 5 minutes
Chill time: 1 hour

1½	cucumbers, peeled and coarsely chopped
3	large firm, ripe golden tomatoes, peeled and coarsely chopped
1	red bell or other sweet pepper, stems removed, seeded and coarsely chopped
2	teaspoons freshly squeezed lemon juice
1	tablespoon extra-virgin olive oil
1	clove garlic, crushed and minced
1½	tablespoons coarsely chopped cilantro leaves
½	teaspoon salt
1	teaspoon freshly ground black pepper
4	½-inch-thick slices Italian-style country bread, toasted and rubbed with whole garlic

Condiments

½	cucumber, peeled, seeded and coarsely chopped
8–10	red cherry tomatoes, quartered
¼	cup coarsely chopped cilantro leaves

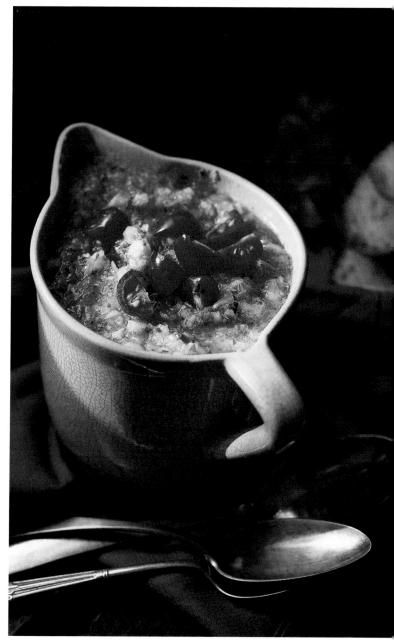

Place cucumbers, tomatoes, peppers, lemon juice and olive oil in a food processor and blend until chunky but not puréed. Pour into a glass bowl. Stir in garlic, cilantro, salt and pepper. Chill for at least 1 hour.

Remove soup from refrigerator and stir. Ladle into 4 soup bowls and serve with condiments.

NUTRITION SCORE
Per serving (1 ½ cups soup): 198 **calories**
26% **fat** (5.7 g fat, .8 g saturated)
60% **carbs** (31.5 g), 3.6 g **fiber**
14% **protein** (6.9 g)

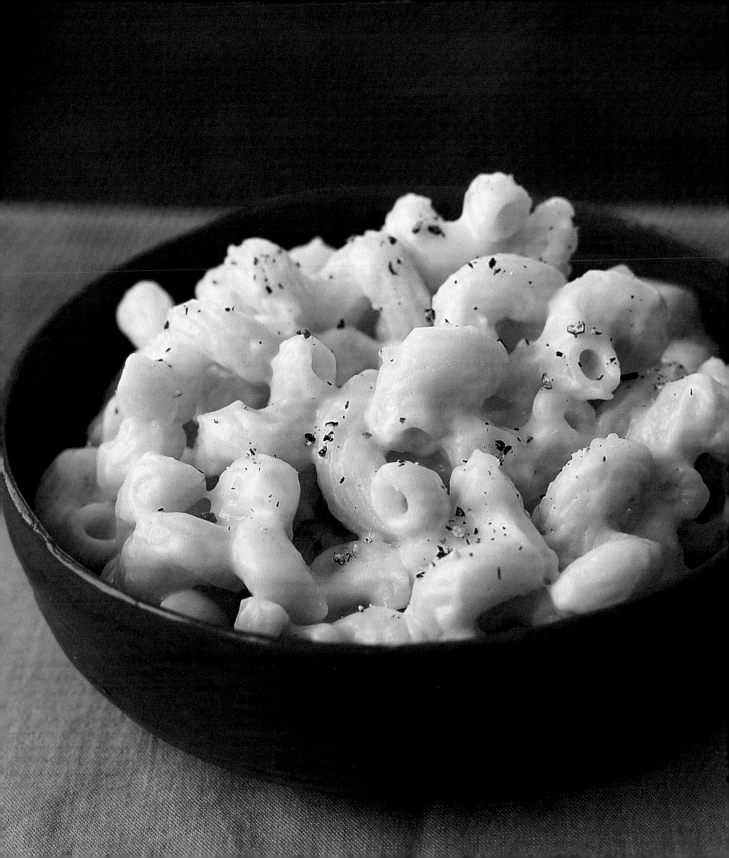

pizzas and pastas

You don't have to miss out on the comfort of pizza and pasta just because you're trying to lose weight. Rich sauces and overuse of cheese are what put traditional pastas and pizzas on a health-conscious eater's forbidden-food list. Our lightened versions load up on vegetables and show you just how painless it is to cut the fat.

recipes

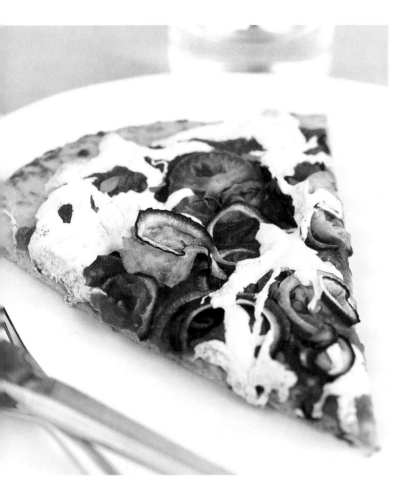

Turkey Sausage and Onion Pizza

Serves 6
Prep time: 8 minutes
Cook time: 12 minutes

- 2 links of 85 percent fat-free (or leaner) Italian turkey sausage
- 1 10-ounce Boboli Thin Pizza Crust
- 1 cup Healthy Choice Garlic & Herb Pasta Sauce
- ½ plum tomato, sliced into 6 thin rounds
- ⅓ cup thinly sliced red onion
- ½ cup shredded part-skim mozzarella cheese
- ¼ teaspoon garlic powder
- ¾ teaspoon fresh oregano (¼ teaspoon if using dry)
- Black pepper to taste

Preheat oven to 450° F.

Place sausage links in a shallow bowl and microwave on high for 2 minutes. (This will precook links and render some additional fat, which can be blotted with a paper towel.)

Place Boboli crust on a pizza pan or baking sheet and spread sauce evenly over crust. Arrange tomato rounds and onion slices on top of sauce. Remove sausages from microwave and slice into ¼-inch-thick rounds, then place over tomatoes and onions. Sprinkle evenly with mozzarella cheese, garlic powder and oregano, then with black pepper.

Bake for 10-12 minutes or until cheese is bubbly.

NUTRITION SCORE
Per serving (1 slice): 261 **calories**
30% **fat** (9 g; 0.4 g saturated)
47% **carbs** (30 g), 2g **fiber**
23% **protein** (15 g)

Fresh oregano contains so much of the antioxidant rosmarinic acid that 1 tablespoon has the same cancer-fighting power as one whole apple.

Mexican Pizza

Serves 4
Prep time: 5 minutes
Cook time: 15 minutes

- 2 large lowfat whole-wheat flour tortillas
- 1 cup Spanish-style canned tomato sauce (such as Hunt's or Goya)
- 3 tablespoons nonfat black bean soup (such as Health Valley)
- ¼ cup chopped scallions
- 3 ounces Perdue Short Cuts fully cooked Italian-style chicken breast pieces
- 3 ounces Sargento Four Cheese Mexican shredded cheese
- ¾ teaspoon fresh oregano (¼ teaspoon if using dry)
- ¾ teaspoon fresh cilantro (¼ teaspoon if using dry)
- ¼ teaspoon garlic powder

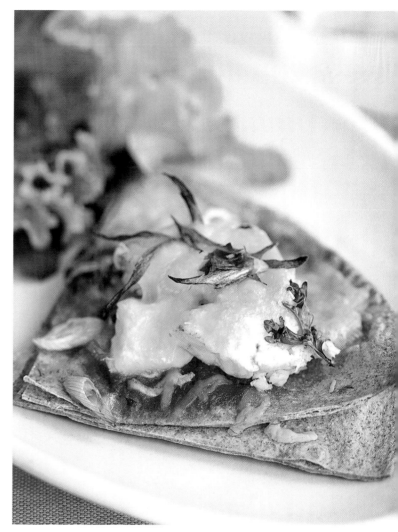

Preheat oven to 450° F. On a flat baking sheet, place one tortilla on top of the other.

Mix tomato sauce and black bean soup together and spread over tortillas. Sprinkle scallions over sauce and arrange chicken pieces on top. Distribute cheese evenly over chicken; then sprinkle with oregano, cilantro and garlic powder. Bake for 10-15 minutes or until cheese melts.

NUTRITION SCORE
Per serving (1 slice): 168 **calories**
41% **fat** (8 g; 5 g saturated)
31% **carbs** (13 g), 6 g **fiber**
28% **protein** (12 g)

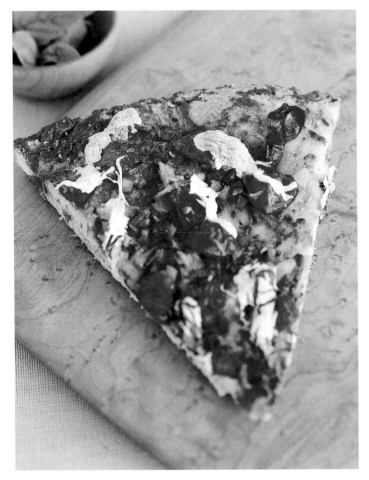

Bruschetta Pizza

Serves 6
Prep time: 5 minutes
Cook time: 15 minutes

- 3 fresh plum tomatoes, diced
- 1 tablespoon canned tomato sauce
- 6 tablespoons diced red onion
- ½ cup fresh basil, lightly chopped
- 2 teaspoons olive oil
- 1 tablespoon balsamic vinegar
- ¼ teaspoon garlic powder
- 1 10-ounce Boboli Thin Pizza Crust
- ¼ cup shredded part-skim mozzarella cheese

Preheat oven to 450° F.

Mix diced tomatoes with tomato sauce in a bowl. Add onions, basil, olive oil, vinegar and garlic powder.

Mix well and spread over Boboli crust placed on a flat baking sheet or pizza pan. Sprinkle cheese over top. Bake for 10-15 minutes or until cheese melts.

NUTRITION SCORE
Per serving (1 slice): 202 **calories**
29% **fat** (6 g; 0.44 g saturated)
55% **carbs** (28 g), 2 g **fiber**
16% **protein** (8 g)

Choose fresh basil, which has more flavor than dried. If you must substitute dried versions: 1 teaspoon of dried herbs equals 1 tablespoon fresh; ½ teaspoon dried equals 1½ teaspoons fresh.

Greek Pizza

Serves 2
Prep time: 5 minutes
Cook time: 15 minutes

- ¼ teaspoon olive oil
- ¼ cup diced yellow onion
- ¾ cup defrosted frozen chopped spinach (or fresh spinach, chopped)
- ¼ teaspoon black pepper
- ¼ teaspoon garlic powder
- Salt to taste
- 1 large whole-wheat pita bread
- ¼ cup lowfat feta cheese

Preheat oven to 450° F.

In a nonstick skillet, heat olive oil together with diced onion. Cook 1 minute and add spinach. Mix well and sauté for 3 minutes (or until spinach wilts if using fresh). Add black pepper, garlic powder and salt.

Place pita on a baking sheet or pizza pan. Spread spinach mixture evenly on top of pita. Crumble feta evenly on top of spinach. Bake about 15 minutes. Cut pita in half to get 2 slices.

NUTRITION SCORE
Per serving (1 slice): 227 **calories**
41% **fat** (11 g; 0 g saturated)
39% **carbs** (22 g), 4 g **fiber**
20% **protein** (11 g)

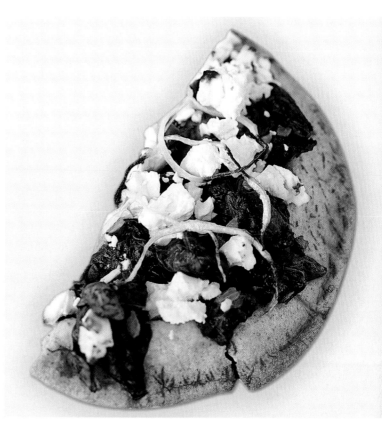

Avoid the temptation to order delivery pizza by stocking your fridge with a variety of washed and prepped healthful toppings. (Try mushrooms, onions, bell peppers and arugula.) That way you can whip up your own creation in less time than it takes for delivery.

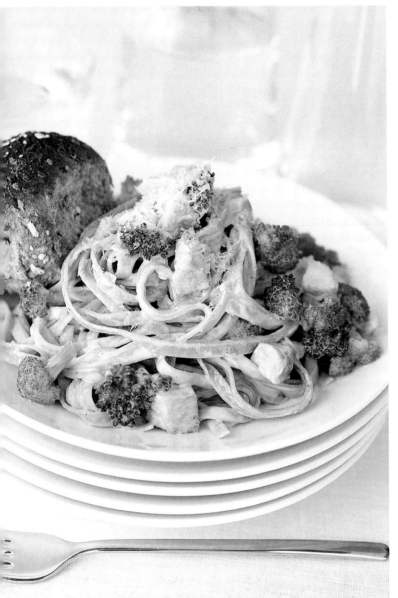

Spinach Fettuccine Alfredo With Chicken and Brocco

Serves 4
Prep time: 5 minutes
Cook time: 15 minutes

- 12 ounces spinach fettuccine
- 2 cups broccoli florets
- 2 teaspoons olive oil
- 1 pound skinless, boneless chicken breasts, cut into 1-inch pieces
- 3 cloves garlic, minced
- 2 tablespoons all-purpose flour
- ½ teaspoon salt
- ¼ teaspoon ground black pepper
- 1½ cups nonfat milk
- 4 tablespoons grated Parmesan cheese, divided
- 4 whole-grain rolls

Cook pasta according to package directions, adding broccoli for the last 30 seconds. Drain and return pasta and broccoli to pot.

Meanwhile, heat oil in a large skillet over medium-high heat. Add chicken and garlic, and cook 3-5 minutes, until chicken is golden brown on all sides. Add flour, salt and black pepper, and stir to coat. Add nonfat milk and 2 tablespoons cheese, and bring to a boil, stirring constantly. Simmer 1-2 minutes, until sauce thickens.

Pour sauce over fettuccine and broccoli and toss to combine. Transfer mixture to individual plates and top with remaining Parmesan. Serve pasta with rolls on the side.

This recipe uses some calorie cutters you can employ in many of your favorite recipes. Coat chicken with flour to create a thick sauce instead of making a butter-flour roux; Use very little olive oil; and opt for skinless chicken breast.

NUTRITION SCORE
Per serving (2 cups, 1 roll): 572 **calories**
17% **fat** (11 g; 3 g saturated)
49% **carbs** (70 g), 8 g fiber
34% **protein** (49 g)

Pasta Primavera With Sun-Dried Tomato Sauce

Serves 4
Prep time: 10 minutes
Cook time: 10 minutes

- 8 ounces whole-wheat pasta spirals
- 1 28-ounce can crushed tomatoes in thick tomato purée
- ½ cup reduced-sodium chicken broth or water
- ½ cup sun-dried tomatoes (packed without oil)
- 2 cloves garlic, chopped
- 2 tablespoons balsamic vinegar
- 1 tablespoon olive oil
- 1 teaspoon dried oregano
- ¼ teaspoon ground black pepper
- 2 cups cauliflower florets
- 1 green bell pepper, seeded and cut into 1-inch pieces
- 1 cup baby carrots, halved
- 1 cup frozen green peas
- ¼ cup chopped fresh basil
- ¼ cup crumbled feta cheese

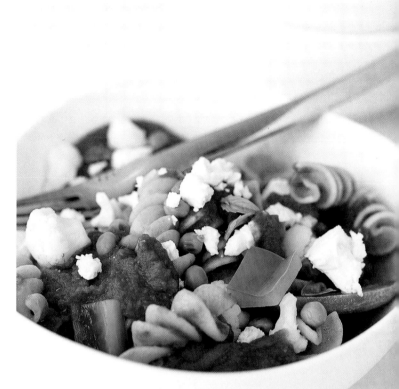

Cook pasta according to package directions. Drain and return to pot.

Meanwhile, purée next 8 ingredients in a blender until smooth. Transfer mixture to a large saucepan and set pan over medium-high heat. Cook until sauce begins to bubble. Add cauliflower, bell pepper, carrots and peas and simmer 5 minutes. Remove from heat and stir in basil. Pour sauce over pasta and toss to combine. Transfer to 4 plates and top with feta cheese.

Take a 30-minute walk before preparing dinner. You'll melt away most of the day's stress and, as a result, be far less likely to overeat.

NUTRITION SCORE
Per serving (2 cups): 426 **calories**
17% **fat** (8 g; 3 g saturated)
66% **carbs** (70 g), 14 g **fiber**
17% **protein** (18 g)

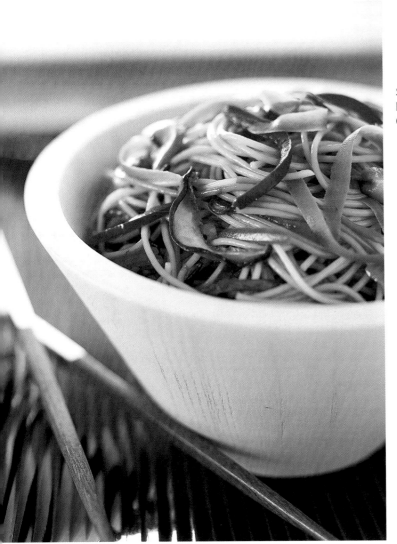

Asian Vegetable Noodles

Serves 4
Prep time: 20 minutes
Cook time: 25 minutes

- ½ pound vermicelli noodles
- 2 tablespoons sesame oil
- 1 teaspoon vegetable oil
- ½ red onion, julienne
- 1 teaspoon grated ginger
- 1 teaspoon minced garlic
- 5 large, fresh shiitake mushrooms (or any kind of fresh mushroom)
- ½ red bell pepper, julienne
- ½ carrot, shredded
- 1 bunch (about 5) scallions, julienne
- ¼ cup reduced-sodium soy sauce
- 1½ tablespoons granulated sugar
- Freshly ground black pepper to taste

Bring 12 cups of water to a boil. Add noodles and boil for 5 minutes. Drain and toss with 1 tablespoon sesame oil. Set aside.

Sauté onion, ginger and garlic in vegetable oil in a small pan for 10 minutes or until soft. Add next 6 ingredients and sauté 5–10 minutes more. Add noodles to pan, toss with vegetables, add remaining sesame oil and black pepper, and heat through, about 2 minutes.

Storage tip: Refrigerate, covered, for up to 5 days.

NUTRITION SCORE
Per serving (1½ cups): 378 **calories**
29% **fat** (12 g; 1.6 g saturated)
63% **carbs** (59 g), 4 g **fiber**
8% **protein** (8 g)

Kasha and Pasta With Lemon Pesto

Serves 2
Prep time: 5 minutes
Cook time: 10-12 minutes

- 4 ounces whole-wheat pasta spirals (or any shape)
- 3 tablespoons medium-granulation kasha (roasted buckwheat)
- 1 egg white or 2 tablespoons refrigerated egg whites
- Cooking spray
- ½ cup fat-free chicken broth
- ¼ teaspoon salt
- ¼ teaspoon ground black pepper
- ¼ cup prepared pesto
- 3 tablespoons fresh lemon juice

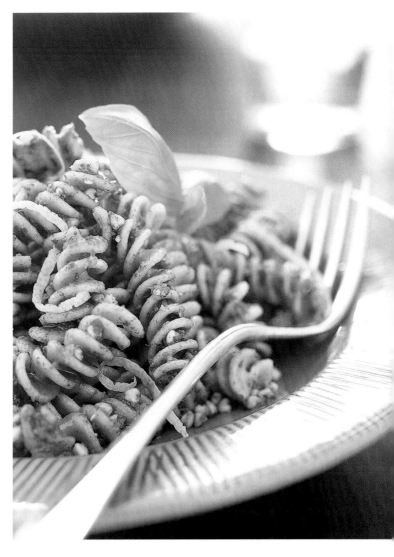

Cook pasta according to package directions. Drain and cover with foil; set aside.

Meanwhile, in a small bowl, combine kasha and egg white. Stir to coat kasha. Spray a small saucepan with cooking spray and set pan over medium heat. Add kasha and cook 2-3 minutes, until egg is cooked and kasha kernels separate. Add broth, salt and pepper; cover and simmer 7 minutes, until liquid is absorbed. Add kasha to pasta and stir.

Whisk together pesto and lemon juice. Pour mixture over pasta and stir to coat. Serve warm or at room temperature.

NUTRITION SCORE
Per serving (1¼ cups): 433 **calories**
31% **fat** (15 g; 3 g saturated)
55% **carbs** (59.5 g), 6 g **fiber**
14% **protein** (15 g)

For a sack lunch, combine leftover kasha-pasta mixture with a 6-ounce can of salmon (drained), ½ cup diced tomato and 1-2 tablespoons balsamic vinegar. Place 2 red lettuce leaves in the bottom of a sealable container; top with mixture; seal and refrigerate until ready to eat.

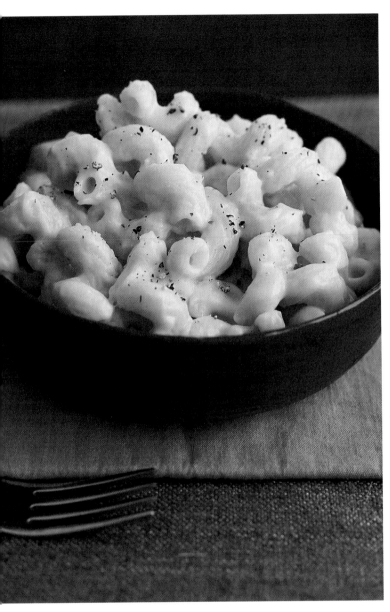

Mac 'n' Cheese

Serves 6
Prep time: 10 minutes
Cook time: 15 minutes

1½ cups dry macaroni
1¼ cups 1 percent milk
  2 teaspoons cornstarch
  ¼ teaspoon salt
  ¼ teaspoon black pepper
  1 cup fat-free finely shredded Cheddar cheese
  1 cup reduced-fat shredded sharp Cheddar cheese

Cook the macaroni according to package directions. Drain well.

Meanwhile, combine ¼ cup of milk with cornstarch. Stir until smooth and lump-free. Combine cornstarch mixture, remaining milk, salt and pepper in a medium saucepan. Cook and stir over medium heat until bubbly and thickened. Remove from heat. Add cheese and stir until melted and smooth.

Add cooked macaroni to the cheese sauce. Toss gently to coat. Cook over low heat for 5 minutes or until heated through. Serve.

NUTRITION SCORE
Per serving (½ cup): 206 **calories**
19% **fat** (4.3 g; 2.8 g saturated)
46% **carbs** (24 g), 1 g **fiber**
35% **protein** (18 g)

Using fat-free Cheddar cheese and reduced-fat sharp Cheddar cheese instead of regular Cheddar saves you 413 calories and 54.8 grams of fat.

Orecchiette With Broccoli Raab and Roasted Tomatoes

Serves 4
Prep time: 10 minutes
Cook time: 8-10 minutes, plus pasta cooking time

 1 28-ounce can whole plum tomatoes, drained
10 ounces orecchiette or other small pasta shells
 1 tablespoon olive oil
 2 cloves garlic, peeled and crushed with flat side of knife
 1 pound broccoli raab (also known as rapini), washed well, cut into 2-inch pieces
 1 tablespoon red wine vinegar
 1 teaspoon freshly ground black pepper

To roast tomatoes, preheat oven to 350° F. Place tomatoes on lightly oiled baking sheet. Roast 90 minutes, turning after 45 minutes, until very soft and slightly blackened. Once cooled, chop tomatoes and set aside.

Cook pasta according to package directions. Drain, reserving ¼ cup of liquid.

In a large nonstick skillet, heat oil over medium heat. Add crushed garlic and cook until slightly golden, 1-2 minutes. Add broccoli raab to skillet; raise heat to high. Cook, tossing constantly, until greens are just wilted, 4-5 minutes. Add tomatoes, cooked pasta, reserved cooking liquid, red wine vinegar and pepper. Toss well. Serve promptly.

NUTRITION SCORE
Per serving (2 cups): 362 **calories**
12% **fat** (5 g; 0.7 g saturated)
53% **carbs** (67 g), 4 g **fiber**
35% **protein** (14 g)

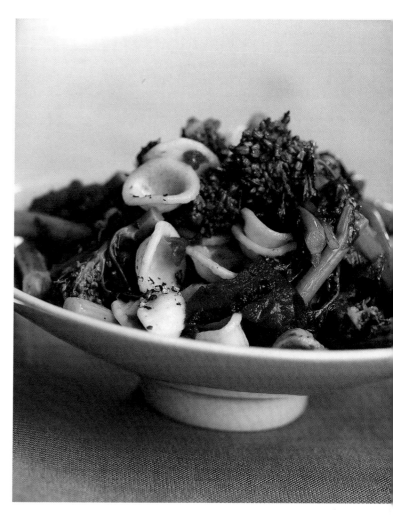

Italian greens give this pasta dish a boost of fiber and vitamin A. You may substitute spinach, arugula or baby broccoli for the broccoli raab.

Pasta With Sweet Potatoes, Shiitakes and Peas

Serves 4
Prep time: 30 minutes
Cook time: 45 minutes

Cooking spray
2 large orange-fleshed sweet potatoes, peeled and cut into 1-inch cubes
1 tablespoon chopped fresh rosemary, or 1 teaspoon dried
4 teaspoons olive oil, divided
12 ounces uncooked bow-tie (farfalle) pasta
1 cup sliced shiitake (or button or cremini) mushrooms
1 cup reduced-sodium chicken or vegetable broth
½ cup nonfat milk
2 tablespoons all-purpose flour
1 cup frozen green peas, thawed
2 tablespoons chopped fresh parsley
Salt and ground black pepper
4 tablespoons grated Parmesan cheese

Preheat oven to 400° F. Coat a large baking sheet with cooking spray.

In a large bowl, combine sweet potatoes, rosemary and 2 teaspoons olive oil. Toss to coat and transfer sweet potatoes to prepared baking sheet. Bake 35 minutes, until tender.

Meanwhile, cook pasta according to package directions. Drain, transfer to a bowl and cover with foil to keep warm.

Heat remaining oil in a large nonstick skillet over medium-high heat. Add mushrooms and sauté 3 minutes, until tender and releasing juice.

Whisk together broth, milk and flour. Add mixture to skillet and simmer 3 minutes, until mixture thickens, stirring constantly. Stir in sweet potatoes, peas and parsley, and heat through. Salt and pepper to taste. Pour mixture over cooked pasta and toss to combine. Spoon mixture onto plates and top with Parmesan cheese.

NUTRITION SCORE
Per serving (2½ cups): 508 **calories**
14% **fat** (8 g; 2 g saturated)
72% **carbs** (91 g), 7 g **fiber**
14% **protein** (18 g)

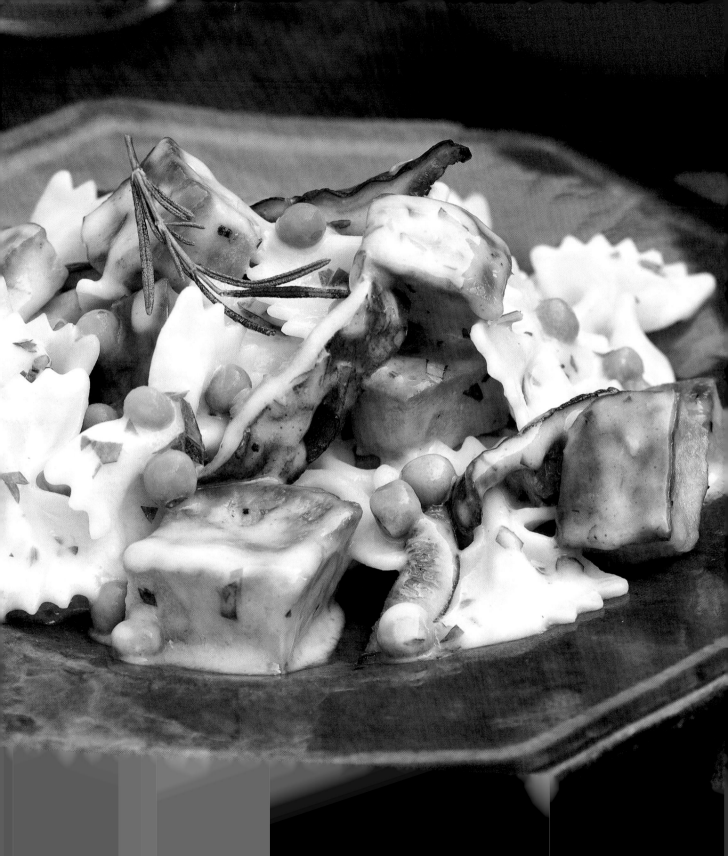

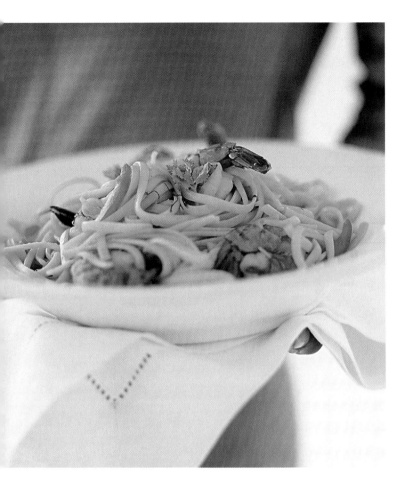

Linguine With Shrimp, Bell Peppers and Saffron-Garlic Sauce

Serves 8
Prep time: 10 minutes
Cook time: 15 minutes

Note: You may substitute diced, cooked chicken breast for the shrimp.

     6 garlic cloves, minced
     4 cups reduced-sodium chicken broth
     1 teaspoon saffron threads
    24 ounces uncooked linguine
     2 pounds medium shrimp, peeled and deveined
     2 green bell peppers, halved, seeded and cut into thin strips
    ¼ cup cilantro
     1 tablespoon soy sauce
    Salt and freshly ground pepper to taste

In a large stockpot, sauté garlic in 1 tablespoon of broth for 2 minutes, until golden. Add remaining broth and saffron. Bring to a boil. Reduce heat, cover and simmer 5 minutes.

Meanwhile, cook pasta according to package directions. Drain and add to broth mixture with the shrimp and bell peppers. Simmer 3 minutes, until shrimp are bright red and cooked through and peppers are tender-crisp. Stir in cilantro and soy sauce. Season with salt and pepper.

NUTRITION SCORE
Per serving (2 cups): 389 **calories**
9% **fat** (3.8 g; 0.7 g saturated)
55% **carbs** (52 g), 3.1 g **fiber**
36% **protein** (34 g grams)

Meal times are prime opportunities to get more water. Switch to a larger glass than you normally use and you'll easily sneak in more H₂0.

Spaghetti With Chunky Tomato Sauce and Olive Tapenade With Crostini

Serves 4
Prep time: 10 minutes
Cook time: 15 minutes

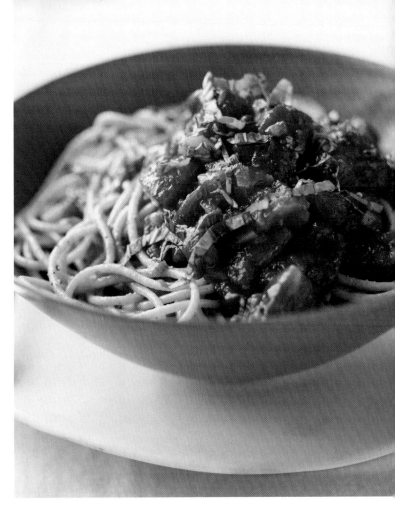

2 teaspoons olive oil

2 shallots, minced

2 cloves garlic, minced

1 28-ounce can diced tomatoes

1 teaspoon dried oregano

½ teaspoon ground black pepper

¼ cup chopped fresh basil

1 ½-pound loaf whole-grain baguette, sliced into
½-inch-thick slices

8 ounces whole-wheat spaghetti

Tapenade

½ cup pitted Greek kalamata olives

¼ cup stuffed green olives (stuffed with pimento)

1 tablespoon drained capers

1 clove garlic, chopped

Preheat oven to 350° F. To make the sauce, heat oil in a medium saucepan over medium heat. Add shallots and garlic and sauté 2 minutes. Add tomatoes, oregano and black pepper and bring mixture to a boil. Reduce heat, partially cover and simmer 10 minutes. Remove from heat and stir in basil.

Meanwhile, arrange bread slices on a baking sheet. Bake 10 minutes, until golden brown. Cook pasta according to package directions. Drain and set aside.

To make the tapenade, in a food processor, combine olives, capers and garlic. Process until almost smooth.

Transfer spaghetti to individual bowls and spoon tomato sauce over top. Top toasted bread with tapenade and serve on the side.

NUTRITION SCORE
Per serving (1 ½ cups pasta with sauce, 2 tablespoons tapenade, 2 slices bread): 402 **calories**
14% **fat** (6 g; <1 g saturated)
71% **carbs** (71 g), 13 g **fiber**
15% **protein** (15 g)

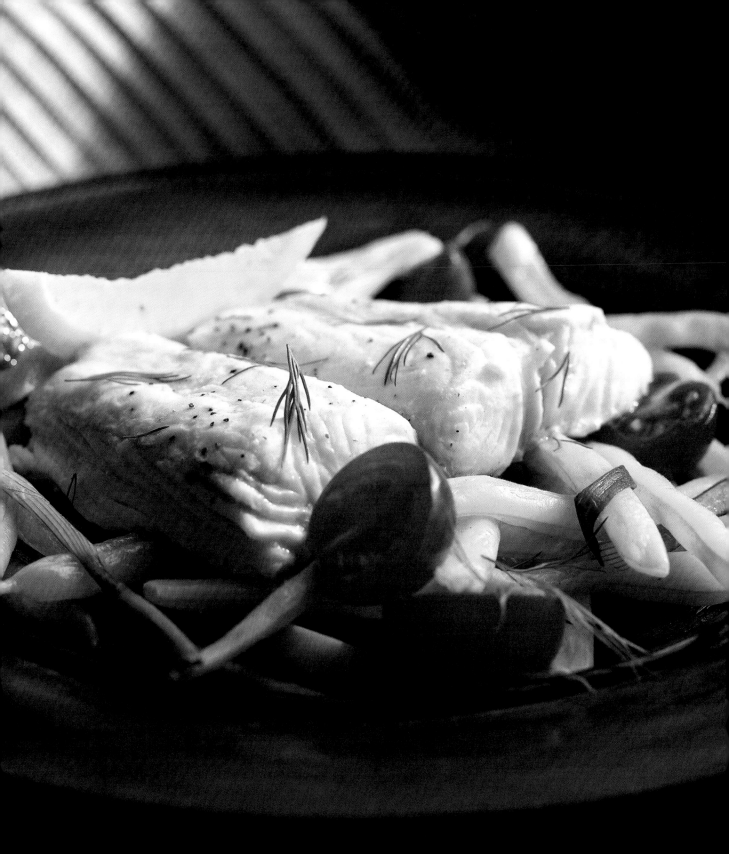

seafood

Fish is high in protein and loaded with heart-healthy omega-3 fats and zinc to boot. But the best reason to enjoy seafood is that it's naturally lowfat, delicious and fast cooking. And it takes well to just about every healthy food preparation, from poaching and steaming to grilling and roasting. In just minutes you can have a healthful dinner with minimum fuss.

recipes

Mercury Alert: Because mercury pollutants concentrate in larger fish, all women of childbearing age, as well as those who are pregnant or nursing, have been warned to avoid eating shark, swordfish, king mackerel and tilefish. The U.S. Food and Drug Administration and the Environmental Protection Agency also caution that women in these groups should eat no more than 12 ounces of all fish and shellfish per week.

Creole Shrimp Kabobs With Couscous

Serves 4
Prep time: 15 minutes
Cook time: 15 minutes

- 1 pound large shrimp, peeled and deveined
- 1 tablespoon Creole seasoning (sold in supermarket spice sections)
- 1 Spanish onion, cut into 2-inch pieces
- 2 green bell peppers, cut into 2-inch pieces
- 16 cherry tomatoes
- 1 cup whole-wheat couscous
- Salt and black pepper to taste

Preheat grill, grill pan or broiler. In a large bowl, toss shrimp in Creole seasoning to coat.

Alternate shrimp and vegetables on skewers. (Soak wooden skewers for 5-30 minutes first.) Grill or broil 5-7 minutes, until shrimp are bright red and cooked through, turning skewers halfway through cooking time.

Meanwhile, bring 1¼ cups water to a boil. Stir in couscous, cover and remove from heat. Let stand 5 minutes. (Add chopped cilantro, thyme and chives if desired.) Season with salt and pepper; serve with kabobs.

NUTRITION SCORE
Per serving (2 kabobs, about 4 shrimp, and ½ cup couscous):
311 **calories**
5% **fat** (1.7 g; 0.3 g saturated)
61% **carbs** (47.5 g), 6 g **fiber**
34% **protein** (26.5 g)

This meal provides zinc from the shrimp, vitamin C from the bell peppers, and beta carotene and lycopene from the tomatoes.

Gingered Salmon With Quinoa and Swiss Chard

Serves 2
Prep time: 5 minutes
Cook time: 10-12 minutes

- ½ cup uncooked quinoa
- ½ cup vegetable broth
- 2 teaspoons minced fresh ginger
- 2 teaspoons fresh lemon juice
- 1 teaspoon finely grated lemon zest
- 1 teaspoon cornstarch
- Cooking spray
- 1 8-ounce salmon fillet, about 1-inch thick
- Salt and ground black pepper to taste
- 2 cups chopped fresh Swiss chard, rinsed well

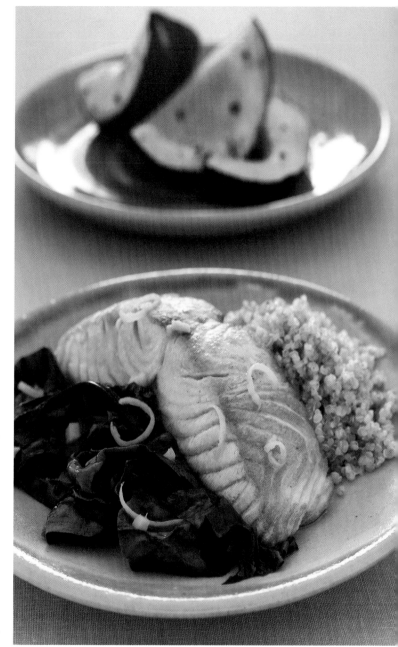

Combine quinoa and 1 cup water in a small saucepan and set pan over medium-high heat. Bring to a boil, reduce heat to low, cover and simmer 10-12 minutes, until liquid is absorbed. Fluff with a fork. Season to taste.

Meanwhile, in a small bowl, whisk together broth, ginger, lemon juice, lemon zest and cornstarch; set aside.

Coat a large nonstick skillet with cooking spray and set pan over medium-high heat. Season both sides of salmon with salt and pepper and place in pan, skin side up. Cook 2 minutes. Flip and cook 2 more minutes. Add broth mixture and simmer 30 seconds. Arrange Swiss chard around salmon, cover pan and cook 1 minute, until greens are wilted and salmon is cooked through. Serve half of salmon and Swiss chard with half of the quinoa on the side.

NUTRITION SCORE
Per serving (3 ounces salmon, ½ cup Swiss chard; ½ cup quinoa):
306 **calories**
26% **fat** (9g; 1g saturated)
36% **carbs** (27.5g), 3 grams of **fiber**
38% **protein** (29g)

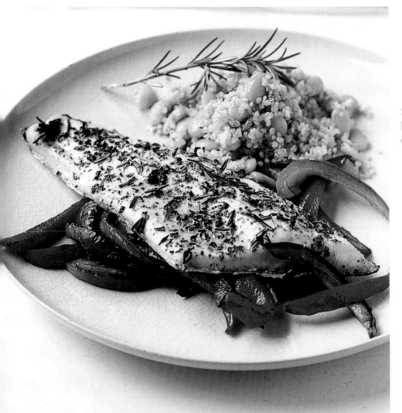

Herb-Crusted Trout With Peppers

Serves 4
Prep time: 7 minutes
Cook time: 10 minutes

Olive-oil cooking spray
1 cup quinoa, uncooked
1 cup frozen lima beans
4 5-ounce trout fillets
2 teaspoons chopped fresh rosemary
2 teaspoons mixed dried herbs (sold as "fines herbes" in the spice aisle)
4 teaspoons fresh lemon juice
1 red bell pepper, seeded and sliced
1 green bell pepper, seeded and sliced
Salt and ground black pepper to taste

Preheat broiler. Coat a large baking sheet with cooking spray. Set aside.

In a medium saucepan, combine quinoa and 2 cups water. Set pan over high heat and bring water to a boil. Add lima beans, reduce heat to low, cover and cook 10 minutes, until liquid is absorbed. Season with salt and black pepper.

Meanwhile, salt and pepper both sides of trout. Transfer trout to prepared baking sheet, flesh side up, and spray the fish with cooking spray. Top each fillet with rosemary and fines herbes, then with lemon juice. Arrange peppers alongside fish and place pan under broiler, 5-6 inches from heat source. Broil 5 minutes, until fish is fork-tender. Serve trout and peppers with quinoa on the side.

NUTRITION SCORE
Per serving (1 trout fillet, ½ cup quinoa mixture): 378 **calories**
24% **fat** (10 g; 2 g saturated)
43% **carbs** (41 g), 6 g **fiber**
33% **protein** (31 g)

Herb-Crusted Trout With Peppers is loaded with heart-healthy omega-3 fatty acids, antioxidants, potassium and fiber.

Poached Salmon With Dill Cream and Lemon Kasha

Serves 4
Prep time: 15 minutes
Cook time: 15 minutes

- 1 cup uncooked kasha
- 1 medium lemon
- 1 teaspoon lemon zest
- 1 pound thick salmon fillets
- 1 bunch fresh asparagus
- ½ cup nonfat sour cream
- 3 tablespoons chopped fresh dill
- 1 tablespoon Dijon mustard
- Salt and black pepper to taste

In a covered saucepan, simmer kasha in 2 cups water for 10-12 minutes (add water as needed), until kernels are tender and liquid is absorbed. Add juice from lemon and 1 teaspoon zest; set aside.

Meanwhile, in a large pot, just cover salmon with cold water. Bring to a boil; immediately remove from heat. Let stand 10 minutes.

Trim asparagus ends; blanch stalks in boiling water for 2 minutes, until crisp-tender. Drain, rinse in cold water; set aside.

In a small bowl, whisk together sour cream, dill and Dijon mustard. Remove salmon from water; add salt and pepper. Serve warm or chilled with dill cream, asparagus and kasha.

NUTRITION SCORE
Per serving (1 4-ounce fillet, 2 tablespoons dill cream, ½ cup kasha, 5 asparagus spears): 364 **calories**
21% **fat** (8.5 g; 1 g saturated)
45% **carbs** (41 g), 6 g **fiber**
4% **protein** (31 g)

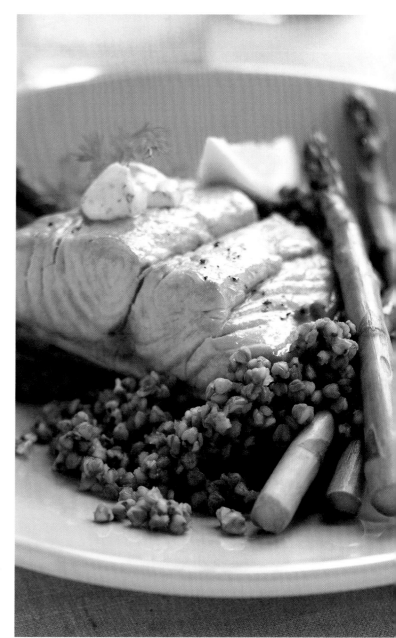

New research shows eating healthy fats such as the omega-3 fatty acids found in salmon makes you feel full longer, avoid bingeing and lose weight permanently.

Grilled Swordfish With Peach and Black-Bean Salsa

Serves 4
Prep time: 8 minutes
Cook time: 6-8 minutes

- 2 peaches or nectarines, pitted, diced into ½-inch pieces (1½ cups)
- 1 kiwi, peeled and diced (½ cup)
- ½ red bell pepper, diced (½ cup)
- 15 ounces canned black beans, rinsed and drained
- ⅓ cup cilantro, chopped
- 2 scallions, sliced
- 2 teaspoons honey
- ½ teaspoon salt
- ¼ teaspoon Tabasco
- Juice of 1 lime, divided
- 4 swordfish* fillets, 4 ounces each
- 4 whole-grain rolls

Preheat grill or grill pan. To make salsa, in a medium bowl, toss first 9 ingredients with half of lime juice. Set salsa aside.

Drizzle remaining juice over fish. Grill 6-8 minutes, until done, turning halfway through. Serve with salsa and rolls.

NUTRITION SCORE
Per serving (4 ounces fish, ¾ cup salsa, 1 whole-grain roll):
397 **calories**
20% **fat** (9 g; 2 g saturated)
38% **carbs** (41 g), 7 g **fiber**
42% **protein** (42 g)

Swordfish are in danger of extinction. Pacific halibut, mahi-mahi and albacore tuna are good environmentally correct substitutes here.

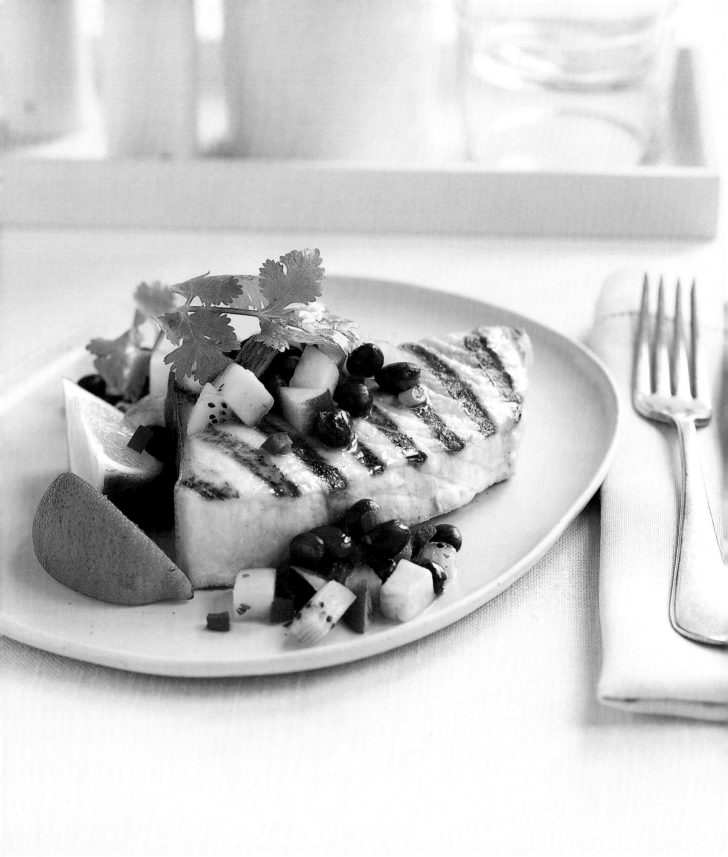

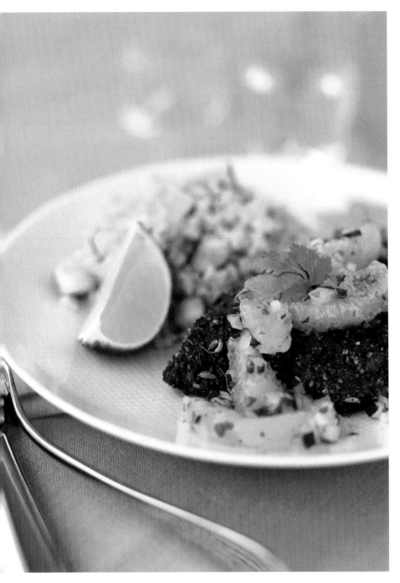

Jerk-Seared Tuna With Clementine Salsa

Serves 4
Prep time: 15 minutes
Cook time: 4-8 minutes

- 4 4-ounce yellowfin tuna steaks (preferably sushi grade)
- 2 teaspoons Caribbean jerk seasoning (McCormick)
- 2 teaspoons olive oil
- 2 cups instant brown rice
- 1 teaspoon dried oregano
- 1 medium zucchini, diced
- Salt and ground black pepper to taste
- 1 cup clementine sections (about 6-8 clementines)
- ¼ cup minced red onion
- 2 tablespoons fresh lime juice
- 2 tablespoons chopped fresh cilantro

Sprinkle both sides of tuna steaks with jerk seasoning. Heat oil in a large nonstick skillet over medium-high heat. Add tuna and cook 2 minutes per side for medium rare (3-4 minutes per side for well done).

In a medium saucepan, bring 2½ cups of water to a boil over high heat. Add brown rice and oregano, reduce heat to low, cover and simmer 5 minutes. Add diced zucchini, remove from heat, cover and let stand 5 minutes, until liquid is absorbed. Fluff with a fork and season with salt and black pepper.

Meanwhile, in a medium bowl, combine clementine sections, onion, lime juice and cilantro. Mix well, and salt and pepper. Serve tuna with salsa spooned over top and rice-zucchini mixture on the side.

To get perfect clementine sections, use a sharp knife to cut away the outer skin and white portion; then cut on both sides of the sections to remove the flesh. If clementines are not available, substitute tangerines or oranges.

NUTRITION SCORE
Per serving (3 ounces tuna, ¼ cup salsa, ½ cup rice-zucchini mixture): 412 **calories**
21% **fat** (10 g; 1.7 g saturated)
49% **carbs** (50 g), 5 g **fiber**
30% **protein** (31 g)

Sautéed Shrimp With Grapefruit and Avocado

Serves 4
Prep time: 10 minutes
Cook time: 10 minutes

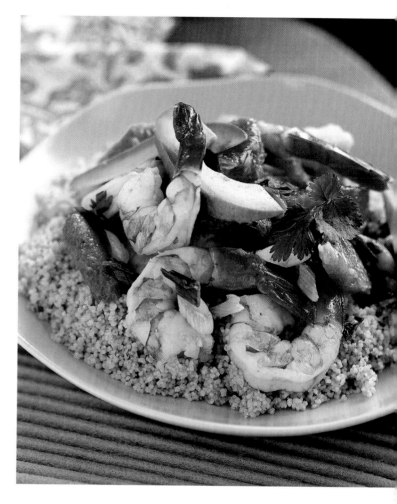

    2 medium white or pink grapefruit
    1 cup whole-wheat couscous, uncooked
    2 teaspoons olive oil
    2 green onions, chopped
    1 clove garlic, minced
    1 teaspoon ground cumin
    1 pound fresh or frozen large shrimp, peeled and
      deveined
    ¼ cup chopped fresh cilantro
    2 tablespoons fresh lime juice
    ¼ teaspoon salt
    ¼ teaspoon ground black pepper
    1 ripe avocado, peeled, pitted and sliced

Peel grapefruit and, using a serrated knife, cut out individual sections so that no white pith remains. Set aside. Bring 1¼ cups of water to a boil in a medium saucepan. Add couscous, cover and remove from heat. Let stand 5 minutes, until liquid is absorbed.

Meanwhile, heat oil in a large skillet over medium-high heat. Add green onions and garlic and cook 1 minute. Sprinkle in cumin and cook 1 minute, until fragrant. Add shrimp and cook 3 minutes, just until bright pink and cooked through, stirring frequently. Stir in grapefruit sections, cilantro, lime juice, salt and pepper. Transfer couscous to individual plates, top with shrimp mixture and garnish with avocado slices.

Both white and pigmented grapefruit are sweet, juicy and delicious. Just remember to choose heavy, firm grapefruit with smooth skins and avoid any with a rough, puffy rind.

NUTRITION SCORE
Per serving (1 cup shrimp mixture, ½ cup couscous, ¼ avocado):
445 **calories**
24% **fat** (12 g; 1.7 g saturated)
52% **carbs** (58 g), 11 g **fiber**
24% **protein** (27 g)

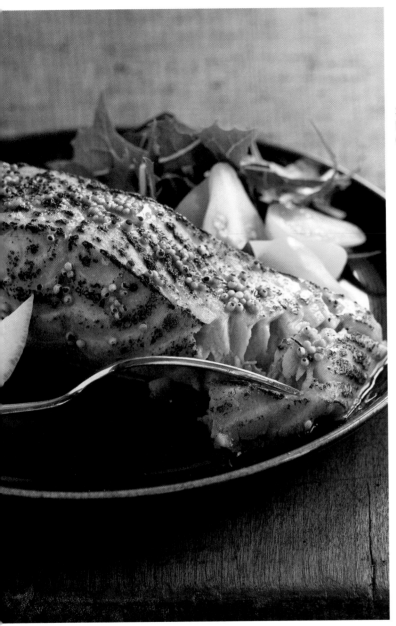

Double Mustard Maple Salmon

Serves 4
Prep time: 10 minutes, plus 20 minutes to marinate
Cook time: 15 minutes

- 2 teaspoons olive oil
- ½ cup yellow mustard seeds
- 3 tablespoons Dijon mustard
- 3 tablespoons real maple syrup
- 1 teaspoon balsamic vinegar
- ¼ teaspoon coarse salt
- ¼ teaspoon freshly ground pepper
- 4 6-ounce salmon fillets

Heat oil in a small nonstick skillet over low heat. Add mustard seeds; stir to coat with oil. Cover and cook until seeds begin to pop. Turn off heat but keep skillet covered until popping stops, about 1 minute. Transfer mustard seeds to a shallow dish and blend together with mustard, maple syrup, vinegar, salt and pepper. Add salmon fillets and turn to coat with mustard mixture. Marinate in refrigerator for 20 minutes.

Prepare broiler. Remove salmon from marinade; reserve marinade. Place salmon on a foil-lined baking pan and carefully spoon mustard seeds from marinade over each salmon fillet. Broil 5 minutes; cover fish lightly with a piece of aluminum foil (to prevent seeds from scorching). Cook 5 minutes more, or until fish flakes easily when tested with a fork.

NUTRITION SCORE
Per serving (1 fillet): 330 **calories**
40% **fat** (14.7 g; 1.8 g saturated)
18% **carbs** (14.7 g), 0.3 g **fiber**
42% **protein** (34.4 g)

Eat slowly to let satiety register – it takes your stomach 20 minutes to send "full" signals to the brain. You'll save 100 calories each time you stop eating when you're almost full instead of eating until you're stuffed.

Pepper-Seared Tuna With Cool Mango Relish

Serves 4
Prep time: 8 minutes
Cook time: 4 minutes

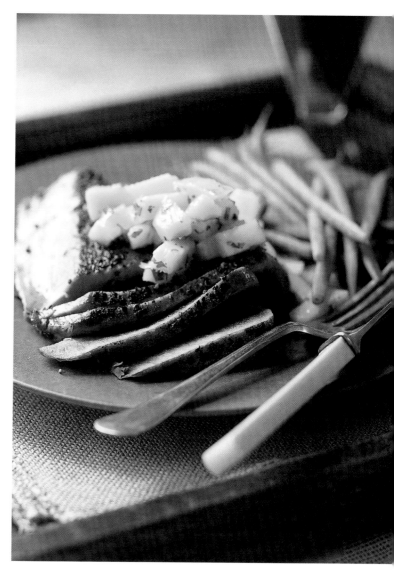

- 2 mangoes
- 6 tablespoons chopped fresh cilantro, plus whole leaves for garnish
- Salt
- ½ teaspoon black pepper, coarsely ground
- 4 6-ounce fresh tuna steaks
- Cooking spray

Peel mangoes and dice the flesh into ¼-inch pieces. Transfer to a small bowl. Add chopped cilantro and a pinch of salt and mix well. Place mango relish in the refrigerator to chill for at least 30 minutes.

Lightly press coarsely ground black pepper into one side of each tuna steak. Sprinkle with salt to taste. Place the fish, pepper-side down, in a large skillet coated with cooking spray. Cook on both sides over medium-high heat until the fish is seared on the outside but still pink in the center. Cut seared tuna on the bias into ½-inch-thick slices.

Mound mango relish in the center of each plate. Arrange tuna slices so they overlap and form a circle around the relish. Garnish with whole fresh cilantro leaves.

NUTRITION SCORE
Per serving (1 tuna steak, ½ cup mango relish): 252 **calories**
7% **fat** (2 g; 0.4 g saturated)
29% **carbs** (18 g), 2 g **fiber**
64% **protein** (40 g)

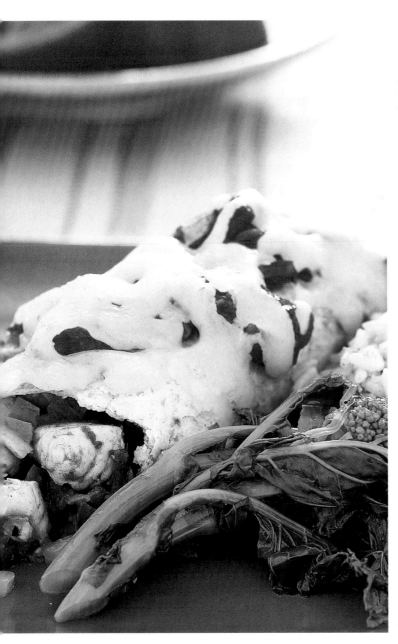

Trout Enchiladas

Serves 2
Prep time: 15 minutes
Cook time: 24 minutes

- 1 8-ounce trout fillet, skinned and cut into ½-inch cubes
- 2 tablespoons fat-free Italian dressing (vinaigrette style)
- 1 tablespoon all-purpose flour
- Cooking spray
- ½ cup minced onion
- 1 green bell pepper, minced
- 1 cup prepared salsa
- ¼ cup chopped fresh cilantro
- 2 8-inch whole-wheat tortillas
- ¼ cup reduced-fat shredded Mexican cheese blend or reduced-fat Cheddar cheese

Combine trout cubes and fat-free Italian dressing in a shallow dish and stir to coat fish with dressing. Let stand 15 minutes. Add flour and toss to coat.

Preheat oven to 350° F. Spray a baking dish (such as an 8-inch-square baking pan) with cooking spray and set aside.

Spray a large nonstick skillet with cooking spray and set pan over medium-high heat. Add onion and green pepper and sauté 2 minutes, until soft. Add trout and cook 2 minutes, until fish is opaque, stirring constantly. Stir in ½ cup of the salsa and cilantro and mix well. Remove from heat.

Spoon fish mixture onto whole-wheat tortillas, roll up and place seam-side down in prepared pan. Spoon remaining salsa over top and sprinkle with shredded cheese. Bake, uncovered, 20 minutes, until cheese melts.

NUTRITION SCORE
Per serving (1 enchilada): 445 **calories**
40% **fat** (20 g; 5 g saturated)
28% **carbs** (31 g), 15 g **fiber**
32% **protein** (34 g)

Poached Chilean Sea Bass With Garlicky Bread Crumbs

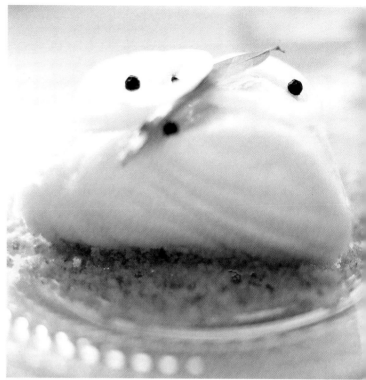

Serves 4
Prep time: 15 minutes
Cook time: 18-20 minutes

- 1½ teaspoons salt
- ½ teaspoon whole black peppercorns
- 1 large onion
- 3 bay leaves
- ¼ cup white-wine vinegar
- 4 thick Chilean sea bass fillets (about 2 pounds total weight)
- 2½ tablespoons olive oil
- 2 medium garlic cloves
- ¾ cup seasoned bread crumbs
- 1 tablespoon freshly squeezed lemon juice

Pour 8 cups of water into a deep 12-inch nonstick skillet. Add salt and peppercorns. Peel onion and cut into thin slices. Add to water, along with bay leaves and vinegar. Bring to a boil and continue to boil for 5 minutes. Lower heat to medium-high. Add fish. The water should just cover the fillets. Cook for 6 minutes on one side; then carefully turn over and cook 6-8 minutes on the other side, until fish is opaque. (Do not overcook. Cooking time depends on the thickness of the fish.)

Meanwhile, heat olive oil in a medium-sized nonstick skillet. Push garlic cloves through a garlic press and add to oil. Cook 15 seconds over low heat; do not brown. Add bread crumbs, stirring constantly. Cook for 1-2 minutes until golden-brown and crispy. Add lemon juice and stir to incorporate.

Remove fish and onions with slotted spatula, draining any liquid and discarding bay leaves. Place on a serving plate and mound fish with bread crumbs. Serve immediately.

 Poaching gently simmers fish or poultry in water infused with broth, wine, vinegar, juices, herbs or other seasonings to add flavor. The best part is that you don't need to add any fat for flavor.

NUTRITION SCORE
Per serving (1 fillet): 400 **calories**
30% **fat** (14 g; 2 g saturated)
25% **carbs** (28 g), 5 g **fiber**
45% **protein** (46 g)

Chilean sea bass are in danger of extinction. Pacific halibut, mahi-mahi and albacore tuna are good environmentally correct substitutes here.

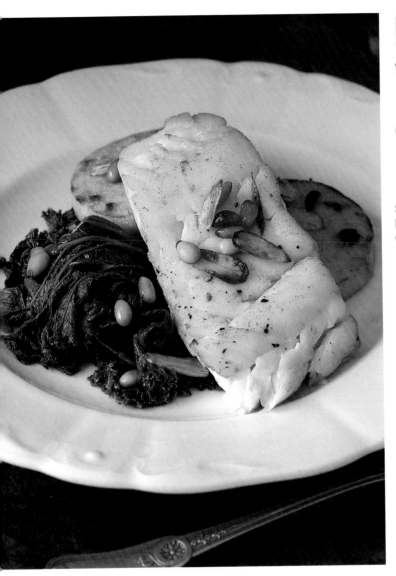

Pan-Seared Cod With Garlic Greens and Parmesan Polenta Toasts

Serves 4
Prep time: 5 minutes
Cook time: 10-13 minutes

½ 24-ounce package precooked, fat-free polenta
2 tablespoons Parmesan cheese
Cooking spray
4 teaspoons olive oil, divided
Salt and pepper to taste
4 5-ounce cod fillets
2 cloves garlic, minced
2 tablespoons pine nuts
1 pound mustard greens, stemmed
2 tablespoons dry white wine

Preheat oven to 425° F. Cut polenta crosswise into 8 ½-inch-thick slices; sprinkle with grated cheese. On a baking sheet coated with cooking spray, bake 8-10 minutes. Cover with foil; set aside.

Heat 2 teaspoons olive oil in a large skillet over medium-high heat. Salt and pepper both sides of cod; add to skillet. Cook 1-2 minutes per side, until fork-tender. Cover with foil and set aside.

Add remaining oil to skillet; sauté garlic and nuts 1 minute. Add greens and wine; cover and steam 1 minute. Serve.

NUTRITION SCORE
Per serving (1 cod fillet, 2 polenta slices, ½ cup greens):
273 **calories**
29% **fat** (8.8 g; 2 g saturated)
29% **carbs** (19.8 g), 3 g **fiber**
42% **protein** (28.7 g)

Ceviche of Scallop and Salmon

Serves 4
Prep time: 10 minutes, plus 24 hours to marinate

1¼ cup fresh sea scallops, sliced
¾ cup ½-inch-diced skinless salmon fillet
1 shallot, minced
½ cup tomato juice
1 tomato, seeded, diced small
¼ cup fresh lemon juice (about
   1 medium lemon)
¼ cup diced red bell pepper
½ tablespoon extra-virgin olive oil
1 teaspoon paprika
1 tablespoon chopped fresh cilantro (reserve
   4 sprigs for garnish)
2 teaspoons sugar
 Salt and pepper to taste
4 lemon wedges for garnish

In a medium bowl, combine all ingredients. Cover with plastic wrap; refrigerate for 24 hours (in a refrigerator that is set no warmer than 40° F), until fish is an opaque white.

Using a slotted spoon, drain liquid and divide fish between 4 plates. Garnish with lemon wedges and cilantro sprigs and serve.

NUTRITION SCORE
Per serving (¼ recipe before draining): 141 **calories**
31% **fat** (4.9 g; 0.7 g saturated)
23% **carbs** (7.8 g), 0.6 g **fiber**
46% **protein** (16.3 g)

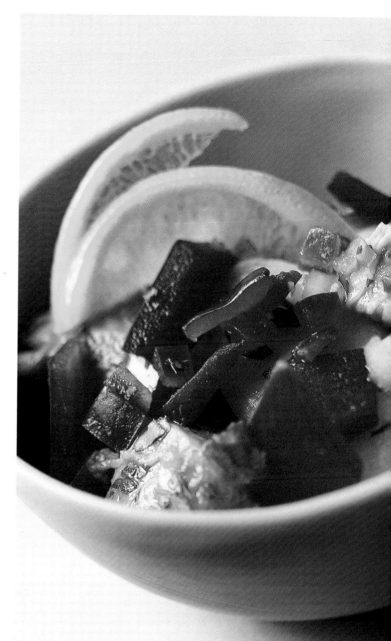

In this Mexican dish, the acid in the lemon juice "cooks" the fish, turning it opaque and killing most bacteria. However, you must start with the freshest fish from a reputable merchant and use scrupulously clean utensils. Drain most of the oil along with the other liquids before serving in order to reduce the fat content.

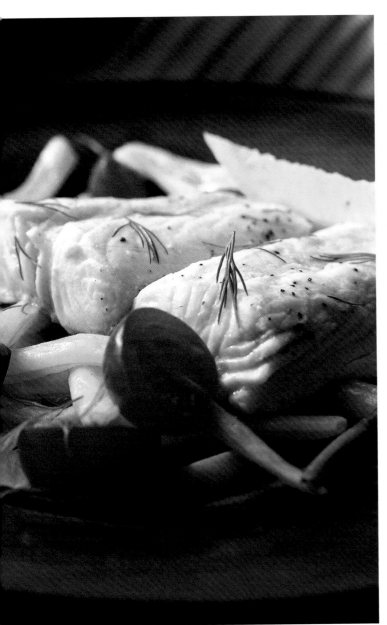

Steamed Halibut With Cherry Tomatoes and Fresh Wax Beans

Serves 4
Prep time: 10 minutes
Cook time: 10-12 minutes

1½ pounds halibut, skin removed and cut into 4 equal portions

4 8-by-10-inch pieces of aluminum foil

1½ cups fresh wax beans (about 1½ pounds unshelled)

½ pint cherry tomatoes, halved

4 green onions, trimmed and cut lengthwise into fourths, then halved, creating matchsticks

2 teaspoons finely chopped fresh dill

½ teaspoon salt

½ teaspoon freshly ground black pepper

2 teaspoons extra-virgin olive oil

Preheat oven to 425° F. Place each piece of fish in the center of a sheet of foil and surround with beans, tomatoes and green onions; sprinkle with dill, salt and pepper and drizzle with olive oil. (Make sure to divide all the ingredients evenly among the 4 servings.) Fold the lengthwise edges of the foil up toward each other to create a tent; then fold the edges over twice to make an airtight seam. Fold the ends inward to seal the edges. (There should be plenty of space between the foil and fish.)

Bake fish packets for about 10-12 minutes, or until fish is no longer opaque and flakes easily.

NUTRITION SCORE
Per serving (1 fish packet): 277 **calories**
20% **fat** (6.3 g; 0.9 g saturated)
24% **carbs** (14 g), 3.7 g **fiber**
56% **protein** (38.9 g)

Monkfish With Black Pepper, Scallions and Jasmine Rice

Serves 4
Prep time: 5 minutes
Cook time: 16 minutes

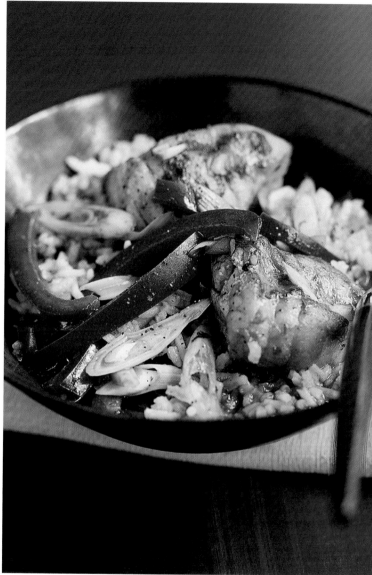

  1 cup uncooked jasmine rice, long-grain white rice or brown rice
6 ½ cups water, divided
  2 teaspoons olive oil
  1 pound monkfish fillet, cut into 2-inch chunks
  1 red bell pepper, thinly sliced
  2 tablespoons hoisin sauce
  ½ teaspoon ground black pepper
  ½ cup thinly sliced green onions

Combine rice and 6 cups water in a medium saucepan. Bring to a boil. Reduce heat; simmer 8-10 minutes, until rice is tender. Drain and set aside.

Meanwhile, place wok or large skillet over medium-high heat. Once hot, add olive oil and swirl to coat pan. Add monkfish chunks and stir-fry 2 minutes. Add red pepper slices and stir-fry 1 minute. Add ½ cup water, hoisin sauce and black pepper and simmer 3 minutes, until fish is fork-tender.

Remove from heat and add sliced green onions. Spoon rice onto 4 dinner plates. Spoon monkfish mixture over top and serve.

NUTRITION SCORE
Per serving (3 ounces fish, ¼ cup red pepper, 2 tablespoons black pepper sauce, ½ cup rice): 303 **calories**
12% **fat** (4 g; <1 g saturated)
61% **carbs** (46 g), 2 g **fiber**
27% **protein** (20.4 g)

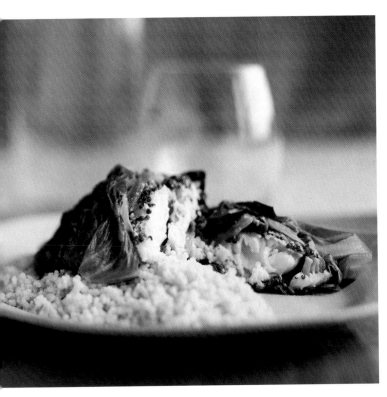

Romaine-Wrapped Tilapia With Red Onion and Capers

Serves 4
Prep time: 10 minutes
Cook time: 15 minutes

- 4 large romaine lettuce leaves
- 4 5-ounce tilapia fillets (substitute halibut, if desired)
- Salt and ground black pepper to taste
- 4 teaspoons grainy, coarse mustard
- 4 slices red onion
- 4 teaspoons drained capers
- 1 cup uncooked whole-wheat couscous
- Cooking spray

It's helpful to carefully monitor what you eat and how much you exercise. Keeping a daily log will help you achieve your weight-loss and fitness goals.

Preheat oven to 400° F. Spray a large, shallow baking dish with cooking spray.

Place romaine leaves on paper towels and sprinkle with water. Cover leaves with another paper towel and microwave on high for 10 seconds, until leaves are tender.

Arrange leaves on a flat surface and top each leaf with a single tilapia fillet (place fish crosswise on leaf). Season the top of fish with salt and black pepper; then spread with 1 teaspoon mustard. Place onion slice and 1 teaspoon capers on top of mustard. Fold over one side of romaine leaf to cover fish, and then fold over the other side. Place wrapped fish seam-side down in prepared baking dish and cover with foil. Bake 15 minutes, until fish is fork-tender.

Meanwhile, to make the couscous, bring 1¼ cups of water to a boil in a medium saucepan. Add couscous and remove from heat. Let stand 5 minutes, until liquid is absorbed. Serve wrapped fish with couscous on the side.

NUTRITION SCORE
Per serving (1 wrapped fish fillet, ½ cup couscous): 318 **calories**
11% **fat** (4 g; 0 g saturated)
60% **carbs** (48 g), 8 g **fiber**
29% **protein** (23 g)

Apricot-Shrimp Stir-Fry

Serves 4
Prep time: 10 minutes
Cook time: 10 minutes

- 2 cups instant brown rice
- 2 teaspoons peanut oil
- 2 cloves garlic, minced
- 2 teaspoons minced fresh ginger
- 1 pound large raw shrimp, peeled and deveined
- 2 fresh apricots, pitted and thinly sliced
- 1 cup snow peas, ends trimmed
- ½ cup reduced-sodium chicken or vegetable broth
- 2 tablespoons apricot preserves
- 1 tablespoon reduced-sodium soy sauce
- ¼ teaspoon ground black pepper

Cook rice according to package directions. Set aside.

Meanwhile, heat oil in a large wok or nonstick skillet over high heat. Add garlic and ginger and cook 1 minute. Mix in shrimp and apricots and cook another minute, until shrimp are just pink. Add remaining ingredients and simmer 5 minutes more, until shrimp are cooked through and liquid reduces slightly, stirring occasionally. Spoon shrimp mixture over rice just before serving.

NUTRITION SCORE
Per serving (1 cup shrimp mixture, ½ cup rice): 332 **calories**
13% **fat** (5 g; <1 g saturated)
57% **carbs** (47 g), 4 g **fiber**
30% **protein** (25 g)

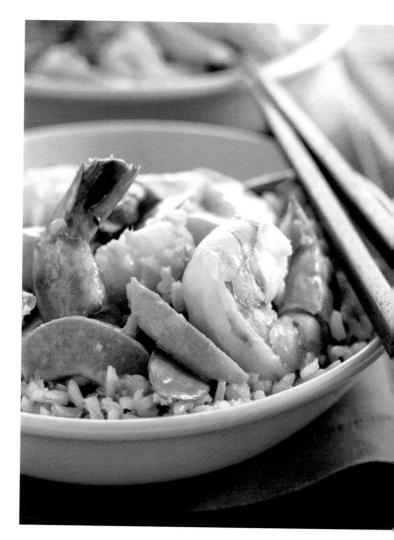

Select firm apricots and leave them on your counter for a few days, until they're slightly tender. Once they're ripe, store them in the refrigerator. If you can't find fresh apricots for this recipe, substitute ¼ cup dried apricots, thinly sliced.

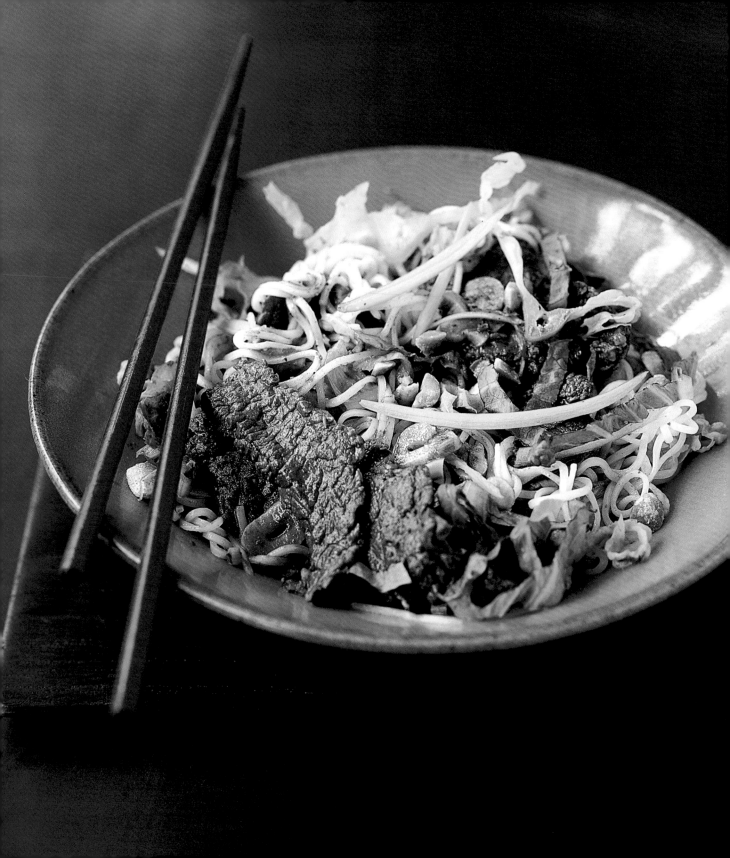

meat and poultry

Meat-based meals needn't be taboo for the health-minded. With the right choice of cut and the proper preparation, you can limit saturated fat and enjoy satisfying dishes like Classic Roast Chicken, Shepherd's Pie With Root Vegetables and Pork Medallions in Cranberry Chutney With Barley.

recipes

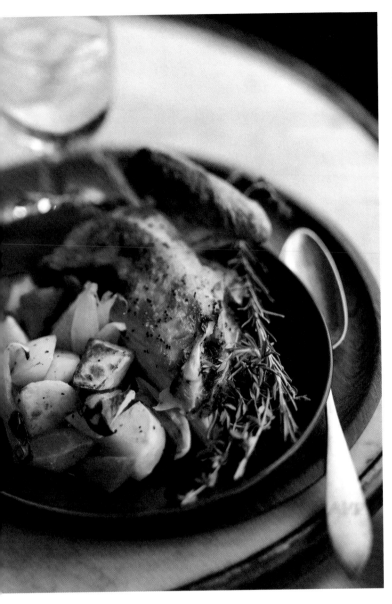

Classic Roast Chicken With Vegetables

Serves 2 (with leftovers)
Prep time: 20 minutes
Cook time: 45 minutes

 1 whole fryer chicken (3½–4 pounds), backbone, giblets and cavity fat removed (*Remove backbone with poultry shears or ask your butcher to do it. This lets the chicken lie flat and cuts roasting time in half.*)

Dash kosher salt

Dash cracked black pepper

 1 pound carrots, peeled, cut into 1-inch chunks

 1 large yellow onion, peeled, cut into 1-inch chunks

 1 pound (4–5 medium) Yukon Gold potatoes, peeled, cut into 1-inch chunks

 2 tablespoons virgin olive oil

Preheat broiler. Set rack to lowest position. Season chicken generously on all sides with salt and pepper. Cook chicken, skin side up, on rack for 20 minutes.

Put carrots, onion and potatoes in a plastic bag and add oil, salt and pepper. Close bag and shake to coat. Add vegetables to pan with chicken and cook for 20–25 more minutes, until chicken's internal temperature reaches 165° F with an instant-read digital thermometer and vegetables are golden brown and fork tender. Serve immediately.

Most overeating happens late in the afternoon or evening when energy levels and mood are low. Up your energy quotient by listening to music, taking a 30-minute nap or going for a brisk 10-minute walk.

NUTRITION SCORE
Per serving (3–4 ounces skinless chicken meat, 1 cup roasted vegetables): 293 **calories**
34% **fat** (11 g; 2.3 g saturated)
29% **carbs** (21 g), 3 g **fiber**
37% **protein** (27 g)

Country Oven-Fried Chicken

Serves 6
Prep time: 8 minutes
Cook time: 45 minutes

   1 cup buttermilk
   2 teaspoons hot sauce (optional)
   6 6-ounce skinned chicken breast halves
   3 cups Corn Chex or cornflakes
   ¾ cup self-rising flour
   2 teaspoons Creole or Cajun seasoning
  Cooking spray

Combine buttermilk and hot sauce in a heavy-duty resealable plastic bag. Add chicken and seal bag. Chill at least 4 hours; turn bag occasionally.

Preheat oven to 400° F. Crush cereal into crumbs in a food processor. Pour into a shallow dish; stir in flour and seasoning. Remove chicken from buttermilk, letting excess drip off. Dredge chicken in cereal mixture. Arrange pieces, bone side down, on a cookie sheet or shallow baking pan coated with cooking spray.

Coat tops of chicken lightly with cooking spray. Bake on bottom shelf of oven for 20 minutes. Use a wide metal spatula to carefully loosen and turn chicken. Coat other sides with cooking spray and bake 15 minutes.

Loosen and turn chicken again, coat top side with cooking spray again, and bake 10-15 minutes or until juices run clear when chicken is pierced.

NUTRITION SCORE
Per serving (1 chicken breast half): 302 **calories**
6% **fat** (2 g; 0.6 g saturated)
38% **carbs** (25 g), 0.7 g **fiber**
56% **protein** (42 g)

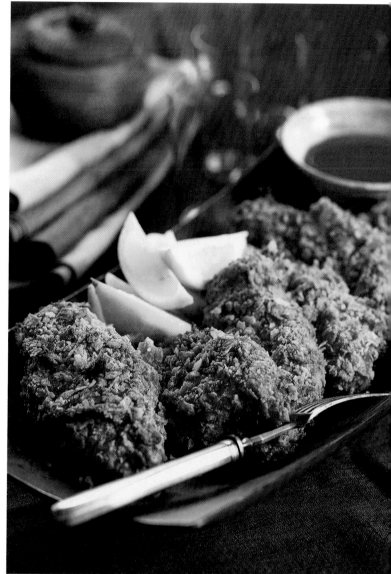

 You also can use this recipe to make delicious, lowfat chicken fingers. Simply batter skinless, boneless chicken as directed above, and bake for 20 minutes per side.

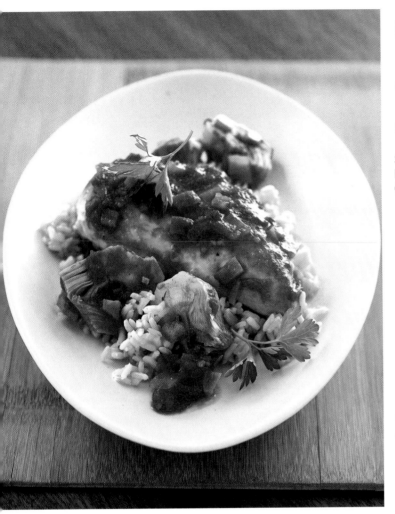

Chicken With Artichoke Hearts and Tomatoes

Serves 4
Prep time: 5 minutes
Cook time: 8 minutes

- 2 cups instant brown rice
- 4 skinless, boneless chicken breast halves, rinsed well and patted dry
- Salt and ground black pepper to taste
- 2 teaspoons olive oil
- 1 14.5-ounce can diced tomatoes with green pepper and onion
- ¼ cup sun-dried tomato pesto
- 1 14-ounce can artichoke hearts in water, drained and quartered

Cook rice according to package directions, without adding fat or salt.

Meanwhile, season both sides of chicken with salt and pepper. Heat oil in a large skillet over medium-high heat. Add chicken and cook 1 minute per side, until golden brown and seared. Using tongs, remove chicken from pan; set aside.

Add canned tomato mix to pan; simmer 1 minute, stirring constantly and incorporating any brown bits from bottom of pan. Stir in pesto and artichokes. Return chicken to pan. Cover; simmer 5 minutes, until chicken is cooked through. Serve chicken and sauce on cooked rice.

Searing (pan-frying in very little oil to create a golden crust) locks in flavor and moisture, and leaves flavorful morsels clinging to the bottom of the pan that are incorporated into a sauce once liquids are added.

NUTRITION SCORE
Per serving (1 chicken breast half, ½ cup sauce, ⅔ cup rice):
433 **calories**
27% **fat** (13 g; 2 g saturated)
41% **carbs** (44 g), 4 g **fiber**
32% **protein** (35 g)

Mu Shu Chicken

Serves 4
Prep time: 20 minutes
Cook time: 5-6 minutes

- 4 dried black Chinese mushrooms or dried shiitake mushrooms
- ⅓ cup fat-free chicken or vegetable broth
- 1 tablespoon reduced-sodium soy sauce
- 2 teaspoons cornstarch
- 2 teaspoons sesame oil
- 2 cloves garlic, minced
- 1 tablespoon minced fresh ginger
- 1 pound skinless, boneless chicken breasts, cut into ¼-inch-thick strips
- 4 cups shredded green cabbage or packaged cole slaw mix
- 1 carrot, cut into matchstick
- 1 small zucchini, cut into matchstick
- 2 green onions, sliced diagonally into ¼-inch pieces
- 8 6-inch whole-wheat or spinach tortillas
- ¼ cup hoisin sauce

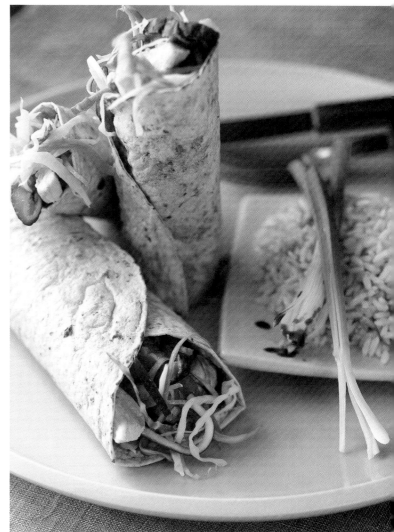

Soak dried mushrooms in ½ cup warm water for 20 minutes. Drain, reserve mushroom liquid, remove and discard any stems and thinly slice caps. Whisk together broth, soy sauce and cornstarch; set aside.

Heat oil in a wok or large skillet over high heat. Add minced garlic and ginger and stir-fry for 30 seconds. Add chicken and stir-fry for 2-3 minutes, until no longer pink. Add cabbage, carrot, zucchini, green onions, reserved mushrooms and mushroom liquid and stir-fry for 1 minute, until cabbage wilts. Add cornstarch mixture and simmer 1 minute, until liquid thickens. Remove from heat.

Wrap tortillas in plastic and heat in the microwave for 15 seconds to soften. Spoon 1½ teaspoons of hoisin sauce on each tortilla, add chicken and vegetable mixture and roll up.

NUTRITION SCORE
Per serving (2 tortillas, 1 cup chicken and vegetable filling):
390 **calories**
14% **fat** (6 g; 1 g saturated)
50% **carbs** (49 g), 21 g **fiber**
36% **protein** (35 g)

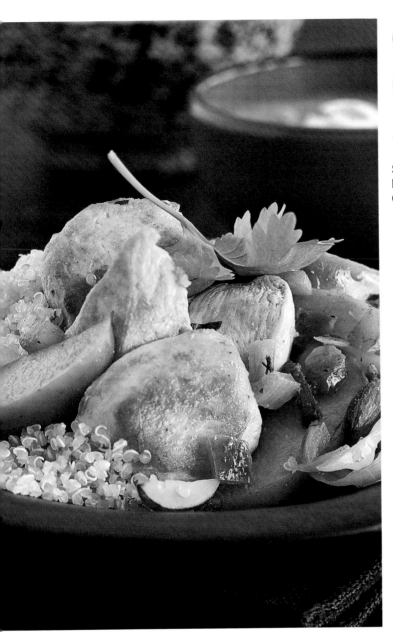

Curried Chicken With Cabbage, Apples and Almonds

Serves 4
Prep time: 20 minutes
Cook time: 16 minutes

- 6 teaspoons olive oil
- ½ cup chopped red onion
- ¼ cup slivered almonds
- 2 cloves garlic, minced
- 1 pound skinless, boneless chicken breasts, cut into 2-inch pieces
- 2 teaspoons curry powder
- ½ teaspoon ground coriander
- ½ teaspoon salt
- ¼ teaspoon ground black pepper
- 1½ cups reduced-sodium chicken broth
- 2 cups green cabbage, cut into 2-inch pieces
- 2 Yellow Delicious apples, cored and diced
- ¼ cup chopped fresh cilantro
- 1 cup quinoa, cooked according to package directions

Heat olive oil in a large nonstick skillet over medium heat. Add onion, almonds and garlic and sauté 2 minutes, until nuts are golden. Add chicken and sauté 3 minutes, until golden brown on all sides.

Add curry powder, coriander, salt and pepper. Stir to coat. Add broth; bring to a boil. Add cabbage; reduce heat to medium-low and simmer 10 minutes, until chicken is cooked through and liquid is reduced. Add apples and simmer 1 minute to heat through. Remove from heat and stir in cilantro. Serve over quinoa.

NUTRITION SCORE
Per serving (1 ½ cups chicken mixture, ½ cup quinoa):
409 **calories**
27% **fat** (12 g; 2 g saturated)
40% **carbs** (41 g), 7 g **fiber**
33% **protein** (34 g)

Turkey With Peanuts and Green Beans

Serves 4
Prep time: 8 minutes
Cook time: 12 minutes

- 1 pound boneless, skinless turkey breast cut into 2-inch cubes
- 1 teaspoon sesame oil
- ½ teaspoon garlic powder
- ¼ teaspoon cayenne pepper
- 1 cup fresh green beans, stemmed (substitute frozen, if desired; no thawing necessary)
- 3 tablespoons water
- 1 cup instant brown rice, uncooked
- 2 teaspoons canola oil
- ½ cup roasted, unsalted peanuts
- ¼ cup nonfat chicken broth
- 1 tablespoon soy sauce (or reduced-sodium soy sauce)

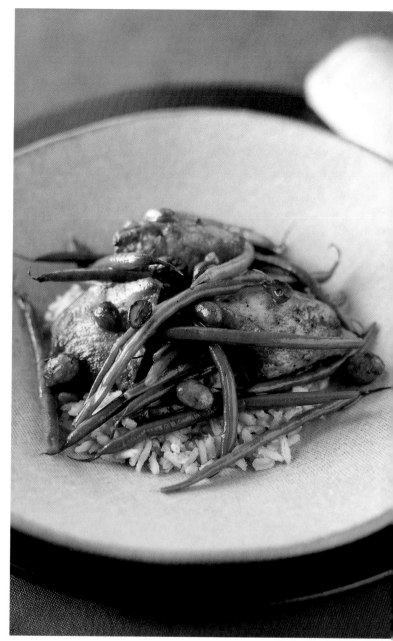

In a small bowl, mix together turkey, sesame oil, garlic powder and cayenne pepper. Coat well and set aside.

Place fresh green beans and water in a microwave-safe dish. Cook on high for 30 seconds. Remove and drain water. (Skip this step if using frozen green beans.) Meanwhile, prepare instant brown rice according to package instructions.

Heat a large nonstick frying pan (or wok) over medium heat and add canola oil. Add turkey mixture and cook, stirring frequently with a wooden spoon for 5 minutes. Add peanuts and stir-fry for 30 seconds. Next, add the green beans and stir-fry for 1 more minute. Pour in chicken broth and soy sauce and cook until liquid evaporates, about 5 minutes. Divide rice among 4 plates and top rice with turkey-peanut mixture.

NUTRITION SCORE
Per serving (1 cup turkey mixture, ½ cup cooked brown rice):
423 **calories**
26% **fat** (13 g; 2 g saturated)
41% **carbs** (44 g), 4g **fiber**
33% **protein** (35 g)

Pine-Nut-Crusted Chicken Cutlets With Angel-Hair Pasta

Serves 4
Prep time: 5-7 minutes
Cook time: 7-8 minutes

- 6 tablespoons seasoned dry bread crumbs
- 2 tablespoons finely chopped pine nuts
- 4 skinless, boneless chicken breast halves, flattened between 2 pieces of plastic wrap until ½ inch thick
- 2 teaspoons olive oil
- 8 ounces uncooked angel-hair or capellini pasta
- 1 14-ounce can diced tomatoes seasoned with basil, garlic and oregano

In a shallow dish, combine bread crumbs and pine nuts. Add chicken and turn to coat both sides. Heat oil in a large nonstick skillet over medium-high heat. Add chicken and cook 3 minutes per side, until golden brown. Reduce heat to medium, cover and cook 1-2 more minutes, until chicken is cooked through.

Meanwhile, cook pasta in a large pot of rapidly boiling water until tender, about 2-3 minutes. Drain and toss with diced tomatoes. Serve chicken with pasta on the side.

NUTRITION SCORE
Per serving (1 chicken breast, 1¼ cup pasta mixture): 464 **calories**
18% **fat** (9.3 g, 2 g saturated)
49% **carbs** (57 g), 3 g **fiber**
33% **protein** (38 g)

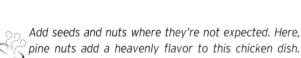

Add seeds and nuts where they're not expected. Here, pine nuts add a heavenly flavor to this chicken dish. For variety, try substituting almonds.

Grilled Hoisin Pork Chops With Pineapple and Green Onion Relish

Serves 8
Prep time: 10 minutes
Cook time: 15 minutes

8 1-inch-thick pork chops (about 4 ounces each)

Hoisin Marinade

1 cup hoisin sauce
3 tablespoons rice wine vinegar
2 tablespoons soy sauce
4 garlic cloves, minced
1 teaspoon sesame oil
½ teaspoon ground black pepper

Pineapple and Green Onion Relish

1 small pineapple, peeled and diced (about 2 cups)
1 small jalapeño pepper, seeded and minced
2 tablespoons fresh lime juice
2 tablespoons chopped fresh cilantro
2 green onions
Olive-oil cooking spray
½ teaspoon salt
½ teaspoon ground black pepper

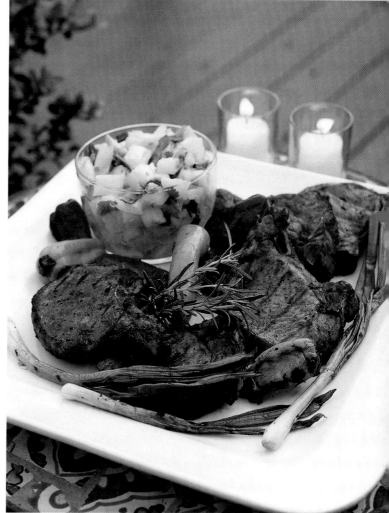

Whisk together all ingredients for hoisin marinade in a large, shallow baking dish. Add pork chops and turn to coat both sides. Cover with plastic and refrigerate until ready to use.

To prepare the pineapple-grilled green onion relish, combine pineapple, jalapeño, lime juice and cilantro. Toss gently and refrigerate until ready to use.

To grill the pork chops, remove from marinade (discard marinade) and grill 6-7 minutes per side for medium-well meat. While the pork chops are grilling, spray green onions with olive-oil spray and season with salt and pepper. Grill until just golden, about 4 minutes. Remove from grill and slice crosswise into ¼-inch pieces. Add to pineapple mixture. Serve with grilled pork chops.

NUTRITION SCORE
Per serving (1 pork chop, ¼ cup relish): 203 **calories**
18% **fat** (4 g; 1.4 g saturated)
57% **carbs** (29 g), 1 g fiber
25% **protein** (12.6 g)

Chicken Saté With Rice and Peas

Serves 4
Prep time: 5 minutes
Cook time: 5-7 minutes

- 1 pound skinless, boneless chicken breasts, cut into thin strips
- Salt and ground black pepper to taste
- ¼ cup reduced-sodium chicken broth
- ¼ cup reduced-fat creamy peanut butter
- 1 tablespoon reduced-sodium soy sauce
- 2 cups cooked instant white or brown rice
- 1 cup frozen green peas, thawed

Sauté chicken in a large nonstick skillet over medium-high heat until golden brown on all sides and cooked through, about 3-5 minutes (or grill or broil it). Season with salt and pepper.

In a small saucepan, combine broth, peanut butter and soy sauce. Simmer 2 minutes, until hot, stirring with a wire whisk (or microwave on high for 1 minute).

Cook rice according to package directions. Remove from heat and stir in peas. If desired, season with salt and pepper.

Serve chicken strips atop rice mixture, with peanut sauce on the side.

NUTRITION SCORE
Per serving (1 chicken breast, sliced into strips; 2 tablespoons peanut sauce; 1 cup rice mixture): 450 **calories**
18% **fat** (9 g; 2 g saturated)
49% **carbs** (54 g), 3 g **fiber**
33% **protein** (37 g)

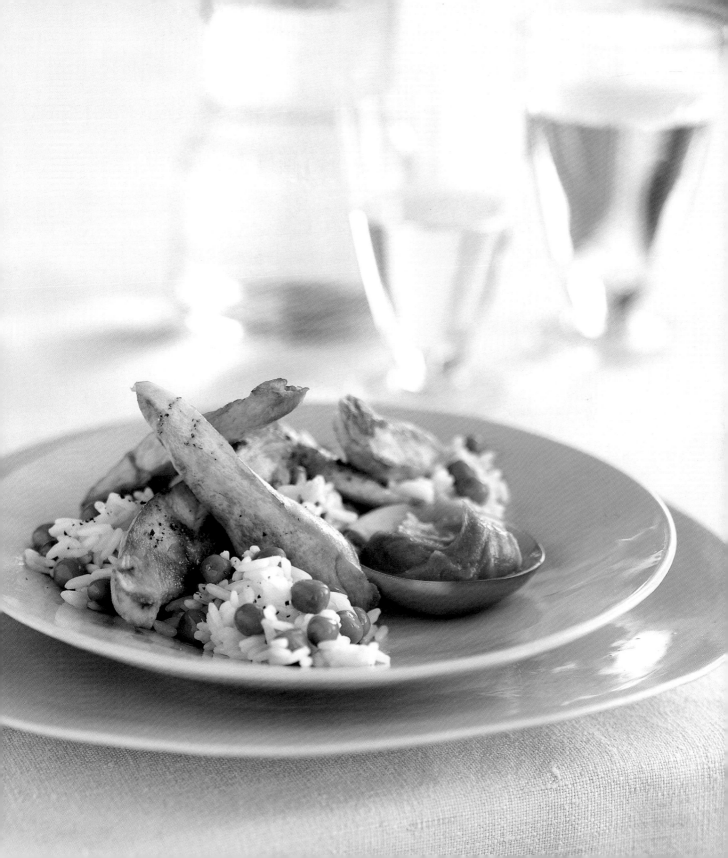

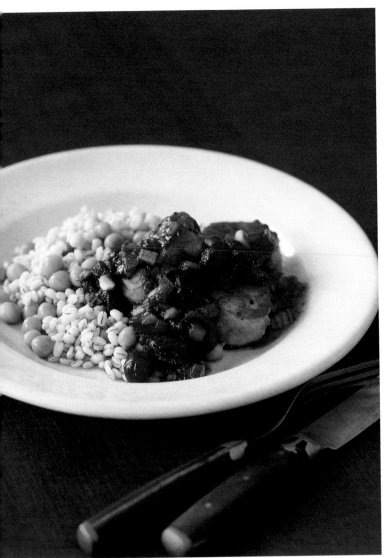

Pork Medallions in Cranberry Chutney With Barley

Serves 4
Prep time: 5 minutes
Cook time: 10-12 minutes

- 1 cup quick-cooking barley
- 2 cups reduced-sodium, nonfat chicken broth or water
- ¾ cup frozen green peas
- Salt and pepper to taste
- 2 teaspoons peanut or olive oil
- 2 8-ounce pork tenderloins, cut crosswise into 1-inch-thick slices
- ⅓ cup chopped red onion
- 1 cup canned whole-berry sweetened cranberry sauce
- 1 tablespoon cider vinegar
- ½ teaspoon ground ginger

In a saucepan, add barley to boiling broth (or water). Cover, reduce heat; simmer 8 minutes. Add peas. Cook 2 minutes, until liquid is absorbed and barley is tender. Season with salt and pepper.

Heat oil in a large skillet. Salt and pepper both sides of pork and sauté 2 minutes per side. Remove pork; set aside.

In juices in skillet, sauté onion for 2 minutes. Add remaining ingredients. Return pork to pan; simmer 2 minutes. Serve.

Don't get stuck on rerun meals. Eating the same safe low-calorie foods every day can deprive you of nutrients. In time, the few foods you're eating will no longer feel satisfying, and you'll compensate by eating more or adding impulse foods to your diet.

NUTRITION SCORE
Per serving (3 ounces pork, ⅓ cup chutney, 1 cup barley and peas):
455 **calories**
15% **fat** (7.5 g; 2 g saturated)
57% **carbs** (65 g), 11 g **fiber**
28% **protein** (32 g)

Curried Lamb Patties With Chutney

Serves 4
Prep time: 10 minutes
Cook time: 10 minutes

- 1   pound lean lamb, ground
- 1   (10-ounce) package frozen chopped spinach, thawed and squeezed dry
- ⅔   cup fresh whole-wheat bread crumbs (about 2 slices of bread)
- 2   cloves garlic, minced
- ½   teaspoon coarse salt
- ⅓   cup purchased mango chutney
- 1   teaspoon curry powder
- 1   teaspoon ground ginger
- ¼   teaspoon cayenne pepper

Cooking spray

Combine all ingredients except cooking spray in a medium bowl; stir well to blend. Divide mixture into 4 equal portions and shape into ½-inch-thick patties. Prepare grill or broiler. Place patties on grill rack or broiler pan coated with cooking spray. Cook for approximately 5 minutes on each side or until cooked through.

NUTRITION SCORE
Per serving (1 patty): 287 **calories**
28% **fat** (8.8 g; 3.1 g saturated)
33% **carbs** (24.3 g), 4.5 g **fiber**
39% **protein** (27.8 g)

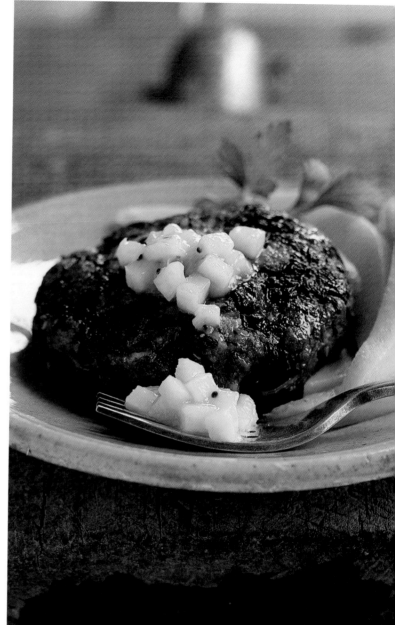

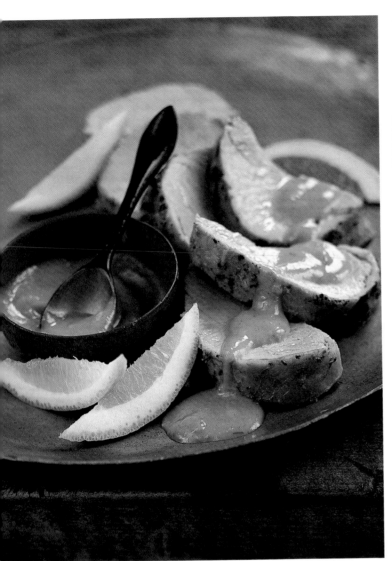

Peanut-Orange Pork Tenderloin

Serves 4
Prep time: 12 minutes
Marinating time: 1 hour
Cook time: 23 minutes

- ⅓ cup orange marmalade
- ¼ cup orange juice
- 2 tablespoons reduced-fat peanut butter
- 1 tablespoon Dijon mustard
- 1 teaspoon ground cumin
- 1 teaspoon vegetable oil
- ½ teaspoon coarse salt
- ¼ teaspoon chili paste
- 1 pound pork tenderloin, trimmed of fat

Blend first 8 ingredients in a food processor until smooth. Pour into a shallow dish. Add pork; turn to coat. Refrigerate 1 hour. Preheat oven to 400° F.

Place pork on a foil-lined baking sheet (reserve marinade); roast 10 minutes a side. In a saucepan lightly boil remaining marinade for 3 minutes.

Slice pork in thin slices. Serve with warm peanut-orange sauce.

NUTRITION SCORE
Per serving (3 ounces pork, 1½ tablespoons sauce): 275 **calories**
28% **fat** (8.7 g; 2.2 g saturated)
34% **carbs** (24 g), 1.7 g **fiber**
38% **protein** (26 g)

Saigon Beef With Noodles

Serves 4
Prep time: 5 minutes
Cook time: 10 minutes

- 10 ounces uncooked Chinese noodles (mein)
- 2 teaspoons roasted peanut oil
- 4 garlic cloves, minced
- 1 pound top round, trimmed of fat and sliced against the grain into thin strips
- ½ cup water
- Salt and ground black pepper to taste
- 2 cups thinly shredded romaine lettuce
- ¼ cup dry-roasted peanuts, chopped

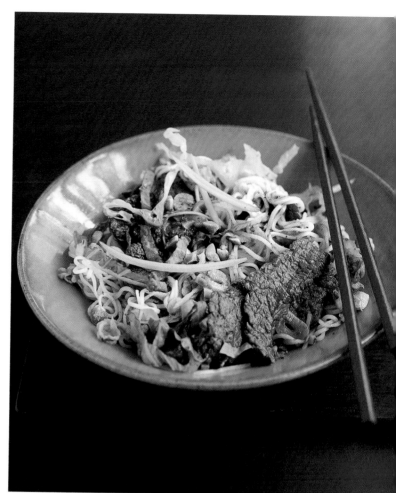

Bring a large pot of water to a boil. Add Chinese noodles and cook 3 minutes, until just tender. Drain and set aside.

Meanwhile, set wok or large skillet over medium-high heat. Once hot, add oil and swirl to coat pan. Add garlic and stir-fry 1 minute. Add beef and stir-fry 3 minutes, until browned on all sides, stirring constantly. Add ½ cup water and simmer 2 minutes. Remove from heat and season with salt and pepper.

Divide noodles among 4 dinner plates. Top with lettuce and then beef mixture. Sprinkle peanuts over top and serve.

NUTRITION SCORE
Per serving (3 ounces beef, ¾ cup noodles, ½ cup romaine lettuce, 1 tablespoon peanuts): 482 **calories**
25% **fat** (13.6 g; 3 g saturated)
45% **carbs** (54 g), 2 g **fiber**
30% **protein** (36 g)

Lean beef is an excellent source of protein and iron. For the leanest meat, choose cuts with the words round *or* loin *in them, such as* eye round, top round, round tip, sirloin *and* tenderloin.

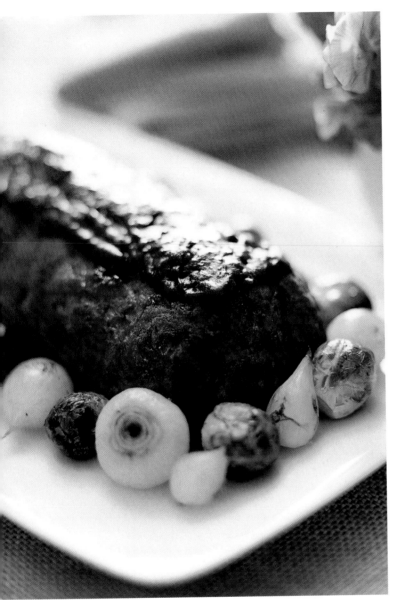

Barbecue Turkey Meatloaf

Serves 6
Prep time: 10 minutes
Cook time: 1 hour

Cooking spray
1¼ pounds ground turkey
⅓ cup plain bread crumbs
1 cup chopped onion
⅓ cup plus ¼ cup barbecue sauce
1 tablespoon Worcestershire sauce
2 egg whites
1 teaspoon salt
¼ teaspoon pepper

Preheat oven to 350° F. Lightly coat a 13-by-9-inch baking pan or baking sheet with cooking spray.

In a large bowl, combine the turkey, bread crumbs, onion, ⅓ cup barbecue sauce, Worcestershire sauce, egg whites, salt and pepper. With your hands or a spoon, mix well until thoroughly combined.

Place meatloaf mixture in the center of a cookie sheet or large baking pan and shape into a 10-by-4-inch loaf by hand. Spread the remaining ¼ cup barbecue sauce evenly over the top of the loaf. Bake 1 hour and let stand 5 minutes before draining fat and slicing.

NUTRITION SCORE
Per serving (2 1-inch slices): 190 **calories**
16% **fat** (3.5 g; 0.9 g saturated)
41% **carbs** (17.7 g), 0.7 g **fiber**
43% **protein** (18.7 g)

Preparing this meatloaf on a baking sheet or large baking pan allows the fat to drain away from the loaf. You also can use this technique for meats like roasts and briskets. Leave at least 3 inches of space around the meat.

Shepherd's Pie With Root Vegetables

Serves 4
Prep time: 10-15 minutes
Cook time: 40 minutes

- 2 Idaho potatoes, peeled and cut into 2-inch chunks
- 1 celery root (celeriac), about ¼ pound, peeled and cut into 2-inch chunks
- ½ cup fat-free sour cream
- 2 tablespoons all-purpose flour
- 1 teaspoon dried thyme
- ½ teaspoon salt
- ¼ teaspoon ground black pepper
- 2 teaspoons olive or vegetable oil
- 1 cup chopped onion
- 1 cup sliced button mushrooms
- 1 pound boneless beef round or chuck, cut into 2-inch cubes
- 1 cup fat-free beef broth
- 1 tablespoon Dijon mustard
- 2 medium carrots, peeled and chopped
- ¼ cup chopped fresh parsley

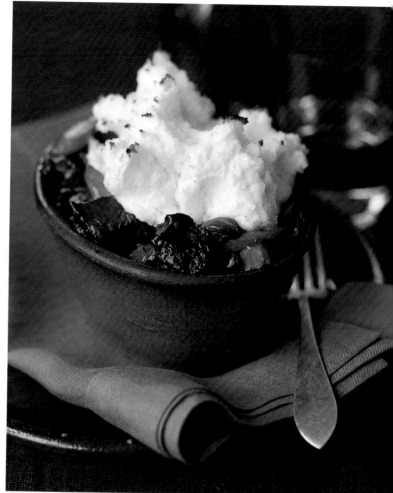

Preheat oven to 400º F. Combine potatoes, celery root and enough water to cover them in a medium saucepan; set pan over high heat. Bring to a boil, reduce heat to medium-high and simmer 10 minutes, until vegetables are fork-tender. Drain and transfer to a food processor or large bowl. Add sour cream and process or, using a potato masher, mash vegetables until smooth; set aside.

Meanwhile, in a small bowl, combine flour, thyme, salt and pepper; set aside.

Heat oil in a large saucepan over medium-high heat. Add onion and mushrooms and sauté 2 minutes, until mushrooms release juice. Add beef and sauté 5 minutes, until browned on all sides. Add flour mixture and stir to coat.

Whisk together broth and mustard in a small bowl. Add to pan along with the carrots. Bring mixture to a boil. Remove from heat and transfer to a deep, 9-inch pie plate or shallow baking dish.

Top beef mixture with potato purée and, using the back of a spoon,

smooth the surface while making decorative swirls. Place pie plate on a baking sheet.

Bake 30 minutes, until top is golden. Sprinkle the top with parsley before serving, if desired.

NUTRITION SCORE
Per serving (2 cups): 352 **calories**
24% **fat** (9.2 g; 2.5 g saturated)
40% **carbs** (35 g), 4 g **fiber**
36% **protein** (32 g)

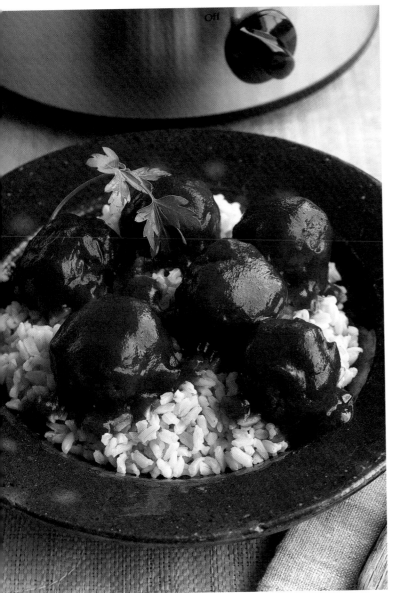

Sweet 'n' Sour Turkey Meatballs

Serves 4
Prep time: 10 minutes
Cook time: 8-10 hours (in a slow cooker)

- 1 pound ground turkey breast
- ¼ cup dry bread crumbs
- 2 tablespoons chopped fresh parsley
- 2 tablespoons minced onion
- 1 egg
- 1 16-ounce can jellied cranberry sauce
- ⅓ cup ketchup
- ¼ cup Heinz chili sauce
- 2 cups instant brown rice
- 1 10-ounce package fresh spinach leaves, steamed

In a large bowl, combine turkey, bread crumbs, parsley, onion and egg. Mix well and shape the mixture into 24 meatballs. Set aside.

In a slow cooker (6-quart size or larger), combine cranberry sauce, ketchup and chili sauce. Mix well. Gently stir in meatballs. Cover and cook on low for 8-10 hours.

Cook rice according to package directions. Serve meatballs and sauce over rice. Serve spinach on the side.

NUTRITION SCORE
Per serving (6 meatballs, ½ cup sauce, ½ cup rice, ½ cup spinach):
521 **calories**
9% **fat** (5 g; <1 g saturated)
70% **carbs** (91 g), 6 g **fiber**
21% **protein** (27 g)

The slow cooker, aka crock pot, is making a comeback. It's a stress-free way to prepare dinner. Just put the ingredients in the pot before you go to work, and when you return at day's end, a healthy meal awaits you.

Marinated Beef Kabobs With Veggies

Serves 6
Prep time: 15 minutes
Marinating time: 4-6 hours
Cook time: 5-8 minutes

- 3 pounds sirloin tri-tip beef fillets or skinless, boneless chicken breasts
- 1 medium-large onion
- 2 cups plain nonfat yogurt
- 2 tablespoons finely chopped cilantro
- 1 teaspoon ground cumin
- ½ teaspoon freshly ground black pepper
- 2 medium zucchini, sliced into 1-inch-thick pieces
- 1 medium red bell pepper, chopped into 1-inch squares
- 1 medium yellow bell pepper, chopped into 1-inch squares
- 12 medium button mushrooms
- 3 plum tomatoes, quartered
- 1 medium onion, sliced into 1-inch squares
- ½ teaspoon salt

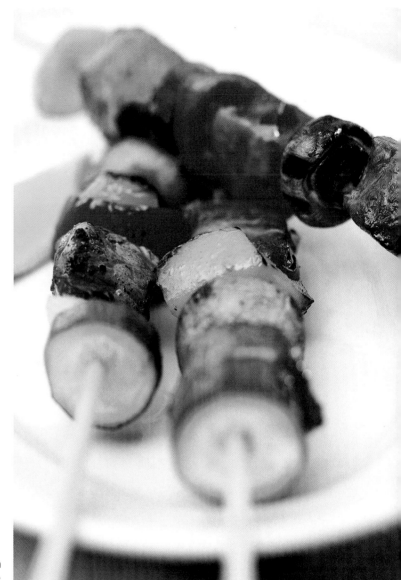

Trim any visible fat from beef. Cut beef into 48 1½- to 2-inch cubes. Peel onion, cut in half and grate on the large holes of box grater, until there is a heaping ¼ cup of grated onion and onion juice. Pour yogurt into a large bowl and add onion and its juice. Stir in cilantro, cumin and black pepper. Add beef and mix thoroughly. Cover and refrigerate. Marinate for 6 hours, turning once or twice. (If using chicken, marinate for 4 hours. Do not exceed the recommended marinating time because the acid in yogurt will "cook" the protein in the meat and make it tough.)

Heat outdoor grill or preheat broiler. Skewer meat onto 12-inch metal or bamboo skewers. (If using bamboo skewers, soak them in water for at least 15 minutes so they are thoroughly saturated.) Alternate meat with vegetables until skewer is nearly full. Grill or broil for 3 minutes on each side. (If using chicken, cook for 2 minutes on each side.) Sprinkle lightly with salt.

NUTRITION SCORE
Per serving (2 kabobs): 550 **calories**
23% **fat** (10 g; 4 g saturated)
21% **carbs** (18 g), 4 g **fiber**
56% **protein** (52 g)

Broiled Flank Steak With Orange-Glazed Carrots and Sweet Potatoes

Serves 4
Prep time: 10 minutes
Cook time: 15 minutes

 2 large sweet potatoes, peeled and cubed

24 baby carrots

 1 11-ounce can mandarin oranges in light syrup, undrained

 2 tablespoons water

 1 tablespoon reduced-sodium soy sauce

 1 cup quinoa

    Cooking spray

 1 pound flank steak, trimmed of fat

    Salt and ground black pepper

 2 teaspoons Worcestershire sauce

 2 garlic cloves, minced

 4 cups broccoli florets

 2 teaspoons water

Blanch sweet potatoes in boiling water for 8 minutes, until fork-tender. Drain and return potatoes to pan. Add carrots, oranges (with liquid), water and soy sauce. Cook over medium heat, uncovered, 5-6 minutes, until carrots are tender and liquid is absorbed.

Meanwhile, cook quinoa according to package directions.

Preheat grill or broiler. Coat a baking sheet with cooking spray. Score flank steak by making a few $1/8$-inch-deep slices, crosswise, on both sides. Rub Worcestershire sauce and garlic on both sides. Broil 5 minutes per side for medium-rare. Transfer to cutting board; let stand 10 minutes.

Place broccoli in a microwave-safe dish, add 2 teaspoons water and cover with plastic. Microwave on high 3-5 minutes, until broccoli is crisp-tender.

Cut steak diagonally, across the grain, into thin slices. Serve with sweet-potato mixture, broccoli and quinoa.

NUTRITION SCORE
Per serving (3 ounces steak, 1 cup sweet-potato mixture, $1/2$ cup broccoli, $1/2$ cup quinoa): 490 **calories**
21% **fat** (11 g; 4 g saturated)
50% **carbs** (61 g) 8 g **fiber**
29% **protein** (36 g)

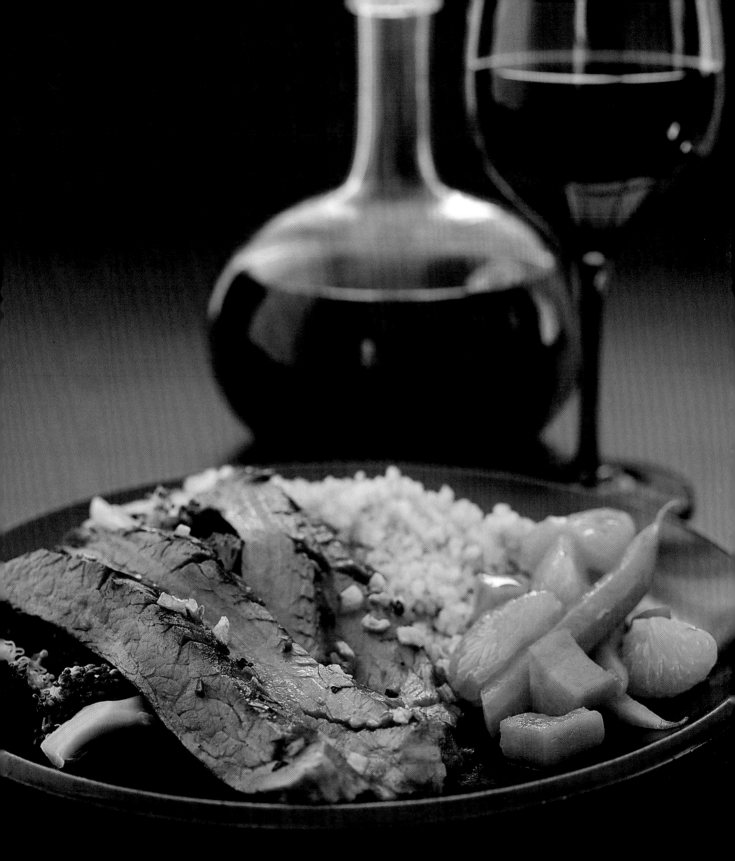

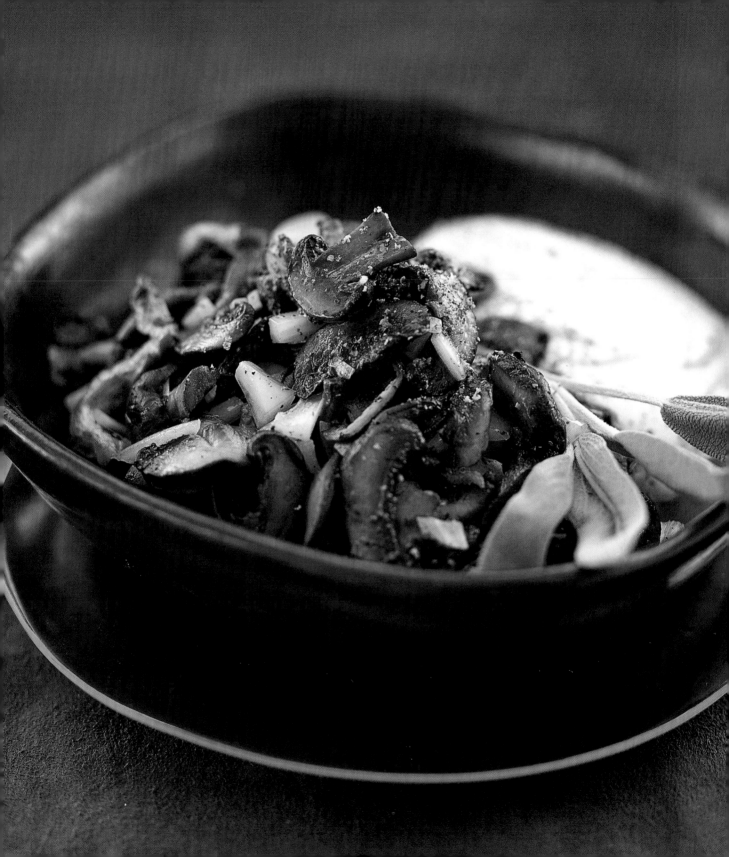

sides

Side dishes usually take a back seat to their main course cousins. But these innovative sides are tasty enough to be the main attraction, something vegetarians will appreciate. Broccoli Bake, Creamy Wild Mushrooms With Sage, and Black-Bean and Zucchini Pancakes are hearty enough to stand on their own, while Celery-Root-Spiked Mashed Potatoes and Mediterranean-Style Green Beans are the perfect foil for tofu, meat and poultry entrees.

recipes

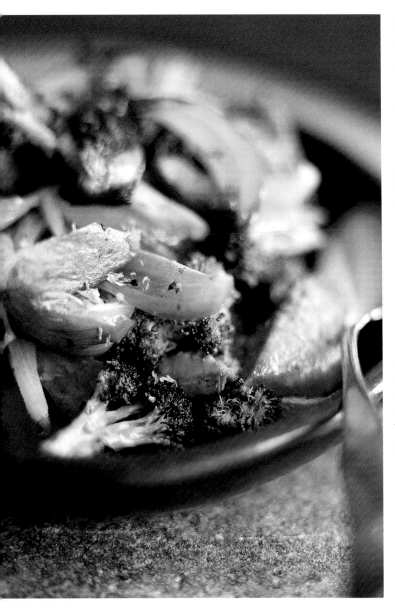

Soft-Roasted Winter Vegetables With Herbs

Serves 4
Prep time: 12 minutes
Cook time: 45 minutes

  4 cups broccoli florets
  2 yams, trimmed and cut into bite-size chunks
  1 red onion, peeled and cut into bite-size pieces
1½ tablespoons olive oil
  1 teaspoon dried Italian herb seasoning
     Salt and freshly ground black pepper to taste

Preheat oven to 375° F. Place vegetables in a roasting pan. Add oil, herbs, salt and pepper, and toss well to mix. Shake roasting pan to scatter vegetables evenly. Roast, turning vegetables with a spatula occasionally, for 45 minutes, or until soft and browned.

NUTRITION SCORE
Per serving (1 cup): 140 **calories**
35% **fat** (6 g; 0.7 g saturated)
54% **carbs** (21 g), 5 g **fiber**
11% **protein** (4 g)

The isothiocynanates in cruciferous vegetables like broccoli stimulate the liver to break down pesticides and other carcinogens.

Broccoli Bake

Serves 6
Prep time: 10 minutes
Cook time: 40-45 minutes

2 10-ounce packages frozen broccoli spears, thawed and drained
1 10.75-ounce can reduced-fat condensed cream of mushroom soup
½ up low-fat mayonnaise
¼ cup evaporated skim milk
¼ cup shredded reduced-fat sharp Cheddar cheese
2 egg whites, slightly beaten
¼ cup bread crumbs
1 tablespoon light butter
Cooking spray

Preheat oven to 350º F. Coat a 10-by-10-inch pan with cooking spray. Lay broccoli evenly in pan.

In a medium bowl, combine soup, mayonnaise, evaporated milk, cheese and egg whites until well mixed. Pour over broccoli.

Using a fork, combine bread crumbs with melted light butter in a small bowl until thoroughly mixed. Sprinkle over soup and broccoli mixture. Bake 40-45 minutes or until golden.

NUTRITION SCORE
Per serving (⅙ of recipe): 144 **calories**
30% **fat** (4.7 g; 2.5 g saturated)
50 % **carbs** (18 g), 2 g **fiber**
20% **protein** (7 g)

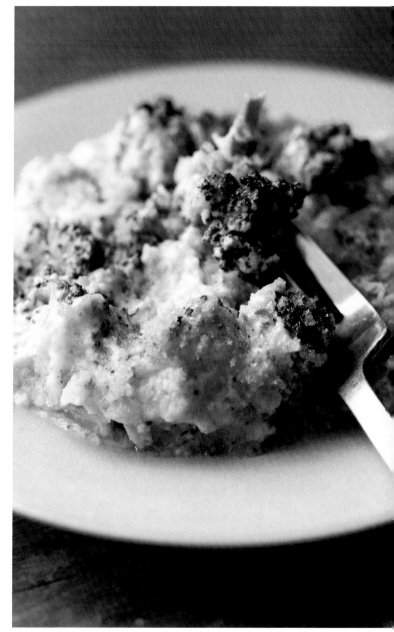

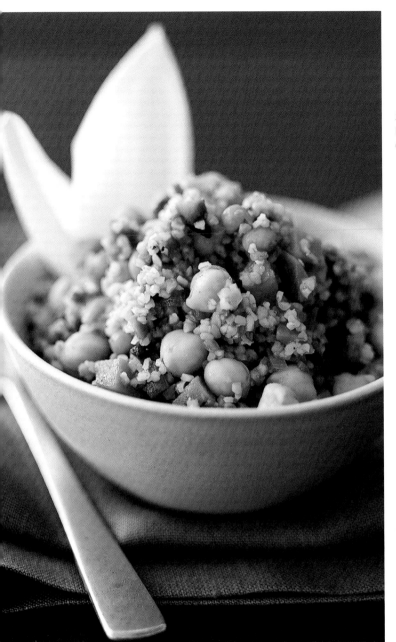

Bulgur-Portobello Pilaf

Serves 4 (with leftovers)
Prep time: 20 minutes
Cook/stand time: 20 minutes

  1 tablespoon virgin olive oil
  ½ large yellow onion, finely diced
  Pinch kosher salt
  ½ teaspoon ground cumin
  ½ teaspoon curry powder
  2 medium portobello mushrooms (about 3 ounces), finely diced
1¼ cups fat-free, low-sodium chicken broth
  2 tablespoons tomato paste
  1 cup coarse bulgur
  1 15-ounce can chickpeas, drained and rinsed
  ½ cup frozen peas and carrots

Heat oil in a 3-quart saucepan on medium-high heat. Add onion; stir to coat. Cook 5 minutes. Add spices and mushrooms; reduce heat to medium. (If mixture gets dry, add 1 tablespoon broth.) Cover and cook 5 minutes more.

Raise heat to high, add broth and tomato paste; stir until paste dissolves and mixture boils. Stir in remaining ingredients. Turn off heat, cover; let stand 15 minutes, until liquid is absorbed.

NUTRITION SCORE
Per serving (1 ½ cups): 229 **calories**
16% **fat** (4 g; 0.5 g saturated)
69% **carbs** (39.5 g), 10 g **fiber**
15% **protein** (8.5 g)

Fried Rice With Carrots, Tomato and Pine Nuts

Serves 4
Prep time: 10 minutes
Cook time: 10 minutes

- 2 teaspoons dark sesame oil
- 4 green onions, minced and divided in half
- 4 cloves garlic, minced and divided in half
- 1 16-ounce container firm light tofu, drained and cut into 1-inch pieces
- 1 cup uncooked instant brown rice
- 1 cup diced carrots
- 1 medium tomato, diced
- 2 tablespoons reduced-sodium soy sauce
- 2¼ cups reduced-sodium chicken broth or water
- 2 teaspoons olive oil
- 2 tablespoons pine nuts
- 6 cups chopped fresh kale leaves (substitute chopped fresh or frozen spinach, if desired)
- Salt and ground black pepper to taste

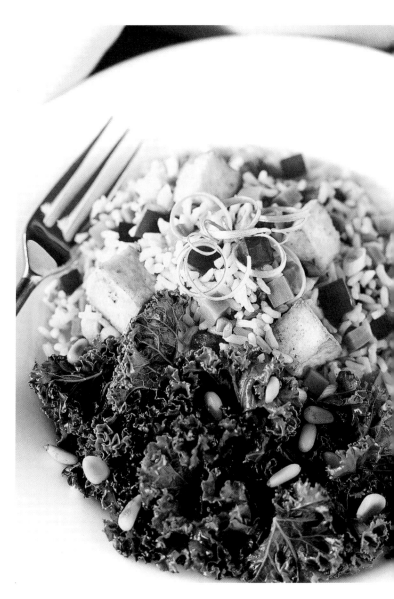

Heat sesame oil in a medium saucepan over medium-high heat. Add half of the green onions, half of the garlic and all of the tofu and sauté 3-5 minutes, until tofu is golden on all sides. Add rice, carrots, tomato and soy sauce and stir to coat.

Add chicken broth and bring mixture to a boil. Reduce heat to low, cover and simmer 5 minutes, until liquid is absorbed. Remove from heat and stir in remaining green onions.

Meanwhile, heat olive oil in a large skillet over medium-high heat. Add pine nuts and remaining garlic and cook 1 minute. Add kale (don't worry about there not being enough room in the pan; the kale will wilt quickly) and cook 1 minute, until leaves wilt, stirring frequently. Remove from heat; season with salt and black pepper.

Serve fried rice with kale on the side.

NUTRITION SCORE
Per serving (1¼ cups fried rice, ½ cup kale mixture):
330 **calories**
26% **fat** (10 g; 1 g saturated)
57% **carbs** (47 g), 5 g **fiber**
17% **protein** (14 g)

Barley Medley

Serves 4
Prep time: 10 minutes
Cook time: 45 minutes

    1 cup pearl barley
    5 cups fat-free vegetable or chicken broth, or water
    2 tablespoons fresh lemon juice or more to taste
    2 teaspoons olive oil
    2 teaspoons dried oregano
    1 cup vine-ripened tomatoes, diced
    1 cup cucumber, diced with skin on
    1 medium carrot, diced
    1 medium onion, minced
    ½ cup fresh parsley leaves, chopped
       Salt and ground black pepper to taste

Combine barley and broth in a large saucepan. Set pan over high heat and bring to a boil. Reduce heat to low, cover and cook 45 minutes, until barley is tender.

Drain any excess water and transfer barley to a large bowl. Add lemon juice, olive oil and oregano and toss to combine. Add vegetables and parsley; toss again. Season with salt and pepper. Serve warm or chilled.

NUTRITION SCORE
Per serving (1½ cups): 248 **calories**
11% **fat** (3 g; ‹1 g saturated)
75% **carbs** (46.5 g), 10 g **fiber**
14% **protein** (8.6 g)

Your diet should include five to seven servings of grains daily, with most of these coming from whole grains. You can easily achieve this by adding barley to soups, salads, risotto or any dish in which you normally use converted rice.

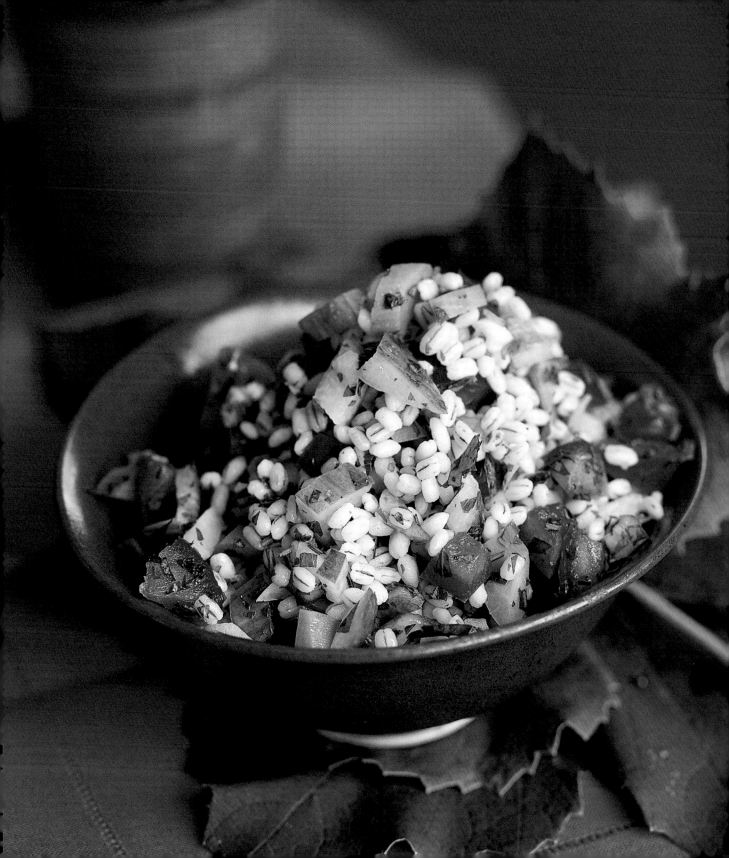

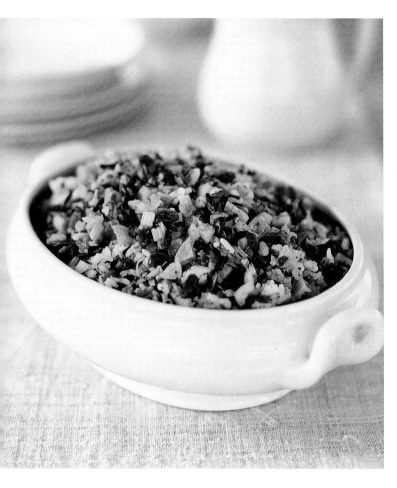

Rice Stuffing With Apples, Rosemary and Bacon

Serves 10
Prep time: 25 minutes
Cook time: 1 hour

　1　cup wild rice
2⅔　cups fat-free, salt-free chicken broth
3⅜　cups plus 1 tablespoon water
　⅓　cup country (thick-cut) bacon, finely diced
　3　cups onion, finely diced
　3　cups celery, finely diced
　¼　cup plus 2 tablespoons chopped mixed herbs
　　 (such as rosemary, sage, thyme, oregano and
　　 Italian parsley)
　　 Coarse-grained salt to taste
　1　cup white rice
1¾　cup currants
　½　cup dried apricots, diced
　¾　cup dried cherries, chopped
　¾　cup dried cranberries, chopped
　3　cups apples, diced with peel on
　½　cup chopped Italian parsley

NUTRITION SCORE
Per serving (½ cup): 342 **calories**
5% **fat** (1.9 g; 0.5 g saturated)
84% **carbs** (75.6 g), 6.8 g **fiber**
11% **protein** (9.4 g)

In a 4-quart microwaveable bowl, cook wild rice, broth and 1½ cups water 30 minutes in microwave on high; stir. Cook 15 minutes more on medium-low.

Meanwhile, in a 10-inch nonstick skillet, fry bacon over medium-high heat until crispy, 3–5 minutes. Drain on paper towels. Cook onion, celery in bacon drippings and 1 tablespoon water, covered over medium heat for 20 minutes. Turn off heat. Stir in bacon, mixed herbs and salt. Set aside.

When wild rice has cooked 45 minutes, add white rice, remaining water and fruit. Microwave on high 10 minutes; stir. Cook on medium-low for 15 minutes more. If making in advance, cool and refrigerate in a tightly covered container. Reheat 2–3 minutes on medium-high; add parsley and more salt.

White Beans With Garlic and Basil

Serves 4
Prep time: 20 minutes
Cook time: 30 minutes

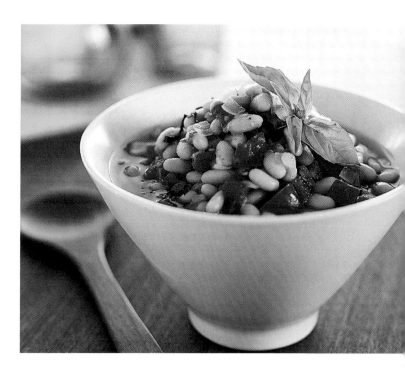

     1 tablespoon olive oil
1 ½ yellow onions, chopped
4-8 garlic cloves, peeled and minced to taste
  12 ounces canned chopped tomatoes, drained
     Salt to taste
  24 ounces canned cooked cannelloni beans, rinsed
     and drained
     2 cups fat-free chicken broth
     1 large handful fresh basil (about 10 leaves)
     Juice from 1 lemon (¼ cup)
     Freshly ground pepper to taste

Heat oil in a large, heavy soup pot. Sauté onion and garlic over low to medium heat until soft, about 10-15 minutes. Add tomatoes and salt, and simmer about 10 minutes; add the beans and broth. Simmer 5-10 minutes more. Just before serving, add basil, lemon juice and pepper, and stir well to combine. Enjoy immediately, or let flavors blend at room temperature overnight.

To ensure a balanced meal, pretend your dinner plate is divided into four quarters. Each quarter should be filled with one of these: grains, vegetables, legumes and/or fruits and meat or protein. This way you'll get a mix of nutrients, controlled portion sizes and decreased fat and calories.

NUTRITION SCORE
Per serving (1 heaping cup): 270 **calories**
13% **fat** (4 g; ‹1 g saturated)
64% **carbs** (43 g),11 g **fiber**
23% **protein** (16 g)

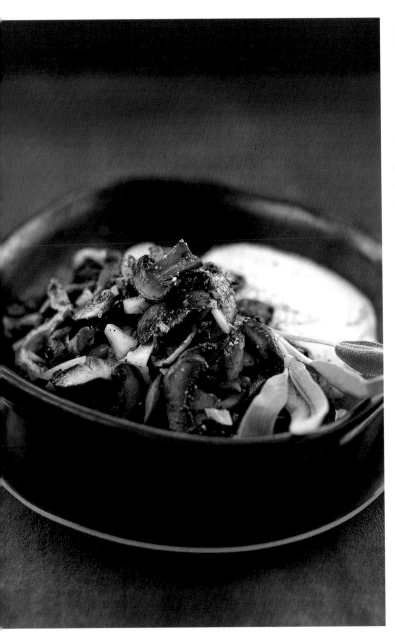

Creamy Wild Mushrooms With Sage

Serves 6
Prep time: 5 minutes
Cook time: 13 minutes

1¼	pounds wild mushrooms, such as portobello caps and oyster mushrooms, sliced
1	teaspoon olive oil
1	small onion, peeled and chopped (about 1 cup)
½	teaspoon ground sage
¼	cup reduced-fat sour cream
⅛	teaspoon grated nutmeg
	Salt and freshly ground black pepper to taste

Trim mushrooms (such as cutting stems off oyster mushrooms) as necessary.

Place oil in a large nonstick skillet over high heat. Add onion, sage and mushrooms; sauté for about 13 minutes. Stir in sour cream and nutmeg. Season with salt and pepper.

NUTRITION SCORE
Per serving (½ cup): 50 **calories**
36% **fat** (2 g; 0.8 g saturated)
42% **carbs** (6 g), 1 g **fiber**
22% **protein** (3 g)

When shopping for mushrooms, look at the gills on the underside of the mushroom cap. The tighter they are, the fresher they are. Open and very dark gills betray old produce.

Celery-Root-Spiked Mashed Potatoes

Serves 4
Prep time: 10 minutes
Cook time: 20 minutes

2 large baking potatoes, peeled and cut into
 2-inch pieces
1 cup celery root, peeled and diced
2 cloves garlic, peeled
⅓ cup nonfat sour cream
1 tablespoon butter
Salt and ground black pepper to taste

Combine potatoes, celery root and garlic in a large saucepan and
add enough water to cover. Place pan over high heat and bring to
a boil. Reduce heat to medium and simmer 20 minutes, until potatoes and celery root are fork-tender. Drain and return to pan.

Add sour cream and butter and beat or mash until smooth (or
until desired consistency). Season with salt and black pepper.

NUTRITION SCORE
Per serving (½ cup): 175 **calories**
16% **fat** (3 g; 2 g saturated)
74% **carbs** (32 g), 3 g **fiber**
10% **protein** (4 g)

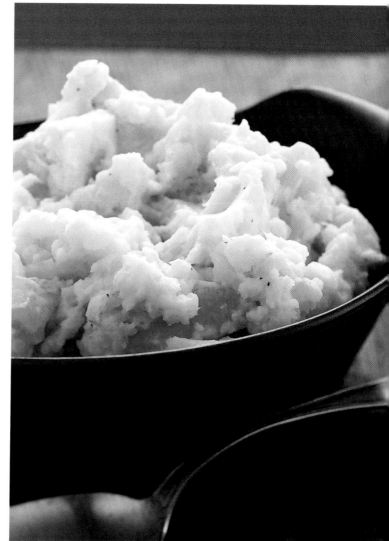

*Celery root, also known as celeriac or celery knob, is a
close relative of regular celery. It's grown for its root,
whose gnarly brown skin covers a soft, white flesh with a
superior texture (no strings) and the sweet flavor of celery. You can eat it raw (in salads or dunked in dips) or toss
it into stir-fries.*

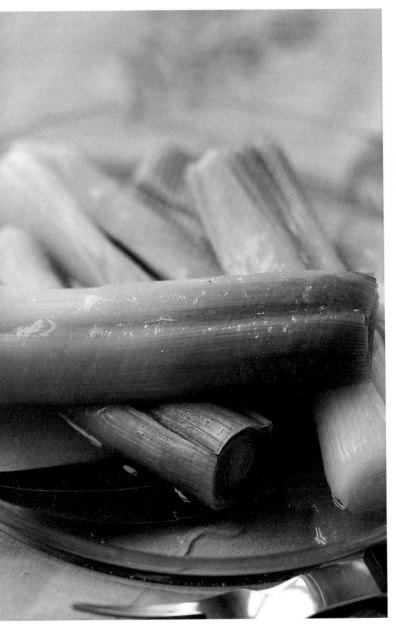

Braised Leeks in Orange-Fennel Dressing

Serves 6
Prep time: 15 minutes
Cook time: 28 minutes
Chill time: 4 hours

- 6 leeks (about 3 pounds), trimmed of all but 2 inches of greens
- 1 teaspoon salt, divided
- ½ lemon, cut in 2 pieces
- 2 bay leaves
- 2 cups orange juice
- 1 small vine-ripe tomato (5 ounces), seeded and halved crosswise
- ¼ teaspoon crushed fennel seeds
- ⅛ teaspoon fresh ground black pepper
- ½ tablespoon olive oil

Cut leeks in half lengthwise to within 1½ inches of root end. Rinse under running water, being careful to rinse out all sand between layers of leaves.

Combine leeks, ¾ teaspoon salt, lemon and bay leaves in large skillet or Dutch oven. Add water to cover and bring to boil. Reduce heat, cover and simmer for 15-20 minutes, or until tender; turn leeks halfway through cooking. Drain and place in serving bowl just large enough to hold them (11 inches by 7 inches).

Meanwhile, combine orange juice, tomato halves, fennel, pepper and remaining salt in same skillet. Boil 8 minutes or until reduced to 1 cup, pressing down on tomatoes to flatten. Discard tomato skins. In a blender, process mixture and oil until smooth. Pour over leeks so that they are almost submerged in juice. (Note: If leeks are not submerged, place all in food storage bag, push out air and seal bag.)

Cool to room temperature and refrigerate at least 4 hours. Let stand at room temperature for 1 hour before serving.

NUTRITION SCORE
Per serving (1 cup): 221 **calories**
24% **fat** (5.8 g; 0.8 g saturated)
70% **carbs** (41.5 g), 3.9 g **fiber**
6% **protein** (3.4 g)

Carmelized Sweet Potatoes and Pearl Onions

Serves 8
Prep time: 10 minutes
Cook time: 1 hour

- 6 medium sweet potatoes (about 2½ pounds), peeled, halved lengthwise and cut into ½-inch-thick slices
- 1 16-ounce package frozen small, whole onions, thawed
- 3 tablespoons light brown sugar
- 2 tablespoons maple syrup
- 1 tablespoon butter or margarine, melted
- ½ teaspoon salt

Preheat oven to 375° F. In a large bowl, combine sweet potatoes and onions; set aside. Whisk together sugar, maple syrup, butter and salt until well blended. Pour mixture over sweet potatoes and onions and stir to coat. Transfer mixture to an 11-by-7-inch baking dish. Place in oven and roast for 1 hour, stirring every 15 minutes, to ensure even browning.

NUTRITION SCORE
Per serving (1 cup): 234 **calories**
8% **fat** (1 g)
87% **carbs** (43.2 g), 3.2 g **fiber**
5% **protein** (4 g)

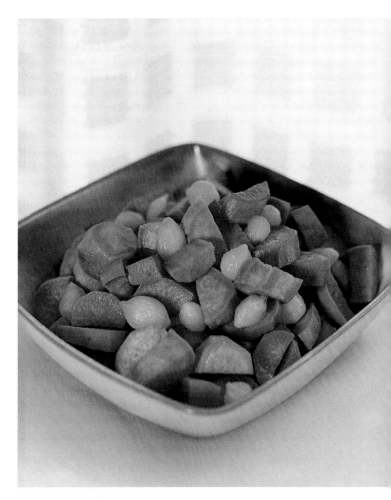

Black-Bean and Zucchini Pancakes

Serves 4
Prep time: 7 minutes
Cook time: 8 minutes

15	ounces canned black beans, rinsed and drained
2	egg whites
1	teaspoon chopped roasted garlic (jarred)
1	teaspoon ground cumin
1	zucchini, shredded (1⅓ cups)
⅓	cup plain dried whole-grain bread crumbs
2	teaspoons olive oil, divided
½	cup chipotle (or your favorite salsa)
2½	tablespoons reduced-fat sour cream

In a medium bowl, mash beans, egg whites, garlic and cumin to a coarse texture (there should be a mixture of mashed and nearly whole beans). Stir in zucchini and bread crumbs.

Heat large nonstick skillet over medium-high heat. Add 1 teaspoon of oil. Using ½ of the bean mixture, drop 4 mounds into pan and flatten to about 3½-inch rounds. Cook for 4 minutes, turning halfway during cooking; repeat with remaining mixture. Serve with salsa and sour cream.

NUTRITION SCORE
Per serving (2 4-inch pancakes, 2 teaspoons light sour cream, 2 tablespoons salsa): 140 **calories**
24% **fat** (4 g; 1 g saturated)
51% **carbs** (22 g), 7 g **fiber**
25% **protein** (9 g)

You'll get protein, fiber and folate in the beans; vitamins A and C in the salsa; and potassium in both the zucchini and beans.

Practically Fat-Free Onion Rings

Serves 4
Prep time: 25 minutes
Cook time: 15 minutes

- 3 large onions, sliced ¼ inch thick
- 1 cup buttermilk
- ½ cup all-purpose flour
- 1 teaspoon paprika
- ½ teaspoon salt
- 4 egg whites, beaten
- 1½ cups corn flake crumbs
- Cooking spray

Cut onions into rings. Mix with buttermilk in a large bowl until coated. Set coated onions aside 20 minutes.

Preheat oven to 375° F. Spray a baking sheet with cooking spray. Combine flour, paprika and salt in a shallow dish. Put egg whites in a second shallow dish and cornflakes in a third. Dip each onion ring in the flour, the egg and the cornflakes. Place on sheet, spritz with cooking spray and bake 15 minutes, until brown.

NUTRITION SCORE
Per serving (3-4 onion rings): 245 **calories**
1% **fat** (0.4 g, 0.1 g saturated)
84% **carbohydrate** (53 g), 2.7 g fiber
15% **protein** (9 g)

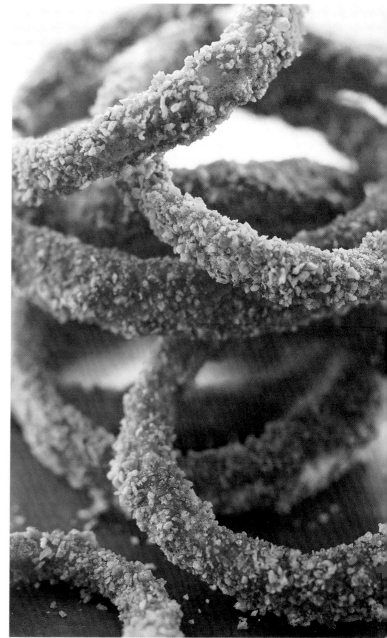

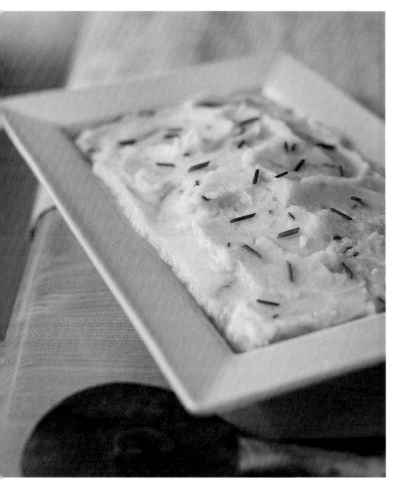

Chunky Squash and Potato Purée With Buttermilk and Chives

Serves 10
Prep time: 20 minutes
Cook time: 25 minutes

2 pounds butternut squash (one medium), cut in half lengthwise, seeds removed
1 teaspoon olive oil
Coarse-grained salt to taste
Cracked black pepper to taste
4-6 cloves garlic, peeled and cut in half lengthwise
2 sprigs thyme
2 pounds Yukon Gold or russet potatoes, peeled and cut into 1½- to 2-inch chunks
1-1½ cups nonfat buttermilk
2 tablespoons chives, minced

NUTRITION SCORE
Per serving (½ cup): 134 **calories**
5% **fat** (0.8 g; 0.3 g saturated)
82% **carbs** (29 g), 3.1 g **fiber**
13% **protein** (4.4 g)

Preheat oven to 375° F. Brush squash's cut surfaces with olive oil. Season with salt and black pepper. Place half the garlic and 1 sprig of thyme on a cookie sheet and cover with a squash half, cut side down. Do the same with the other squash half. Bake until completely soft and tender, about 25-35 minutes.

Meanwhile, in a large stockpot, place potatoes and cover with cold, salted water. Bring water to a boil; then reduce to a simmer and cook until a fork goes through potatoes easily, approximately 25-30 minutes. (Don't overcook or potatoes will become waterlogged.)

Place drained potatoes in a large bowl. Before adding squash, wait until it's cool enough to handle; then scrape squash meat from skin into bowl, using a large spoon. Discard the thyme. Add the other half of garlic to bowl and pour in buttermilk. Purée with a potato masher until desired consistency is reached. Add more buttermilk if necessary. Season again with salt and black pepper. Stir in chives just before serving.

Mediterranean-Style Green Beans

Serves 10
Prep time: 15 minutes
Cook time: 5-8 minutes

- 8 cups water
- 1 teaspoon salt
- 2 pounds green beans, washed, ends removed
- 2 tablespoons extra-virgin olive oil
- Coarse-grained salt to taste
- Cracked black pepper to taste
- 3-4 tablespoons fresh lemon juice (to taste)

Pour water into a large pot. Stir in salt. Bring to a boil. Add green beans and cook to desired degree of tenderness. Strain; then return green beans to the pot. Drizzle beans with olive oil and stir to coat. Season with coarse-grained salt and cracked black pepper and gradually add lemon juice, stirring once more.

NUTRITION SCORE
Per serving (1 cup): 63 **calories**
47% **fat** (3.3 g; 0.5 g saturated)
41% **carbs** (8.4 g), 3.2 g **fiber**
12% **protein** (1.9 g)

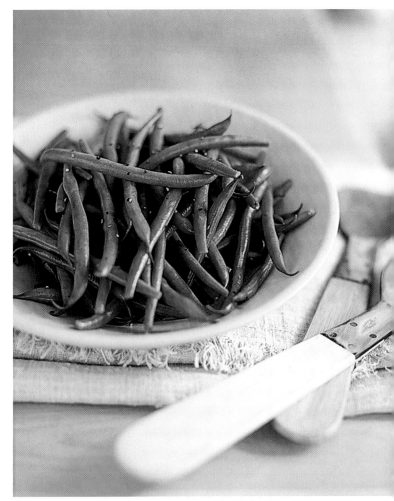

This simple treatment works with a variety of vegetables, including zucchini, brussels sprouts, broccoli and baby potatoes. Just cook to desired tenderness; then dress with oil and lemon.

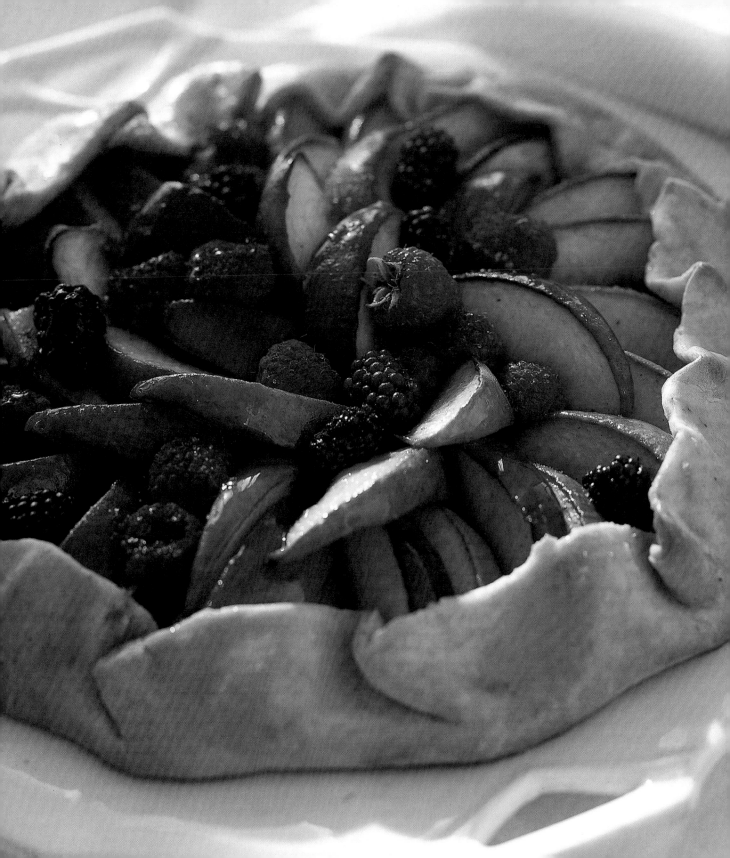

desserts

Yes, there is room for dessert in a healthy diet. Try something familiar yet spectacular such as Hot Mexican Volcanoes and Chocolate-Cherry Pie to Die For. The key is moderation, and a light hand with rich ingredients. For a truly effortless end to your meal, try a simple but stunning fruit-based dessert like Ruby Surprise or Mango Fool.

recipes

The Any Kind of Fresh-Fruit Sorbet

Makes 1 quart, about 7 servings
Prep time: 10 minutes
Chill time: 8-10 hours

Note: This is a standard sorbet recipe – good for all types of fruit.
It's delicious and a great way to use up your overripe fruit.

  4 cups ripe fresh fruit, peeled, pitted (if necessary)
      and coarsely chopped (try mangoes, kiwis,
      pears, strawberries, peaches, papaya, plums or
      cantaloupe)
  1 tablespoon fresh lemon or lime juice
½-¾ cup Sugar Syrup (recipe follows), depending on
      the sweetness of fruit

Place fruit and lemon or lime juice in a food processor fitted with the metal blade and process until smooth.

Pour in the Sugar Syrup gradually; process to blend evenly. Taste for sweetness. If sorbet needs more syrup, pour in a bit more and process again. Repeat if necessary.

Transfer to a medium-sized metal bowl or cake pan. Cover with plastic wrap and place in the freezer. Allow to partially freeze, about 4 hours; ice will form around the edge, but the center will be mushy. If the mixture freezes solid, let it partially thaw at room temperature before proceeding.

Return the mixture to the food processor and reprocess until completely blended, smooth and fluffy, about 1 minute. Immediately scrape the mixture into a plastic freezer container with an airtight lid and refreeze 4-10 hours. Let soften at room temperature slightly before serving, about 15 minutes.

NUTRITION SCORE
The following figures are an average, using fruits listed above.
Per serving (½ cup): 150 **calories**
3% **fat** (0.4 g; 0.03 g saturated)
94% **carbs** (27 g), 2 g **fiber**
3% **protein** (0.8 g)

 Sorbets are traditionally made with ice cream machines, but using a food processor (or blender) and freezing the sorbet in airtight plastic storage containers produces just as fine results – without the fuss.

Sugar Syrup

Makes 1 cup
Prep time: 2 minutes
Cook time: 8 minutes
Chill time: 1 hour

  ⅔ cup granulated sugar
  ½ cup water

In a heavy-bottomed saucepan, combine the sugar and water. Bring to a boil over high heat. As soon as the mixture comes to a rolling boil, remove the pan from the heat. Cool completely before using or store in the refrigerator in a glass jar. Makes enough for 1 batch of sorbet. (Recipe can be doubled or tripled.)

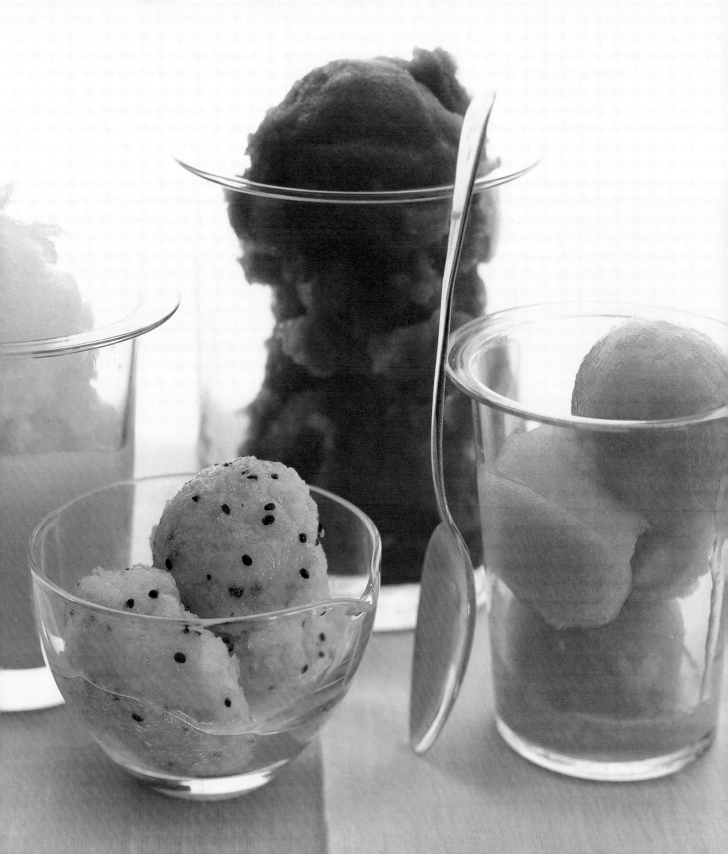

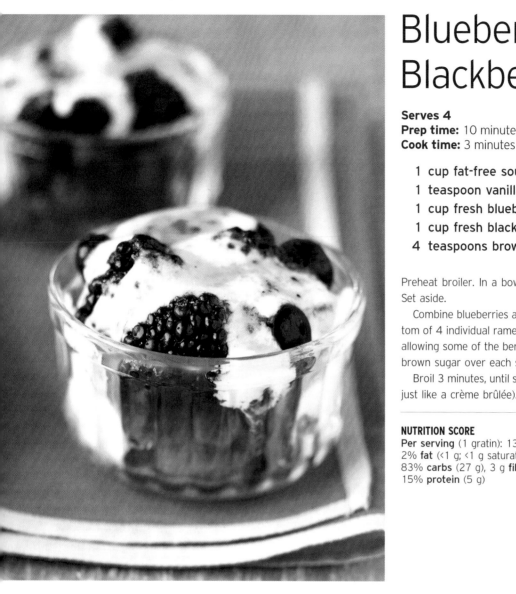

Blueberry and Blackberry Gratin

Serves 4
Prep time: 10 minutes
Cook time: 3 minutes

- 1 cup fat-free sour cream
- 1 teaspoon vanilla extract
- 1 cup fresh blueberries
- 1 cup fresh blackberries
- 4 teaspoons brown sugar

Preheat broiler. In a bowl, whisk together sour cream and vanilla. Set aside.

Combine blueberries and blackberries and place them in the bottom of 4 individual ramekins. Top berries with sour-cream mixture, allowing some of the berries to show through. Sprinkle 1 teaspoon brown sugar over each serving, breaking up any lumps.

Broil 3 minutes, until sugar melts (the top should be caramelized, just like a crème brûlée).

NUTRITION SCORE
Per serving (1 gratin): 130 **calories**
2% **fat** (<1 g; <1 g saturated)
83% **carbs** (27 g), 3 g **fiber**
15% **protein** (5 g)

The use of low- and nonfat dairy products in place of full-fat versions is virtually undetectable in most multiple-ingredient dessert recipes.

Mango Fool

Serves 4
Prep time: 10 minutes
Chill time: 30 minutes

- 2 cups cubed mango (about 3 mangoes)
- 2 tablespoons fresh lime juice
- 1 tablespoon orange juice
- 1¼ cups frozen light nondairy whipped topping (such as Cool Whip), slightly thawed

Purée mango, lime juice and orange juice in a blender or food processor until smooth. Cover and chill 30 minutes (and up to 24 hours).

Transfer the mango mixture to a large bowl and carefully fold in the whipped topping (you can blend thoroughly or leave orange streaks). Spoon Mango Fool into tall glasses and serve.

NUTRITION SCORE
Per serving (1 cup): 155 **calories**
17% **fat** (3 g; 2 g saturated)
81% **carbs** (31 g), 3 g **fiber**
2% **protein** (<1 g)

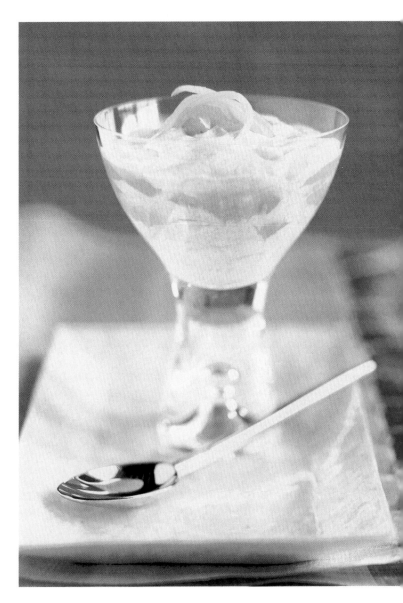

To make your own low-calorie whipped topping, whip evaporated skim milk with a calorie-free sweetener and a dash of vanilla extract.

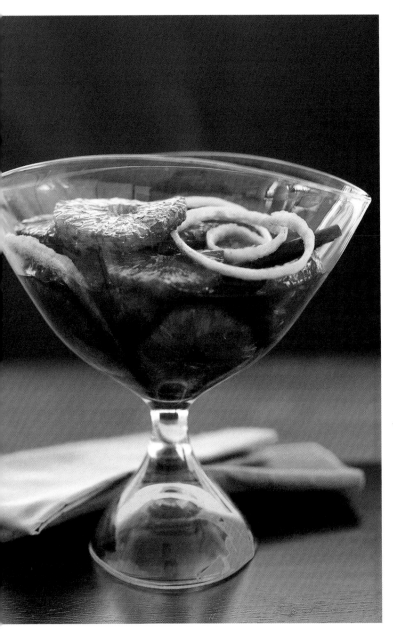

Zinfandel-Mulled Orange Slices

Serves 6
Prep/cook time: 12 minutes
Chill time: 2 hours

1½ cups red Zinfandel wine
¾ cup granulated sugar
½ cup water
4 whole cloves
1 cinnamon stick
Zest of 1 lemon, peeled in a continuous spiral
6 large navel oranges

Bring all ingredients except oranges to a boil in a medium saucepan. Reduce heat to medium-low and simmer for 12 minutes.

Meanwhile, peel oranges and remove white pith. Using a sharp knife, slice oranges into thin rounds, and place in a large bowl. Pour Zinfandel mixture through a strainer over oranges. Refrigerate until cold (about 2 hours).

NUTRITION SCORE
Per serving (1 cup): 231 **calories**
1% **fat** (0.3 g; 0 g saturated)
96% **carbs** (49 g), 5 g **fiber**
3% **protein** (2 g)

Ruby Surprise

Serves 6
Prep time: 8 minutes

- 2 pints fresh raspberries (about 3 cups)
- 3 cups red grapes, rinsed
- 6 tablespoons minced candied ginger
- 6 tablespoons grenadine

For each dessert, arrange ½ cup raspberries and ½ cup grapes in a bowl or glass. Sprinkle 1 tablespoon minced candied ginger over fruit, and then drizzle with 1 tablespoon of grenadine.

NUTRITION SCORE
Per serving (1 cup of fruit, 1 tablespoon of ginger and 1 tablespoon of grenadine): 155 **calories**
5% **fat** (0.8 g; 0.1 g saturated)
92% **carbs** (36 g), 5 g **fiber**
3% **protein** (1 g)

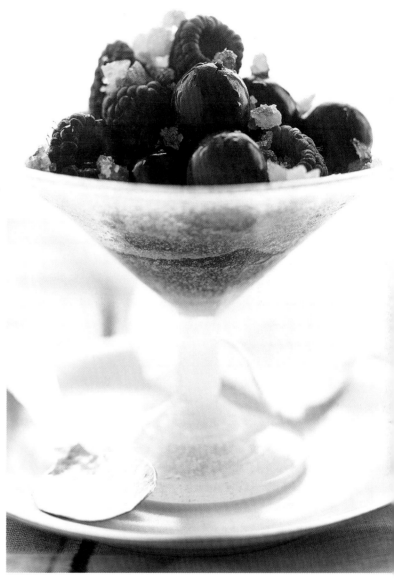

Replace your late-evening trip to the fridge with a relaxation ritual. Light a lavendar-scented candle, slip into a soothing bubble bath or sink into a cushy chair with an inspirational book.

Chocolate Pound Cake With Roasted Strawberries and Yogurt Cream

Serves 6
Prep time: 3 minutes
Cook time: 12 minutes

- 1 tablespoon lightly salted butter
- 24 medium-large strawberries, hulled
- 3 tablespoons granulated sugar
- 6 1-inch-thick slices fat-free chocolate pound cake (such as Entenmann's)
- 2 cups nonfat whipped topping
- ½ cup plain nonfat yogurt

Preheat oven to 450° F. Melt butter in a large oven-safe skillet over high heat. Add strawberries and gently shake skillet to coat berries with butter. Sprinkle sugar over berries and shake skillet again to coat them with sugar. Place skillet in oven, uncovered, and roast for 10 minutes.

While berries cook, lightly toast pound cake until edges are crunchy. Place cake slices on 6 dessert plates. Whisk together nonfat topping and yogurt. Remove berries from oven and spoon 4 berries and some juice over each slice of pound cake. Serve yogurt cream on side.

Roasting fruit with a little sugar intensifies its flavor without adding too many calories. For a variation on this dessert, try using plums, peaches, nectarines or apricots.

NUTRITION SCORE
Per serving (1 slice cake, 4 berries and juice, and about ¼ cup yogurt cream): 197 **calories**
9% **fat** (2 g; 1 g saturated)
84% **carbs** (41.5 g), 2 g **fiber**
7% **protein** (3.6 g)

Raspberry-Peach Galette

Serves 8
Prep time: 20-25 minutes
Cook time: 55-60 minutes

Crust

- 1½ cups all-purpose flour
- 1 tablespoon granulated sugar
- ¼ teaspoon salt
- 3 tablespoons butter or margarine, chilled and cut up
- 5 tablespoons cold water

Raspberry-Peach Filling

- 4 medium ripe peaches, halved, pitted and sliced ⅛ inch thick
- 3 tablespoons granulated sugar
- ¼ teaspoon ground nutmeg
- ½ cup fresh or frozen raspberries, thawed
- 1 egg, lightly beaten

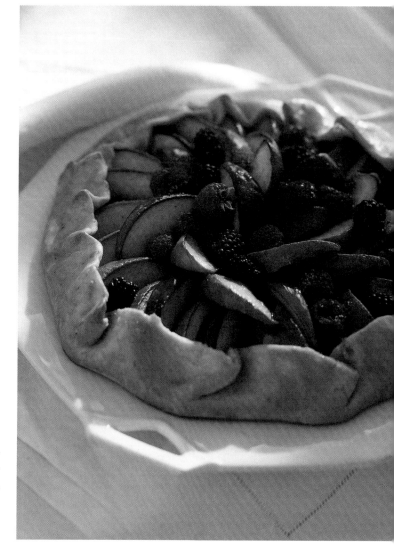

Preheat oven to 425° F. To make crust, in a large bowl or food processor with a metal blade, combine flour, sugar and salt. Add butter or margarine; process or mix with your fingers until mixture resembles coarse meal. Add water, a tablespoon at a time; mix just until dough forms a ball.

Transfer to a large sheet of parchment paper and roll into a 12-inch circle. Transfer (on paper) to a baking sheet and set aside.

To make the filling, in a large bowl, combine peaches, sugar and nutmeg; toss to coat. Arrange peach slices atop dough in slightly overlapping concentric rings, leaving a 2-inch border around the edge. Arrange raspberries on top of peaches. Fold border back over peach mixture and brush the dough with beaten egg.

Bake 15 minutes. Reset oven to 350° F; then bake 40-45 more minutes, until pastry is golden brown. Serve warm.

To remove the pit, cut around the peach on the "seam line," twist the halves in opposite directions and gently pull them apart. (If the pit doesn't come out, make several slices down to the pit, and pull individual slices away until the whole peach is sliced.)

NUTRITION SCORE
Per serving (⅛ of galette): 168 **calories**
29% **fat** (5.4 g; 3 g saturated)
63% **carbs** (26.5 g), 2 g **fiber**
8% **protein** (3.5 g)

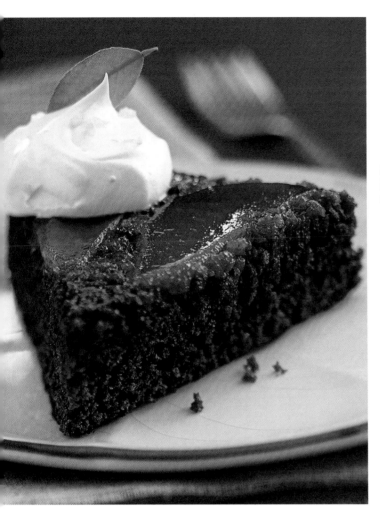

Gingerbread With Pears and Whipped Lemon Topping

Serves 8
Prep time: 35 minutes
Cook time: 40-45 minutes

Cooking spray
½ cup granulated sugar
3 ripe pears, peeled, cored, and sliced lengthwise
1 lemon, juice and zest
4 tablespoons lightly salted butter, softened
½ cup dark brown sugar, packed
1 large egg
½ cup nonfat buttermilk
¼ cup dark molasses
1 cup flour
1½ teaspoons ground ginger
1 teaspoon baking soda
1 teaspoon pumpkin pie spice
¼ teaspoon coarse salt
2 cups nonfat whipped topping

Preheat oven to 350° F. Coat bottom and sides of a 10-inch cake pan with nonstick cooking spray. Sprinkle sugar over bottom of cake pan. Place pears in a medium bowl. Grate zest from the entire lemon. Add ½ teaspoon of zest to pears, along with 1 tablespoon lemon juice; save remaining zest for whipped topping. Arrange pears in pinwheel pattern around bottom of cake pan.

Blend together butter and dark brown sugar in a medium bowl until well mixed. Beat in egg, then nonfat buttermilk and molasses.

Whisk together flour, ginger, baking soda, pumpkin pie spice and salt in a small bowl. Add to buttermilk mixture and stir until blended. Pour batter over pears and gently smooth top with a knife. Bake for 40-45 minutes, or until gingerbread springs back when gently pressed. Let cool on a rack.

To serve, carefully run a sharp knife around the inside edge of cake pan and invert cake onto a serving platter. Cut into 8 wedges.

Gently stir remaining lemon zest into the nonfat whipped topping. Serve each gingerbread wedge with a dollop of whipped lemon topping.

NUTRITION SCORE
Per serving (1 wedge, ¼ cup whipped lemon topping):
307 **calories**
21% **fat** (7 g; 4 g saturated)
75% **carbs** (58 g), 2 g **fiber**
4% **protein** (3 g)

Vanilla-Pistachio Panna Cotta

Serves 6
Prep time: 17 minutes
Cook time: 2 ½ minutes
Chill time: 4 hours

2½ teaspoons plain gelatin
¼ cup evaporated skim milk
3 8-ounce containers nonfat vanilla yogurt
1½ teaspoons pure almond extract
2 10-ounce packages frozen raspberries in syrup, thawed (or frozen strawberries)
1 pint fresh raspberries (or fresh, sliced strawberries)
2 tablespoons shelled pistachio nuts, finely chopped

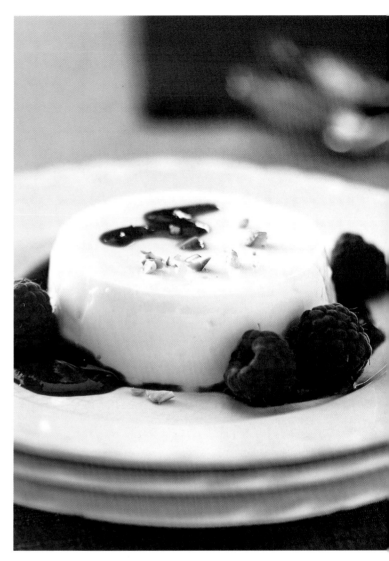

Sprinkle gelatin over evaporated skim milk in a very small saucepan. Set aside.

Whisk together yogurt and almond extract in a small bowl. Place gelatin mixture over very low heat and stir until gelatin just dissolves, about 2½ minutes. Blend into yogurt mixture.

Pour yogurt mixture into 6 ½-cup ramekins that have been rinsed with cold water (to prevent sticking). Seal with plastic wrap and refrigerate for 4 hours, or until set. Place thawed berries and their syrup in a food processor or blender and purée.

To serve, run a sharp knife around inside edge of ramekins and reverse panna cotta onto dessert plates. Spoon some berry purée around each panna cotta. Garnish with fresh berries and a sprinkling of chopped pistachio nuts.

NUTRITION SCORE
Per serving (1 panna cotta, ⅓ cup sauce, 1 teaspoon nuts): 205 calories
9% **fat** (2 g; <1 g saturated)
70% **carbs** (36 g), 9 g **fiber**
21% **protein** (11 g)

Panna cotta (literally, "cooked cream") is a luscious, silky Italian custard. In our eggless version, nonfat vanilla yogurt substitutes for the heavy cream. Also, the chopped green pistachios and red sauce add a colorful seasonal touch. (If fresh raspberries are scarce, you can opt for sliced strawberries instead to make the garnish.)

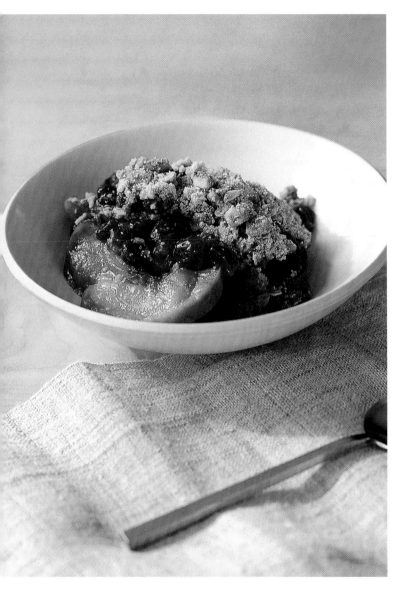

Pear, Apple and Cranberry Crisp

Serves 10
Prep time: 15 minutes
Cook time: 1 hour

Topping

- ½ cup raw walnuts, chopped
- ½ cup old-fashioned oats
- 1 cup plus 2 tablespoons flour
- ½ cup tightly packed light brown sugar
- Dash cinnamon
- 6 tablespoons butter, at room temperature

Filling

- 3 pears
- 2 large apples
- 1 12-ounce bag frozen cranberries
- 3 tablespoons sugar
- 4 tablespoons flour
- ½ teaspoon almond extract
- ⅓ cup apple juice

Preheat oven to 375° F; set rack in the center. To prepare topping, combine walnuts and oats in a medium-sized bowl. Spread onto a cookie sheet: toast in oven for 5 minutes. Return to bowl, add remaining topping ingredients; mix with a fork until pea-size crumbs form. (Can be made up to 1 week ahead and frozen in a plastic bag.)

Cut pears and apples into ¼-inch slices. In a large mixing bowl, stir together fruit, sugar and flour. In a cup, combine almond extract and apple juice; pour over fruit and stir. Bake mixture in a shallow 3-quart baking dish for 30 minutes at 375° F. Cover with foil; refrigerate.

To assemble crisp, allow fruit to reach room temperature. Sprinkle evenly with topping and bake 30 minutes at 375° F.

The tartness of cranberries complements the sweet, tender nature of almost any variety of pear and apple.

NUTRITION SCORE
Per serving (¾ cup): 340 **calories**
34% **fat** (13 g; 5.3 g saturated)
60% **carbs** (54.4 g), 5.5 g **fiber**
6% **protein** (4.7 g)

Mocha Pudding With Crystallized Ginger

Serves 6
Prep time: 15 minutes
Chilling time: 1 hour

- 2 cups light silken tofu
- ½ cup melted milk chocolate
- 1 tablespoon dehydrated coffee or espresso
- 1 teaspoon boiling water
- ½ cup lowfat sour cream
- ½ cup sugar
- 1 teaspoon vanilla
- ½ teaspoon cinnamon
- 2 tablespoons chopped crystallized ginger

Drain tofu and blend in a food processor until smooth. Add melted chocolate. Combine coffee or espresso with 1 teaspoon boiling water and add to tofu. Add sour cream, sugar, vanilla and cinnamon and blend until creamy. Transfer to individual serving cups and sprinkle the ginger on top. Chill thoroughly before serving.

NUTRITION SCORE
Per serving (1 cup): 204 **calories**
26% **fat** (6 g; 3.6 g saturated)
59% **carbs** (30 g), 1g **fiber**
15% **protein** (7.5 g)

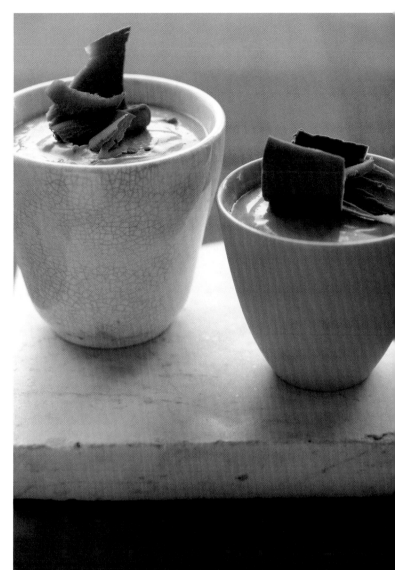

Substitute vanilla- or chocolate-flavored light soy milk for nonfat milk in puddings and pie fillings.

Chocolate-Cherry Pie to Die For

Serves 4
Prep time: 25 minutes
Cook time: 24 minutes

Filling

- 1 24-ounce can or jar of red tart pitted cherries in their juice, drained except for 4 tablespoons
- ¼ teaspoon almond extract
- 8 teaspoons chocolate chips

Topping

- 3 tablespoons slivered almonds
- 3 tablespoons old-fashioned oats (do not use instant)
- ¼ cup plus 2 tablespoons all-purpose flour
- 3 tablespoons light brown sugar
- Dash cinnamon
- 1 tablespoon plus 1 teaspoon cold unsalted butter, cut into tiny cubes

Preheat oven to 375° F. Place cherries, almond extract and chocolate chips for the filling in a medium bowl and stir well, until thoroughly combined. Pour filling into an ungreased, 9-inch glass pie plate.

Combine all the topping ingredients in a blender and pulse until the mixture is the size of small peas. Sprinkle topping over filling. Bake for 24 minutes or until bubbly. Divide into 4 servings and serve hot.

NUTRITION SCORE
Per serving (¼ of recipe): 281 **calories**
32% **fat** (10 g; 4 g saturated)
62% **carbs** (49 g), 2 g **fiber**
6% **protein** (4 g)

Peanut Butter Swirl Brownies

Makes 16 brownies
Prep time: 15 minutes
Cook time: 25 minutes

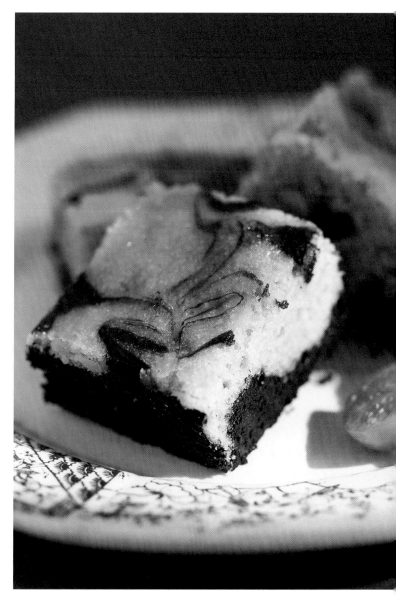

  Cooking spray
½ cup applesauce
⅔ cup granulated sugar
½ cup brown sugar
2 egg whites
1 whole egg
2 tablespoons buttermilk
¾ cup all-purpose flour
½ teaspoon baking powder
¼ teaspoon salt
¼ cup creamy peanut butter
¼ cup peanut butter chips
⅓ cup cocoa powder
⅓ cup semisweet mini chocolate chips

Preheat oven to 350° F. Lightly coat a 9-inch square pan with cooking spray.

In a mixing bowl, using an electric mixer, beat together the applesauce, sugars, eggs and buttermilk. In another bowl, combine flour, baking powder and salt. Add to the egg mixture and mix until blended.

Divide the batter in half. Add peanut butter and peanut butter chips to one portion and cocoa powder and chocolate chips to the other. Spoon the chocolate batter into 8 mounds in a checkerboard pattern into the prepared pan. Spoon 7 mounds of the peanut butter batter, placing it between the chocolate mounds. Using the tip of a knife, swirl the batters.

Bake for 25 minutes or until the edges begin to pull away from the pan and a toothpick inserted in the center comes out clean. Cut into 16 squares and serve.

NUTRITION SCORE
Per serving (1 brownie): 139 **calories**
28% **fat** (4.3 g; 1.3 g saturated)
63% **carbs** (23 g), 1.3 g **fiber**
9% **protein** (3 g)

Hot Mexican Volcanoes

Serves 15
Prep time: 1 hour
Cook time: 25-30 minutes

- ½ cup, minus 1 tablespoon, nonfat sweetened condensed milk
- ¾ cup reduced-fat chocolate chips
- 1 10.1-ounce box reduced-fat devil's food cake mix
- 2 tablespoons instant coffee granules
- 1 teaspoon ground cinnamon
- 1 tablespoon pure chili powder (not chili seasoning), or ⅛ teaspoon cayenne pepper
- 1 cup water
- 1 whole egg
- 3 egg whites
- ¾ cup granulated sugar
- 15 whole macadamia nuts
- ¾ cup confectioners' sugar
- 1½ tablespoons unsweetened cocoa powder
- ¾ teaspoon vanilla extract
- 3-4 tablespoons nonfat milk

In a saucepan, combine condensed milk and chocolate chips and cook over low heat until chocolate melts. Transfer to a bowl. Refrigerate about 30 minutes.

Meanwhile, line 15 muffin pan cups with foil-and-paper liners. In a large mixing bowl, combine cake mix, instant coffee, cinnamon and chili powder or cayenne. Using an electric mixer on low speed, beat in water and whole egg. Increase speed to medium and beat 2 minutes more.

To make meringue, clean beaters thoroughly; then beat egg whites until foamy in a clean nonreactive bowl (do not use aluminum or plastic). Gradually beat in sugar until stiff and glossy.

Preheat oven to 350° F. Remove chocolate mixture from refrigerator and wrap about 1 teaspoon of the mixture around each macadamia nut, shaping it into a ball. Set aside. Fill muffin cups ⅔ full of cake batter. Spoon 1 heaping tablespoonful of meringue on top and smooth out evenly, making sure meringue extends all the way to paper liners and no batter is exposed. Place a chocolate ball in exact center of meringue; do not push in. Bake until a toothpick inserted in the side of a cupcake comes out clean, about 25-30 minutes.

Cool in pans on rack; then carefully loosen meringue with tip of sharp knife and remove cakes from pans. Place on wire racks set over waxed paper and cool completely.

In a small bowl, combine confectioners' sugar, cocoa, vanilla and enough milk to make a glaze of drizzling consistency. Spoon glaze on top of meringue, letting it drip down sides, and serve.

NUTRITION SCORE
Per serving (1 volcano): 247 **calories**
26% **fat** (7 g; 3.8 g saturated)
68% **carbs** (46 g), 1.5 g **fiber**
6% **protein** (3.9 g)

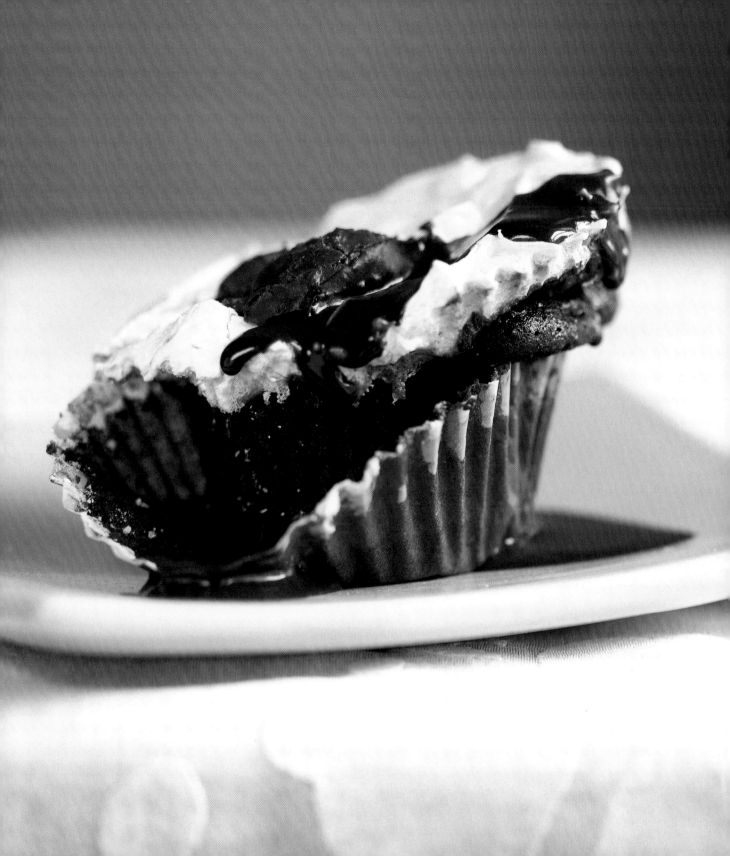

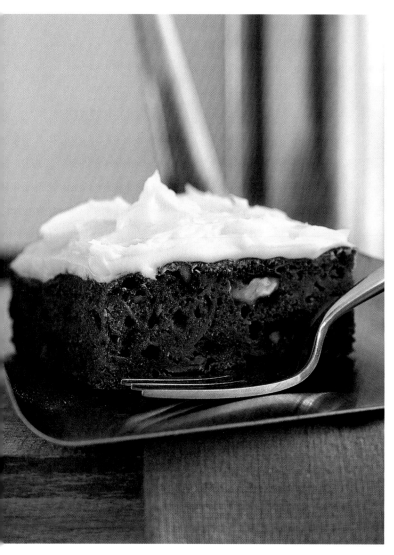

Carrot Cake

Serves 16
Prep Time: 20 minutes
Cook Time: 35-40 minutes

Cake
Cooking spray
1 cup all-purpose flour
1 cup whole-wheat flour
1¾ cups sugar
2 teaspoons cinnamon
2 teaspoons baking soda
1 teaspoon nutmeg
½ teaspoon salt
1 cup applesauce
½ cup buttermilk
6 egg whites
3 cups shredded carrots
⅔ cup chopped walnuts

Cream Cheese Frosting
8 ounces light cream cheese
8 ounces fat-free cream cheese
6 tablespoons light butter
1½ cups powdered sugar
1 teaspoon vanilla

Be cart smart when grocery shopping: Bring a list and stick to it; shop solo and do it when you're well-fed and rested; skip the junk food and soda aisles.

To make the cake, preheat oven to 375° F. Coat a 9-by-13-inch pan with cooking spray.

In a medium bowl, combine flours, sugar, cinnamon, baking soda, nutmeg and salt; set aside. In a large bowl, using an electric mixer, beat together applesauce, buttermilk and egg whites. Add flour mixture to applesauce mixture and beat until combined. Stir in carrots and walnuts. Pour batter into prepared pan.

Bake 40-45 minutes, or until toothpick inserted near the center comes out clean.

To make frosting, beat together cream cheeses until smooth. Add butter and mix well. Beat in sugar and vanilla until well mixed and fluffy. Spread over cooled cake.

NUTRITION SCORE
Per serving: 305 **calories**
24% **fat** (8.8 g; 3.4 g saturated)
65% **carbs** (50 g) 2.5 g **fiber**
11% **protein** (9 g)

Pumpkin Squares

Serves 16
Prep time: 15 minutes
Cook time: 60-65 minutes

Cooking spray
1 29-ounce can pumpkin purée
1½ cups nonfat milk
¾ cup nonfat powdered milk
6 egg whites
¾ cup white sugar
1½ teaspoons cinnamon
1½ teaspoons allspice
1 9-ounce package yellow cake mix
¾ cup chopped walnuts
4 tablespoons light butter
⅓ cup brown sugar

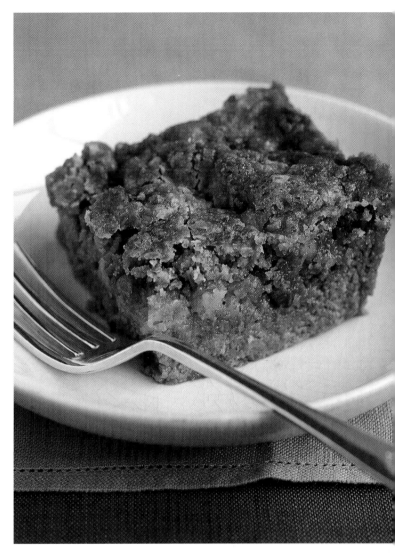

Preheat oven to 350º F. Spray a 9-by-13-inch pan with cooking spray.

In a large bowl, beat together pumpkin and the liquid and powdered milks, using an electric mixer on medium speed. Beat in egg whites, white sugar, cinnamon and allspice until smooth. Pour pumpkin mixture into prepared pan.

Sprinkle dry cake mix evenly over pumpkin mixture. Sprinkle walnuts over the dry cake mix layer.

In a small microwave-safe bowl, combine butter and brown sugar. Microwave on high until melted, about 90 seconds. Stir together until blended. Drizzle brown sugar mixture evenly over the walnut layer. Cover with aluminum foil. Bake 45 minutes. Remove foil and bake an additional 15-20 minutes, or until golden brown and a toothpick inserted comes out clean.

NUTRITION SCORE
Per serving (1 square): 216 **calories**
29% **fat** (7.1 g; 5.3 g saturated)
59% **carbs** (33.5 g), 2.9 g **fiber**
12% **protein** (7 g)

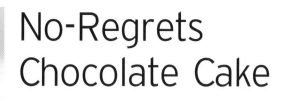

No-Regrets Chocolate Cake

Serves 12
Prep time: 10 minutes
Cook time: 25 minutes

Cooking spray
1¾ cups all-purpose flour
1¾ cups packed light brown sugar
¾ cup cocoa powder
1½ teaspoons baking soda
1½ teaspoons baking powder
¼ teaspoon salt
1¼ cups reduced-fat buttermilk
3 large egg whites
4 tablespoons light margarine, melted
1½ teaspoons vanilla extract
1 cup boiling water
1 tablespoon confectioners' sugar

Preheat oven to 350° F. Lightly coat a 9-by-12-inch baking pan with cooking spray. In a large bowl, combine next 6 ingredients (flour through salt). Mix well with a fork to break up brown sugar. Set aside.

In a large bowl, combine buttermilk, egg whites, melted margarine and vanilla. Mix on low speed until blended. Gradually beat in boiling water. Then slowly add flour mixture and, again, mix on low speed until blended.

Pour batter into prepared pan and bake 25 minutes, or until a toothpick inserted in center comes out clean. Cool cake in pan on a wire rack. Sift confectioners' sugar over top just before slicing into 12 equal squares.

NUTRITION SCORE
Per serving (¹⁄₁₂ of cake): 245 **calories**
11% **fat** (3 g; 1 g saturated)
81% **carbs** (50 g), 2 g **fiber**
8% **protein** (5 g)

Chocolate is packed with polyphenols, the same heart-friendly antioxidants found in red wine and tea. In fact, cocoa contains 2.5 times more polyphenols than a comparable amount of asparagus and beets, and 23 times that found in apples.

Chocolate Chip Cookies

Serves 37
Prep time: 15 minutes
Cook time: 17–19 minutes per sheet

- ½ cup (1 stick) corn-oil margarine, softened
- 1 tablespoon water
- ½ cup dark brown sugar, firmly packed
- ½ cup golden brown sugar, firmly packed
- ½ cup granulated sugar
- 2 egg whites
- 1½ teaspoons vanilla extract
- 1¾ cups all-purpose flour
- 1 teaspoon baking soda
- ½ teaspoon salt
- ½ cup (4 ounces) mini chocolate chips

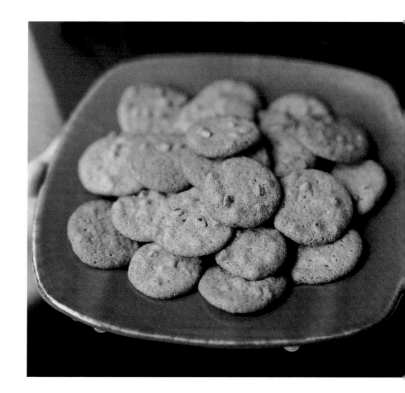

Preheat oven to 350° F. Line cookie sheet with parchment paper and set aside.

In a large bowl, cream together margarine, water and sugars with an electric mixer on a high speed for 2 minutes. Add egg whites and vanilla and mix well. Blend in flour, baking soda and salt. Mix well. Add chocolate chips and blend thoroughly.

Scoop dough in rounded ½-teaspoonfuls and place on prepared cookie sheet about 1 inch apart. Bake until deep golden brown. Cool completely and serve.

(For variety, add ½ cup rolled oats, 1 cup raisins or 1 cup dried cranberries.)

Ignore intense yens for chocolate and you could become so fixated that it's difficult to think of anything else. Give in to your cravings by enjoying the high-fat treat in small doses, such as mini chocolate chips.

NUTRITION SCORE
Per serving (3 cookies): 92 **calories**
33% **fat** (3.4 g; 0.95 g saturated)
63% **carbs** (15 g), 0.3 g **fiber**
4% **protein** (0.9 g)

Warm Rhubarb Compote With Vanilla-Yogurt Timbale

Serves 6
Prep time: 10 minutes
Cook time: 35 minutes
Chill time: 1 hour

  2 cups low-fat vanilla yogurt
1½ pounds fresh rhubarb
 ½ cup best-quality currant jelly

Evenly spoon yogurt into 6 3-ounce paper cups. Place in freezer for about 1 hour, until semi-frozen. (Or, if making in advance, re-move 3-ounce cups of lowfat vanilla frozen yogurt from freezer about 15 minutes before serving.)

Preheat oven to 400° F. Remove green leaves from rhubarb and discard (they're toxic). Cut rhubarb into 1½-inch lengths on the bias. Wash (don't dry).

In a shallow casserole, stir rhubarb and jelly until all pieces are coated. Bake until rhubarb is tender, about 35 minutes, stirring twice. Remove from oven; cool for 5 minutes. Spoon into 6 shallow bowls. Unmold yogurt and serve atop rhubarb.

Although rhubarb is treated like a fruit, botanically this celery-like plant is a veggie. Field-grown rhubarb is available from April to June and has bright red stalks. Hothouse rhubarb is lighter in color and is available year-round. Look for shiny, brightly colored stalks.

NUTRITION SCORE
Per serving (½ cup compote, ⅓ cup yogurt): 162 **calories**
5% **fat** (1 g; <0.5 g saturated)
86% **carbs** (36 g), 1 g **fiber**
9% **protein** (4 g)

Sweet Potato Soufflé

Serves 8
Prep time: 15 minutes
Cook time: 30-35 minutes

Soufflé
Cooking spray
2 cups mashed sweet potatoes
¾ cup granulated sugar
4 egg whites
¼ cup 2 percent milk
2 teaspoons cornstarch
¼ teaspoon cinnamon
¼ teaspoon vanilla extract

Topping
½ cup brown sugar
4 tablespoons light butter
3 tablespoons all-purpose flour
1 8-ounce can crushed pineapple, drained

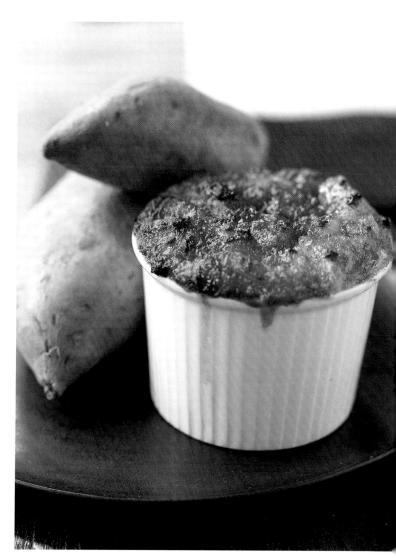

Preheat oven to 350° F.

Spray a soufflé or casserole dish with cooking spray.

In a large bowl, using an electric mixer on the lowest setting, beat together the sweet potatoes and sugar. Add egg whites, milk, cornstarch, cinnamon and vanilla. Beat until fluffy and lump-free. Pour into prepared dish.

In a small microwave-safe bowl, combine the brown sugar and butter. Microwave on high until melted, about 30 seconds. Stir in the flour and pineapple. Drizzle the topping over the sweet potato mixture.

Bake for 30-35 minutes until top of soufflé is bubbly and golden. Serve immediately.

The body converts the beta carotene in one serving of sweet potatoes to more than twice the daily requirement of vitamin A. In addition, sweet potatoes provide nearly as much vitamin E as do fatty nuts and seeds, and supply a nice dose of vitamin C and iron.

NUTRITION SCORE
Per serving (⅛ of recipe): 240 **calories**
11% **fat** (3 g; 0.13 g saturated)
83% **carbs** (50.3 g), 1.3 g **fiber**
6% **protein** (3.7 g)

Index

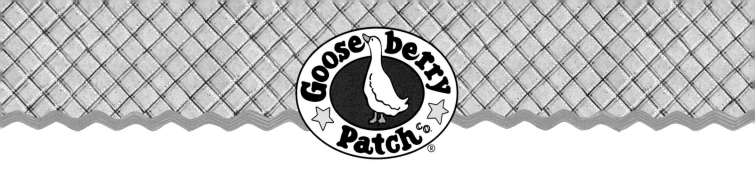

Goose berry Patch

classic
Christmas
recipes

More than 150 recipes plus
memories, tips, ideas & menus
to make the season bright!

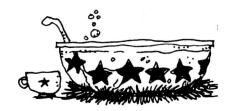

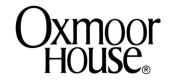

Oxmoor
House

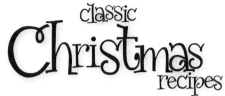

©2010 by Gooseberry Patch
600 London Road, Delaware, Ohio 43015
www.gooseberrypatch.com
©2010 by Oxmoor House, Inc.
P.O. Box 360220, Des Moines, IA 50336-0220

ISBN-13: 978-0-8487-3335-3
ISBN-10: 0-8487-3335-5
Library of Congress Control Number: 2009937187

Printed in the United States of America
Third Printing 2012

Oxmoor House, Inc.
VP, Publishing Director: Jim Childs
Editorial Director: Susan Payne Dobbs
Brand Manager: Terri Laschober Robertson
Senior Editor: Rebecca Brennan
Managing Editor: Laurie S. Herr

Gooseberry Patch Classic Christmas Recipes
Editor: Emily Chappell
Senior Designer: Emily Albright Parrish
Contributing Designer: Allison Sperando
Director, Test Kitchens: Elizabeth Tyler Austin
Assistant Director, Test Kitchens: Julie Christopher
Test Kitchens Professionals: Allison E. Cox, Julie Gunter,
Kathleen Royal Phillips, Catherine Crowell Steele, Ashley T. Strickland
Photography Director: Jim Bathie
Senior Photo Stylist: Kay E. Clarke
Associate Photo Stylist: Katherine Eckert Coyne
Production Manager: Greg Amason

Contributors
Copy Editor: Adrienne Davis
Proofreader: Catherine Fowler
Interns: Chris Cosgrove, Georgia Dodge, Perri K. Hubbard, Christine Taylor
Food Stylists: Ana Kelly, Alyson Haynes, Laura Zapalowski
Test Kitchens Professionals: Connie Nash, Angela Schmidt
Photographers: Lee Harrelson
Photo Stylists: Missie Crawford, Mindy Shapiro

To order additional publications, call 1-800-765-6400 or 1-800-491-0551.

For more books to enrich your life, visit oxmoorhouse.com

To search, savor, and share thousands of recipes, visit myrecipes.com

Cover: New England Turkey & Stuffing (page 54)

Contents

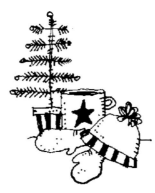

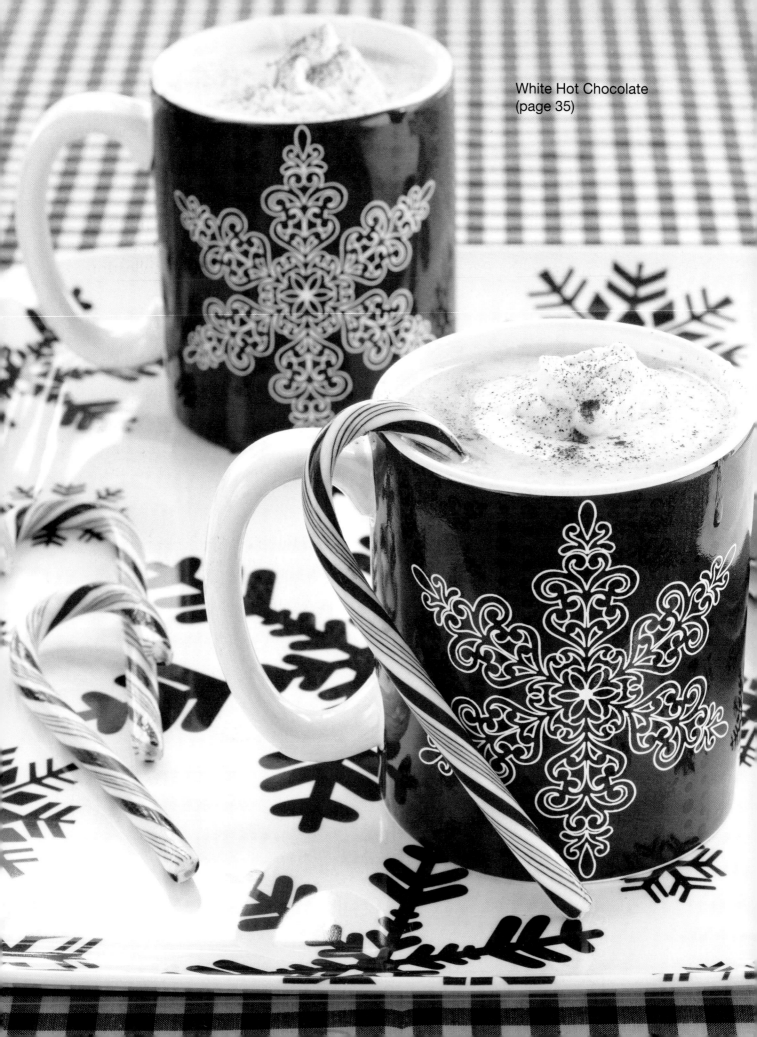

White Hot Chocolate
(page 35)

Dear Friend,

Christmas is best spent gathered together with the ones you love…reminiscing, creating new memories, and enjoying comforting and delicious meals. We'll help you make the most of the holiday season with our latest collection of time-tested, family-favorite recipes, *Gooseberry Patch Classic Christmas Recipes*.

We've shared more than 150 recipes in ten helpful chapters, so you can easily find just what you need to fill out any menu. Turn to page 20 for Rise & Shine…a chapter devoted to breakfast and brunch ideas to help you create the perfect Christmas morning. Or if you're pressed for time, look to In the Nick of Time, beginning on page 36, for quick & easy recipes to make last-minute get-togethers a breeze. And Yuletide Sweets, starting on page 124, is bound to have a dessert to delight everyone's sweet tooth!

In addition, you'll find tips, personal memories from the Gooseberry Patch family, and a few extra pages of recipes and craft ideas, including Lots of Fun for the Little Ones and Gift-Giving & Packaging Ideas. We've also gathered themed meal ideas in our 12 Days of Christmas Menus section.

This year, let us do the planning for you! *Classic Christmas Recipes* has everything you need to get ready for the holiday season, so you can truly enjoy this special time with family and friends.

Wishing you all the joys of Christmas!

JoAnn & Vickie

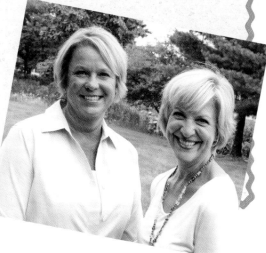

Festive Cheese Ball
(page 12)

Christmas Cheer

Spread a little joy during the holidays with these party-starting
finger foods, dips and beverages. Your guests won't be able to resist
diving into Roasted Red Pepper Salsa or Christmas Shrimp Dip while
they sip on Sonia's Holiday Sangria or Viennese-Style Coffee. These
recipes are sure to keep your crowd coming back for more!

Caramelized Pecans

½ c. sugar   ¾ c. pecan halves

In a heavy saucepan, heat sugar over medium heat until melted (about 4 minutes). Stir constantly to avoid burning sugar. Stir in pecans until well coated. Remove pan from heat. Pour mixture onto wax paper or onto a buttered plate. Cool. If stuck together, break apart. Use whole or coarsely chop for garnish. Makes 1⅓ cups.

Roasted Red Pepper Salsa

Fry up some quartered corn tortillas for your own fresh chips.

2 c. corn
2 tomatoes, diced
7-oz. jar roasted red peppers, drained and chopped
2 green onions, finely chopped
1 jalapeño pepper, seeded and minced
3 T. fresh cilantro, minced

2 T. lime juice
1 T. white vinegar
½ t. salt
¼ t. pepper
¼ t. cumin
2 avocados, pitted, peeled and chopped
multicolored tortilla chips

Gently stir together first 12 ingredients; cover and refrigerate at least 2 hours before serving. Serve with multicolored tortilla chips. Makes 2½ cups.

Christmas Shrimp Dip

You can substitute lobster or crab for the shrimp, and blue cheese makes a tasty difference when substituted for cream cheese!

3-oz. pkg. cream cheese, softened
1 T. mayonnaise
1 c. shrimp, minced
¼ t. Worcestershire sauce
2 t. onion, grated

2 t. parsley, chopped
1½ t. lemon juice
¼ t. salt
3 drops hot pepper sauce
crackers or potato chips

Mix cream cheese with mayonnaise. Add next 7 ingredients and blend thoroughly. Allow mixture to chill for one hour so flavors will blend. Serve with crackers or potato chips. Makes ¾ cup.

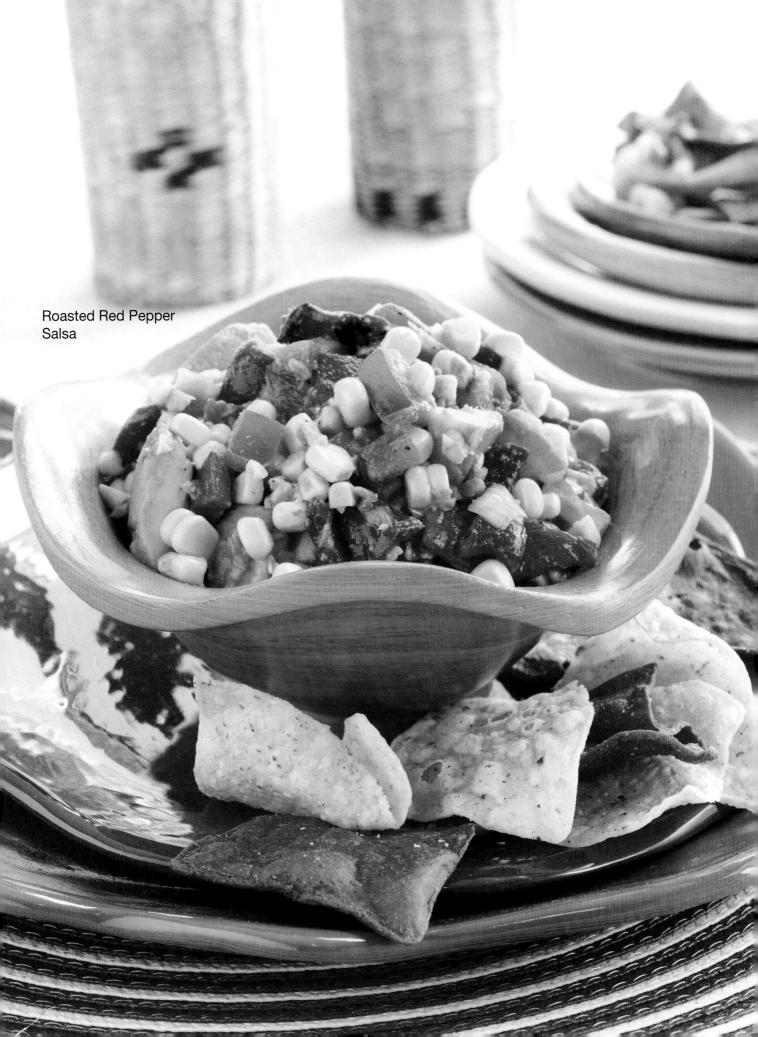

Roasted Red Pepper
Salsa

Garlic-Feta Cheese Spread

This is a real winner!

1 clove garlic, minced
¼ t. salt
8-oz. container feta cheese, crumbled
½ c. mayonnaise
¼ t. dried marjoram

¼ t. dried dill weed, crumbled
¼ t. dried basil, crumbled
¼ t. dried thyme, crumbled
12 oz. cream cheese, softened
crackers, bagel chips or pita bread

Using a fork, mash garlic into a paste; add salt. Using a food processor, blend together feta cheese, mayonnaise, garlic, herbs and cream cheese. Spoon into a crock and chill, covered, for 2 hours. Serve with crackers, bagel chips or slices of pita bread. Makes 1½ cups.

Festive Cheese Ball

(pictured on page 8)

Make ahead of time to allow flavors to blend.

2 (8-oz.) pkgs. cream cheese, softened
2 c. shredded Cheddar cheese
1 T. onion, finely chopped
1 T. pimento, finely chopped
1 T. green pepper, finely chopped
2 t. Worcestershire sauce

1 t. lemon juice
⅛ t. salt
⅛ t. cayenne pepper
½ c. chopped walnuts, toasted
crackers

In a medium bowl, blend cheeses together with a fork. Mix in remaining ingredients except the walnuts and crackers. Place mixture on plastic wrap and shape into a ball; chill thoroughly. Roll in chopped walnuts and serve with assorted crackers or strips of red and green peppers. Makes 4 cups.

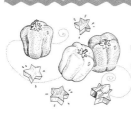

INSTEAD OF USING BOWLS OR DISHES to serve your holiday dips, use red and green peppers as mini containers. They are easy to clean up and very festive.

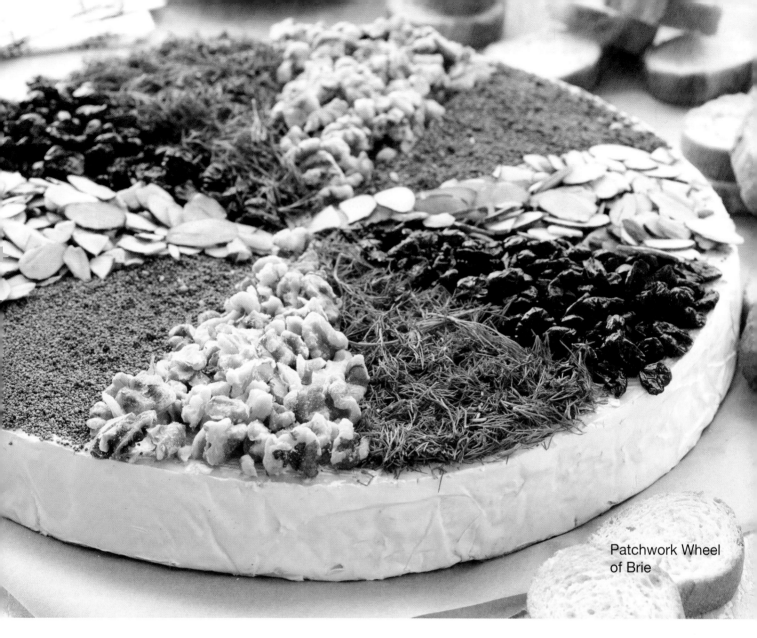

Patchwork Wheel
of Brie

Patchwork Wheel of Brie

5 lb. round of Brie
½ c. sweetened dried cranberries
   or dried currants
½ c. walnuts, finely chopped

½ c. fresh dill or chives, chopped
¼ c. poppy seeds
1 c. sliced almonds, toasted
toasted bread rounds

*A festive centerpiece for
your appetizer table.*

Remove the rind from the top of the cheese by cutting carefully with a sharp knife. Lightly score the top of the cheese into 10 equal pie-shaped sections. Sprinkle half of each of the toppings onto each wedge and press gently until you have decorated all 10 sections. Allow to stand at room temperature for at least 40 minutes before serving. Serve with toasted bread rounds. Serves 20 to 25.

Marinated Olives

These olives are quite spicy and will please anyone who loves to nibble on hot foods!

6-oz. can pitted black olives, drained and rinsed
6-oz. jar pitted green olives, drained and rinsed

1 hot chili pepper, minced
3 cloves garlic, minced
1 t. oregano
1 c. olive oil

Combine olives, chili pepper, garlic and oregano in a jar with a lid. Cover with olive oil. Shake olives gently and let stand at room temperature overnight. Store in refrigerator and use within one week. Makes 2½ cups.

Hot Crab Canapés

"One of Mom's favorites; every time I make it, I think of home."

DeNeane Deskins
Marengo, OH

½ lb. crabmeat, shredded
8-oz. pkg. shredded sharp Cheddar cheese
2 eggs, hard-boiled and finely chopped
¼ c. mayonnaise

2 T. onion, grated
1 T. fresh parsley, minced
⅛ t. garlic powder
salt and pepper to taste
20 slices bread

Combine crabmeat, cheese, eggs, mayonnaise, onion, parsley, garlic powder, salt and pepper; set aside. Cut each slice of bread into 4 squares. Spread each square with crab mixture and place on an ungreased baking sheet. Bake at 350 degrees for 10 to 15 minutes or until lightly golden. Makes 6 dozen.

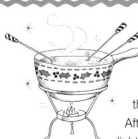

WE HAVE A FAVORITE TRADITION ON CHRISTMAS EVE that makes the evening feel magical. We begin with dinner, which is always served fondue-style. I love this because it doesn't take much time to prepare, and gives me more time with my family. We then go to our Christmas Eve candlelight and communion service. After church, we take the long way home to look at the Christmas lights. Once we're home, we open gifts from all of our out-of-town friends and family. Not only does this help make it easier to wait for Christmas morning, but it also helps clear out from under the tree for Santa's visit! Christmas is such a magical time, it makes me feel so warm and loved.

Kristi Kavicky
Collierville, TN

Marinated Olives

Artichoke-Parmesan Squares

Filled with so many tasty ingredients, this is sure to be a hit when you serve it to family & friends.

1½-oz. pkg. dry vegetable soup mix, divided
½ c. mayonnaise
½ c. sour cream
2 (8-oz.) pkgs. refrigerated crescent roll dough
10-oz. pkg. frozen chopped spinach, thawed and drained

14-oz. can artichoke hearts, drained and chopped
8-oz. can water chestnuts, drained and chopped
4 oz. feta cheese, crumbled
2 to 3 cloves garlic, pressed
½ c. pine nuts, toasted and chopped
¼ c. grated Parmesan cheese

Blend together half the dry soup mix, mayonnaise and sour cream; set aside. (Use remaining soup mix for another recipe.) Unroll packages of crescent dough on a greased 15"x10" jelly-roll pan. Seal perforations of dough and press dough up sides of pan to form a crust. Bake at 375 degrees for 10 to 12 minutes or until golden. Add spinach, artichokes and water chestnuts to mayonnaise mixture; stir in feta cheese and garlic. Fold in pine nuts and spread mixture over crust. Sprinkle with Parmesan cheese. Bake an additional 10 to 12 minutes, or until heated through. Cut into 2-inch squares. Makes about 3 dozen.

Macadamia Cheesy Puffs

Frankly, my dear, these are delicious.

1 c. buttermilk biscuit baking mix
1 c. unsalted macadamia nuts, finely chopped
1 c. Gruyère cheese, shredded

½ c. butter, softened
1 egg, beaten
½ t. ground white pepper

Combine all ingredients and stir until soft dough forms. Drop by tablespoonfuls onto a greased baking sheet. Bake at 375 degrees for 12 to 15 minutes, or until very lightly golden. Cool on pan several minutes; finish cooling on a wire rack. Store in airtight container. Makes 2 dozen.

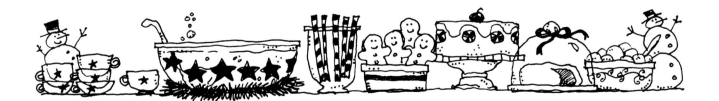

Mushroom Turnovers

8-oz. pkg. cream cheese
1 c. margarine, softened
2 c. plus 2 T. all-purpose flour, divided
4 c. sliced mushrooms, finely chopped
⅔ c. green onions, chopped
2 T. butter or margarine, melted

⅓ c. sour cream
¼ t. thyme
¼ t. salt
1 egg white, beaten
Garnish: sesame seeds

A delicious appetizer to make ahead and freeze.

Blend together cream cheese, margarine and 2 cups flour; chill. Sauté mushrooms and onions in butter for about 3 minutes. Add sour cream, 2 tablespoons flour, thyme and salt; cook for a few more minutes. Roll out half of dough at a time to ⅛-inch thickness and cut with a 2½-inch biscuit cutter or a round cookie cutter. Place a heaping ¼ teaspoon of mushroom mixture in the center of each circle. Fold over and press edges gently with fingers. Transfer turnovers to a lightly greased baking sheet using a spatula; finish sealing edges by pressing with a fork. Brush each turnover with egg white and sprinkle with sesame seeds. Bake at 350 degrees for 20 minutes. Makes about 5½ dozen.

Barbeque Meatballs

1 lb. ground beef
⅓ c. fine bread crumbs
1 egg, slightly beaten
½ t. poultry seasoning

½ c. catsup
2 T. brown sugar, packed
2 T. apple cider vinegar
2 T. soy sauce

"This recipe was given to me by my mother, Nancy Campbell, and is a great appetizer or potluck dish…there are never any left over!"

*Suzanne Carbaugh
Mount Vernon, WA*

Mix ground beef, bread crumbs, egg and poultry seasoning. Shape into about 2 dozen 1½-inch balls. Brown balls slowly in a lightly oiled skillet over medium-high heat; pour off excess fat. In a small bowl, combine catsup, brown sugar, vinegar and soy sauce. Pour over meatballs. Cover and simmer over low heat, stirring constantly, for 15 minutes. Serve warm. Makes 2 dozen.

GIVE YOUR FAVORITE SNACKER A GIANT TIN filled with peanuts, pretzels, chips or party mix. An irresistible treat!

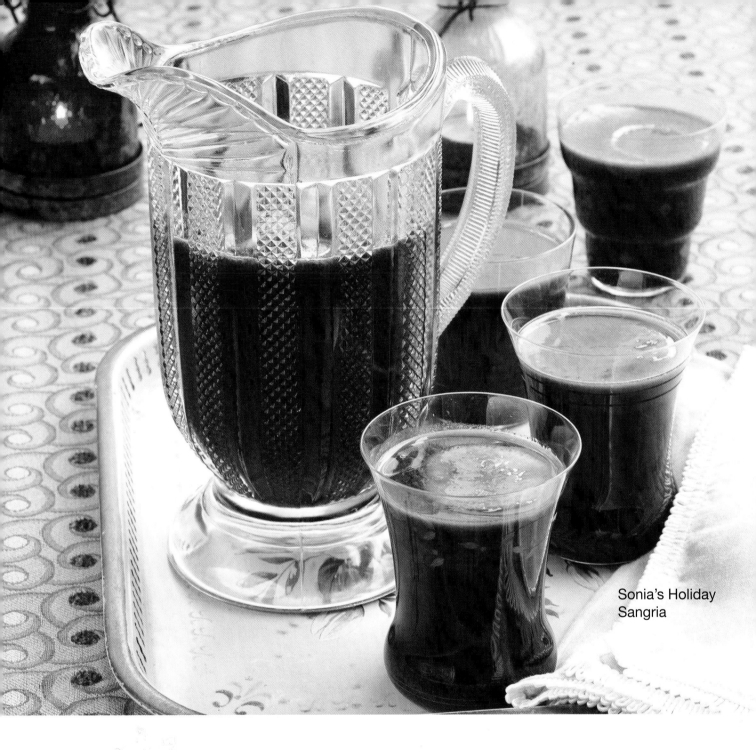

Sonia's Holiday Sangria

Sonia's Holiday Sangria

Use your favorite fresh fruit in this holiday treat.

1 qt. burgundy wine or grape juice
2 c. lemon-lime carbonated drink
⅔ c. strawberry nectar
5½ oz. can frozen orange juice
6-oz. can peach nectar
⅛ t. cinnamon
1 c. fruit, sliced
Garnish: orange, lemon and lime slices

Combine all ingredients in a large container, adding fruit last so it will float on top. Cover and refrigerate for 24 hours, allowing flavors to blend. Serve chilled. Garnish with orange, lemon and lime slices. Makes about 9 cups.

Hot Spiced Wine Punch

1 qt. apple juice
1 qt. cranberry juice
1 qt. water
2 c. sugar
4 (4-inch) cinnamon sticks

12 whole cloves
zest of 1 lemon, cut in strips
2 qts. rosé wine or grape juice
½ c. lemon juice
Garnish: lemon slices

This will be a big hit at your next party.

Combine apple and cranberry juices, water, sugar, cinnamon sticks, cloves and lemon zest in a pot. Bring to a boil. Stir until sugar dissolves. Simmer uncovered for 15 minutes. Add wine and lemon juice. Heat, but do not boil. Serve in punch bowl. (Be sure punch bowl is capable of holding hot punch.) Garnish with lemon slices. Serves 40.

Viennese-Style Coffee

¾ c. ground coffee
6 whole cloves
3 cinnamon sticks, broken
6 whole allspice berries
4 c. water

1 T. chocolate-flavored coffee syrup
1 T. honey
Garnish: whipped cream and freshly grated nutmeg

A wonderful after-dinner drink.

Place coffee, cloves, cinnamon sticks and allspice berries in coffee basket of coffee maker. Fill water reservoir of coffee maker with the water and brew. Add chocolate-flavored coffee syrup and honey to hot coffee. Mix well. Pour into heat-safe wine glasses. Top with whipped cream and freshly grated nutmeg. Serves 6.

Chilled Vanilla Coffee

2 T. instant coffee granules
¾ c. warm water
14-oz. can sweetened condensed milk

1 t. vanilla extract
4 c. ice cubes

For a special treat, serve in frosty holiday glasses.

Dissolve coffee in water; blend in condensed milk and vanilla. Pour mixture into a blender and gradually add ice cubes; blend until smooth. Serve immediately. Serves 4.

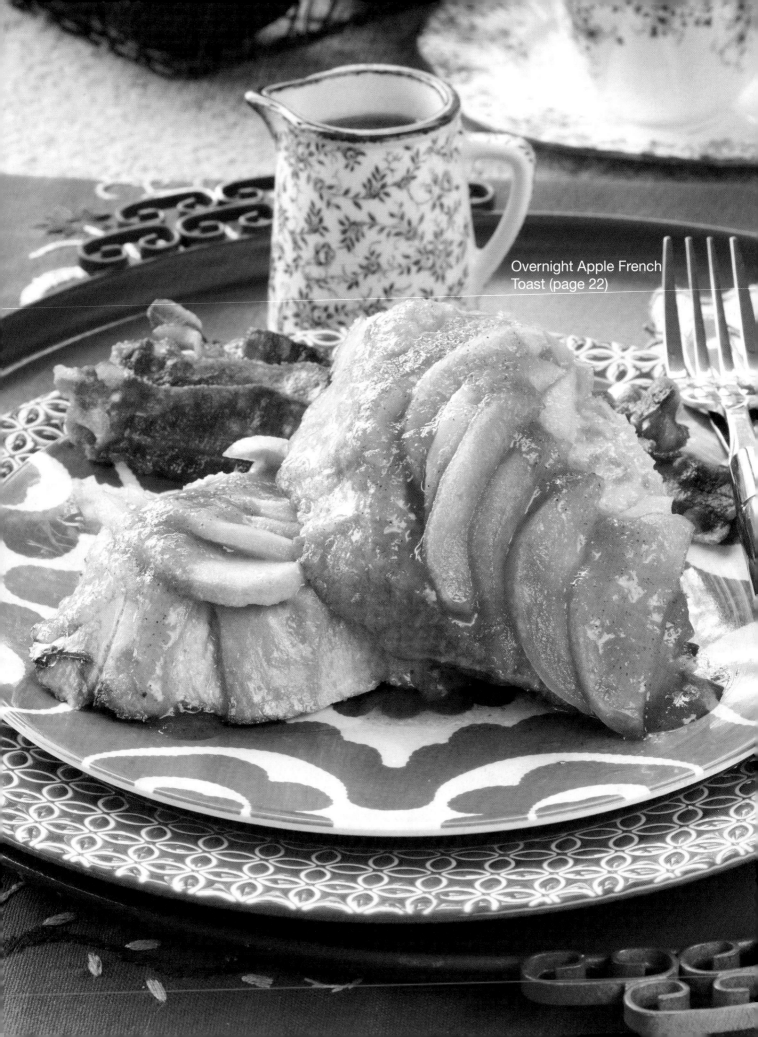

Overnight Apple French
Toast (page 22)

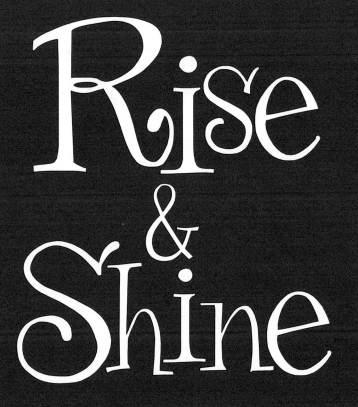

Rise & Shine

Start the day with a delicious breakfast or brunch your whole family will enjoy. Country Breakfast Casserole or Mel's Christmas Morning Casserole are perfect for a house full of holiday guests. If you don't want to spend Christmas morning in the kitchen, try preparing Overnight Apple French Toast the night before!

Country Morning Maple Muffins

...reminiscent of a big bowl of maple & brown sugar oatmeal!

1½ c. all-purpose flour
¾ c. long-cooking oats, uncooked
2 t. baking powder
1 t. salt
½ t. cinnamon
½ c. brown sugar, packaged

¼ c. butter or margarine, softened
1 egg
½ c. milk
½ c. maple syrup
½ t. maple extract
¼ c. chopped pecans

In a small bowl, stir together flour, oats, baking powder, salt and cinnamon. In a separate bowl, beat together brown sugar, butter and egg. Add milk, maple syrup & maple extract to brown sugar mixture until well-blended. Combine flour mixture with brown sugar mixture. Stir in pecans. Spoon into greased muffin cups. Bake at 350 degrees for 20 to 25 minutes. Serve warm. Makes one dozen.

Overnight Apple French Toast

(pictured on page 20)

Serve with bacon or sausage on the side, or fresh orange slices and strawberries.

1 c. brown sugar, packed
½ c. butter
2 T. light corn syrup
4 Granny Smith apples, peeled and
    sliced ¼-inch thick

3 eggs
1 c. milk
1 t. vanilla extract
9 slices day-old French bread

In a small saucepan, combine brown sugar, butter and corn syrup; cook over low heat until thick. Pour into an ungreased 13"x9" pan, arranging apple slices on top of syrup. In a mixing bowl, beat eggs, milk and vanilla. Dip French bread in egg mixture and arrange over top of apple slices. Cover and refrigerate overnight. Remove from refrigerator 30 minutes before baking and uncover. Bake at 350 degrees for 35 to 40 minutes or until the top of the bread is browned. Serve French toast with apple slices up and spoon the warm Sauce on top. Serves 6 to 8.

Sauce:

1 c. applesauce
10-oz. jar apple jelly

½ t. cinnamon
⅛ t. ground cloves

Combine all ingredients in a saucepan and cook over medium heat until jelly is melted.

Warm Country
Gingerbread Waffles

Warm Country Gingerbread Waffles

2 c. all-purpose flour
1 t. cinnamon
½ t. ground ginger
½ t. salt
1 c. molasses

½ c. butter
1½ t. baking soda
1 c. buttermilk
1 egg

Can be served with brown sugar, powdered sugar, hot maple syrup or raspberries.

Combine flour, cinnamon, ginger and salt. Heat molasses and butter until butter melts. Remove from heat and stir in baking soda. Add buttermilk and egg, and then add flour mixture. Cook in a preheated, oiled waffle iron until golden. Makes 9 (4-inch) waffles.

Morning Pecan Casserole

The raisin-cinnamon bread and nutty topping give this a yummy taste.

8-oz. pkg. sausage patties
16-oz. loaf raisin-cinnamon bread, cubed
6 eggs
1½ c. milk
1½ c. half-and-half
1 t. vanilla extract

¼ t. nutmeg
½ t. cinnamon
1 c. brown sugar, packed
1 c. chopped pecans
½ c. butter, softened
2 T. maple syrup

Brown sausage patties on both sides over medium-high heat in a skillet; drain off fat and cut into bite-size pieces. Place bread cubes in a 13"x9" baking dish coated with non-stick vegetable spray; top with sausage pieces. In a large mixing bowl, beat together eggs, milk, half-and-half, vanilla, nutmeg and cinnamon; pour over bread and sausage, pressing sausage and bread into egg mixture. Cover and refrigerate 8 hours or overnight. In a separate bowl, combine brown sugar, pecans, butter and syrup; drop by teaspoonfuls over casserole. Bake at 350 degrees for 35 to 40 minutes or until a toothpick inserted in center comes out clean. Serves 8 to 10.

Jean's Coffee Cake

"This coffee cake recipe is my favorite because it reminds me of my sister. Now that she's no longer with us, I continue the tradition of making this coffee cake each Christmas and it always sparks fond memories of her."

*Deborah Brown
Pasadena, CA*

¾ c. butter, softened and divided
1 c. sugar
3 eggs, lightly beaten
1 t. baking powder
1 t. baking soda

2¼ c. all-purpose flour, divided
1 c. sour cream
2 c. fresh raspberries or frozen, thawed and drained
1 c. brown sugar, packed

In a bowl, beat ½ cup butter and sugar; add eggs, baking powder and baking soda. Add 2 cups flour and sour cream alternately to mixture and fold in raspberries. Pour into a well-buttered Bundt® pan. For topping, combine brown sugar and ¼ cup butter, mixing well. Add ¼ cup flour; mixture will be lumpy. Spread on coffee cake batter; bake at 350 degrees for 35 to 45 minutes, or until a toothpick inserted in center comes out clean. Serves 12.

Cherry Coffee Cake

18¼-oz. pkg. yellow cake mix, divided
2 eggs
⅔ c. warm water
2 pkgs. instant dry yeast

1 c. all-purpose flour
21-oz. can cherry pie filling
5 T. margarine, melted

Mix 1½ cups cake mix with eggs, water, yeast and flour. Beat for 2 minutes. Spread into a greased 13"x9" pan. Top with pie filling. In a separate bowl, mix remaining cake mix with margarine until mixture is crumbly; sprinkle on top of pie filling. Bake at 375 degrees for 35 minutes. Let cool and drizzle with Glaze. Serves 10 to 12.

Glaze:

1 c. powdered sugar
1½ T. water

1 T. corn syrup

Mix all ingredients together and drizzle over warm cake.

"This is a recipe I often serve. Although this can be made ahead, it is wonderful served warm."

*Gloria Kaufmann
Orrville, OH*

Savory Brunch Bread

¼ c. grated Parmesan cheese
3 T. sesame seeds
½ t. dried basil, crushed

1 pkg. 24 unbaked frozen yeast rolls
¼ c. butter or margarine, melted
2 t. real bacon bits

Grease a 10-inch fluted tube pan. In small bowl, combine Parmesan cheese, sesame seeds and basil. Add ⅓ of mix to pan and turn to coat sides. Place 10 frozen rolls in pan and drizzle with half of the butter. Sprinkle with half of the remaining cheese mix and bacon bits. Add remaining rolls. Drizzle with remaining butter and sprinkle with remaining cheese. Cover; let rolls thaw and rise overnight (12 to 24 hours) in the refrigerator. The next day, let stand at room temperature 30 minutes. Bake uncovered at 350 degrees for 20 minutes. Cover with foil and bake 10 to 15 minutes more or until golden. Remove from pan to wire rack; serve warm. Serves 12.

Delicious with your favorite omelet and freshly squeezed orange juice.

Hash Brown Potato Casserole

Always a hit with the breakfast crowd.

½ c. butter
10¾-oz. can cream of mushroom soup
½ c. Cheddar cheese, shredded (or
    pasteurized processed cheese
    spread)

16-oz. container sour cream
¼ c. onion, chopped
32-oz. pkg. frozen shredded potatoes,
    thawed

In a saucepan, heat butter with soup. Blend in remaining ingredients, except potatoes. Stir in thawed potatoes. Place in a 2½-quart buttered casserole. Bake, uncovered, at 350 degrees for 45 minutes to one hour. Serves 10 to 12.

Brunch Baked Eggs

Accompany the eggs with a variety of quick and yeast breads and fresh fruit.

6 c. (24 oz.) Monterey Jack cheese,
    shredded and divided
12-oz. pkg. mushrooms, sliced
½ onion, chopped
¼ c. red pepper, thinly sliced
¼ c. butter or margarine, melted
8 oz. cooked ham, cut into thin strips

8 eggs, beaten
1¾ c. milk
½ c. all-purpose flour
2 T. fresh chives, basil, tarragon,
    thyme or oregano, snipped
1 T. fresh parsley, snipped

Sprinkle 3 cups cheese in the bottom of a lightly greased 13"x9" baking dish. In a saucepan, cook the mushrooms, onion and red pepper in the butter until vegetables are tender but not brown. Drain well. Place vegetables over the cheese. Arrange ham strips over vegetables. Sprinkle remaining 3 cups cheese over ham. Cover and chill in refrigerator overnight. To serve, combine eggs, milk, flour, chives and parsley. Pour over cheese layer. Bake, uncovered, at 350 degrees for 40 to 45 minutes. Let stand 10 minutes. Serves 12.

TRANSFORM ORDINARY ORANGE JUICE into sunrise punch! Freeze cranberry juice cocktail into ice cubes, and then fill your juice pitcher and glasses with cranberry cubes before pouring in the orange juice.

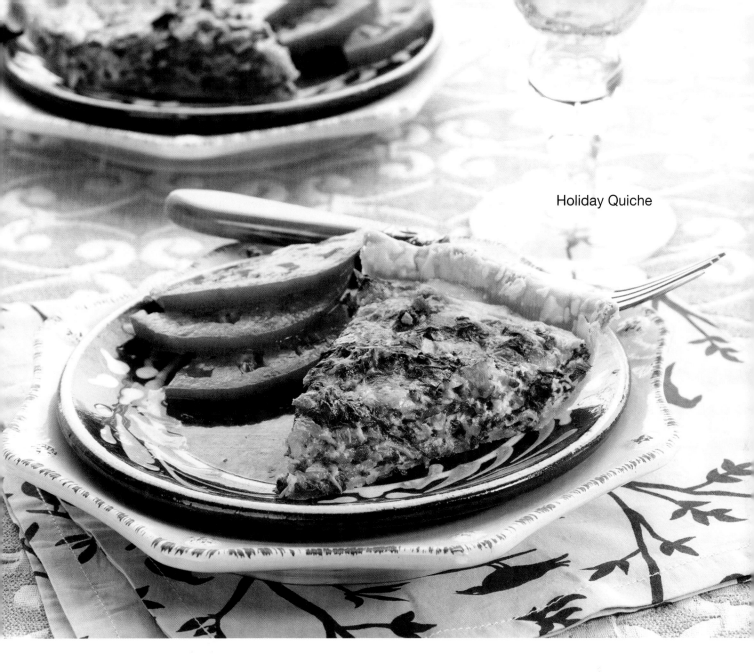

Holiday Quiche

Holiday Quiche

10-oz. pkg. frozen chopped spinach
2 c. shredded sharp Cheddar cheese
2 T. all-purpose flour
1 c. milk
2 eggs, beaten

3 slices bacon, cooked, drained
  and crumbled
⅛ t. pepper
9-inch pie crust
Garnish: tomato slices

*Double the recipe!
Freeze the second
quiche and you have a
quick meal when time is
short!*

Cook the spinach; drain and cool. In a bowl, toss the cheese with the flour. Add spinach and remaining ingredients except crust; mix well. Pour into the pie crust and bake at 350 degrees for one hour. Cool for 10 minutes and slice into pieces. Garnish each slice with a slice of tomato. Serves 6.

Holly's Broccoli Ham &
Cheese Strata

Holly's Broccoli Ham & Cheese Strata

14 slices white or wheat bread, crusts
   trimmed
1½ c. Cheddar cheese, shredded
10-oz. pkg. chopped broccoli, thawed
   and drained
¼ c. onion, chopped
1 c. cooked ham, chopped
1 tomato, peeled, seeded
   and chopped

5 eggs
1 t. seasoned salt
½ t. garlic powder
½ t. prepared mustard
½ t. cayenne pepper
1½ c. milk

A perfect holiday brunch for those you love.

Butter a 13"×9" baking dish. Layer 7 slices of bread on bottom of dish. Sprinkle half of cheese over bread slices. Next, layer thawed chopped broccoli, onion, ham and tomato over cheese. Top with remaining cheese and bread slices. In a mixing bowl, combine remaining ingredients; beat well. Pour egg mixture over layered ingredients in baking dish. Cover and refrigerate at least 3 hours or overnight. Bake, uncovered, at 350 degrees for 40 to 50 minutes, or until a toothpick inserted in center comes out clean. Serves 8 to 10.

Sunrise Ham

1 c. cooked ham, diced
1 c. sliced mushrooms
1 T. butter or margarine, melted
4 eggs
1 c. sour cream
1 c. cottage cheese
½ c. grated Parmesan cheese

¼ c. all-purpose flour
½ t. dill weed
½ t. dry mustard
⅛ t. nutmeg
⅛ t. pepper
1 c. shredded Swiss cheese
½ c. fresh parsley, chopped

Fresh fruit is a refreshing complement to this creamy dish.

Cook ham in a skillet until lightly browned; set aside. Sauté mushrooms in butter until tender; mix with ham and place in a greased 9" deep-dish pie plate. Combine eggs, sour cream, cottage cheese, Parmesan cheese, flour, dill weed, mustard, nutmeg and pepper in a blender; blend until smooth. Sprinkle Swiss cheese and parsley over ham and mushrooms. Pour egg mixture into pie plate. Bake at 350 degrees for 45 minutes or until set; let stand 10 minutes before cutting. Serves 6 to 8.

FOR A COUNTRY FAVORITE, make up a batch of fresh, fluffy biscuits and milk gravy…add sausage, bacon or ham to make it even better!

Country Scramble

"All of our family's favorite breakfast foods in one casserole!"

Dorothy Foor
Jeromesville, OH

2 c. frozen diced potatoes, thawed
1 c. cooked ham, chopped
½ c. onion, chopped
6 eggs, beaten

salt and pepper to taste
1 c. shredded Cheddar cheese
Garnish: fresh chives, minced

In a large skillet, sauté potatoes, ham and onion for 10 minutes or until potatoes are tender. In a small bowl, combine eggs, salt and pepper. Add to potato mixture and cook, stirring occasionally, until eggs are set. Remove from heat and gently stir in cheese. Spoon onto serving platter; sprinkle with chives. Serves 4.

Mel's Christmas Morning Casserole

A whole Christmas day breakfast…baked and ready to go! To save fat, sodium and calories, you can substitute fat-free egg substitute for eggs, low-fat baking mix for regular, use low-fat or skim milk, omit up to ¼ cup cheese and rinse cooked Italian sausage in hot water, draining well before adding.

6 eggs, slightly beaten
½ c. shredded Cheddar cheese
½ c. shredded mozzarella cheese
1 T. dried parsley
1 T. dried, minced onion
1 t. dry mustard

1 t. oregano
1 lb. ground Italian sausage,
   browned and drained
1 c. biscuit baking mix
2 c. milk

On Christmas Eve, mix all ingredients and pour into a lightly greased lasagna pan. Cover and refrigerate overnight. On Christmas morning, bake, uncovered, at 350 degrees for one hour. Serves 10 to 12.

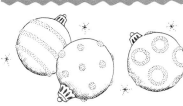

"EACH YEAR, FOR OUR CHRISTMAS DINNER TABLE, we put a special favor at each person's place that they get to keep. Usually it's a handmade ornament for the tree."

Jan Ertola

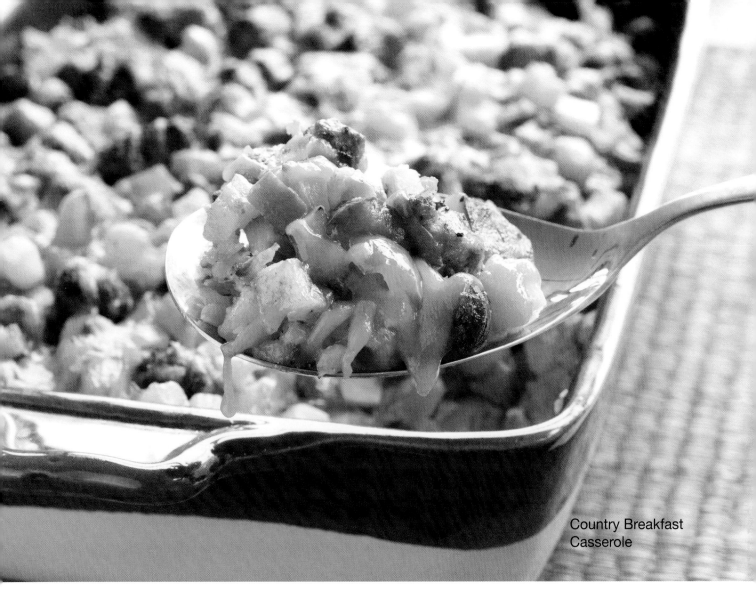

Country Breakfast
Casserole

Country Breakfast Casserole

1 T. oil
4 potatoes, diced
1½ t. salt, divided
1 red pepper, diced
1 green pepper, diced
1 onion, minced
8-oz. pkg. breakfast link sausage,
　chopped, browned and drained

1½ c. egg substitute
1 c. milk
2 T. all-purpose flour
½ t. pepper
1 c. shredded Cheddar cheese

*A small bag of frozen
seasoned hash brown
potatoes can be used
instead of potatoes,
onion and sweet peppers.*

　Heat oil in medium skillet. Fry potatoes and one teaspoon salt in oil until golden.
Add red and green peppers and onion; cook 5 minutes. Spoon into a greased
13"x9" casserole dish and top with sausage. Mix together egg substitute, milk,
flour, ½ teaspoon salt and pepper in mixing bowl. Pour egg mixture over potato
mixture; sprinkle with cheese. Bake, uncovered, at 350 degrees for 30 minutes.
Serves 8.

Escalloped Apples

An old-fashioned dish that goes great with any meal!

½ c. butter
2 c. fresh bread crumbs
5 tart apples, cored, peeled and sliced

½ c. sugar
½ t. cinnamon
¼ t. ground cloves

Melt butter in a saucepan. Add bread crumbs and toast lightly for about 2 minutes; set aside. Toss apples with sugar, cinnamon and cloves. In a greased 8"x8" baking dish, layer half of the apples and half of the toasted bread crumbs. Repeat with the remaining apples and bread crumbs. Bake at 325 degrees, covered, for 45 minutes or until apples are tender. Bake uncovered 15 more minutes. Serves 6.

Hot Fruit Compote

You can make this a day ahead...just bake before guests arrive.

15¼-oz. can pear halves, drained and cut into thick slices
15¼-oz. can peach halves, drained and cut into thick slices
2 (8-oz.) cans pineapple chunks, drained

11-oz. can mandarin oranges, drained
¾ c. brown sugar, packed
½ c. butter, melted
1½ T. cornstarch
1 t. curry powder

Combine fruit and place in a lightly greased 11"x7" baking dish. Combine remaining ingredients in a saucepan and heat, but do not to boil. Pour over fruit. Bake, uncovered, at 325 degrees for one hour. Serves 6.

Eggnog Fruit Salad

This salad can be made the night before.

1 c. chilled eggnog
10.8-oz. pkg. dry whipped topping mix
¼ t. nutmeg, freshly grated
16-oz. can sliced peaches, drained
15¼-oz. can pineapple tidbits, drained

1 apple, chopped
¼ c. maraschino cherries, drained and halved
½ c. fresh or frozen blueberries
½ c. walnuts, chopped

In a small bowl, combine eggnog, topping mix and nutmeg. Beat at high speed with an electric mixer, until soft peaks form (about 5 minutes). Combine fruits and nuts. Fold into eggnog mixture. Cover and chill in refrigerator for several hours or overnight. Stir gently before serving. Serves 6 to 8.

Escalloped Apples

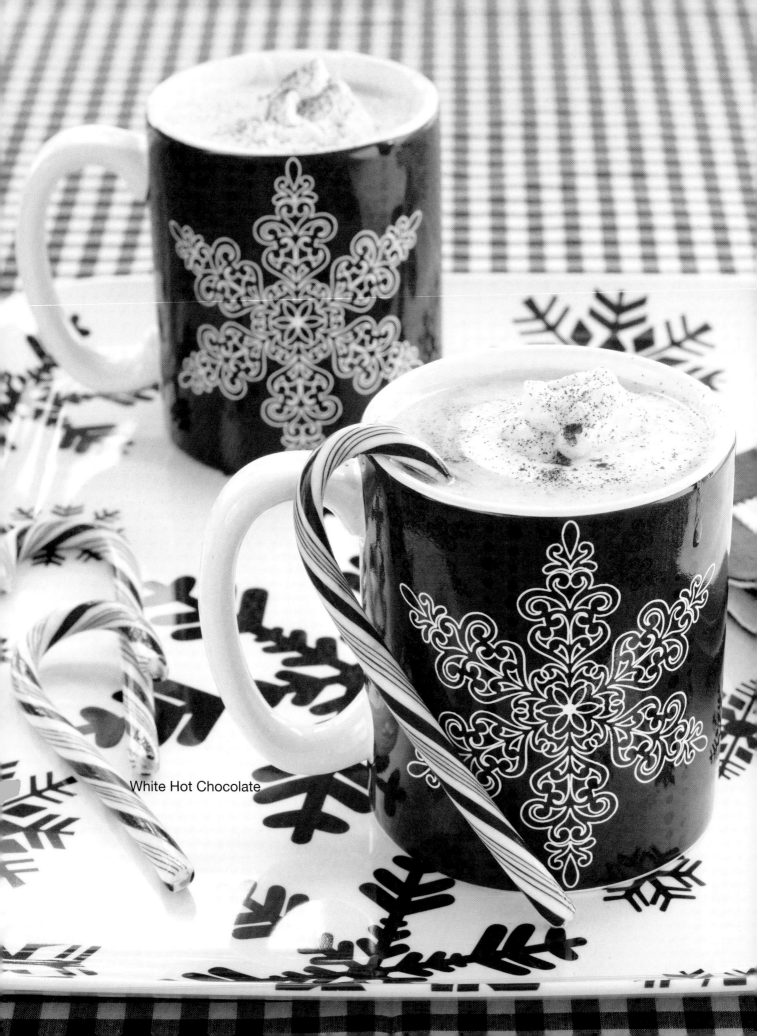

White Hot Chocolate

White Hot Chocolate

3 c. half-and-half, divided
⅔ c. white chocolate chips
3-inch cinnamon stick
⅛ t. nutmeg

1 t. vanilla extract
¼ t. almond extract
Garnish: whipped topping, cinnamon
    and candy canes

Serve in thick mugs with whipped cream, a dash of cinnamon or cocoa powder and a candy cane.

In a saucepan, combine ¼ cup half-and-half, white chocolate chips, cinnamon stick and nutmeg. Whisk over low heat until chips are melted. Remove cinnamon stick. Add remaining half-and-half. Whisk until heated throughout. Remove from heat and add vanilla and almond extracts. Garnish with whipped topping, cinnamon and candy canes. Makes 3 cups.

Tomato Cocktail

46-oz. can tomato juice
1½ T. lemon juice
1 t. sweet onion, grated

1 t. Worcestershire sauce
⅛ t. hot pepper sauce
Garnish: celery sticks

A great beverage to serve while you're putting the finishing touches on brunch.

Combine all ingredients together; chill. Serve each cocktail with a celery stick. Serves 6.

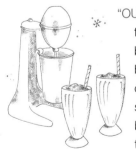

"OUR FAMILY HAS HAD A UNIQUE CHRISTMAS TRADITION for almost thirty years. Every Christmas morning after opening gifts, we share a big country breakfast complete with bacon, sausage, eggs, hash-browns, biscuits and homemade jelly. But the most important thing on our menu is chocolate milkshakes. That's right…chocolate milkshakes, made from scratch and served with breakfast. These have become such a tradition that our grown sons always call in advance to make sure we have ice cream, milk and chocolate syrup on hand to make the shakes. Christmas morning just would not be right in the Hurst household without the chocolate milkshakes!"

Brenda Hurst
Greenwood, IN

Penne Pasta with Tomatoes
(page 38)

In the Nick of time

These quick and easy main dishes will take the stress out
of holiday cooking...and keep your family full and happy!
From traditional recipes like Speedy Chicken Cordon Bleu and
Slow-Cooker Turkey & Dressing to crowd-pleasing Spaghetti
Casserole, you're sure to find a delicious...and fast...meal for
your Christmas get-together.

Penne Pasta with Tomatoes

(pictured on page 36)

"I love this pasta dish in the winter when practically everything is out of season and I'm bored with all my 'family standards.'"

Dana Stewart

6 T. olive oil, divided
1½ c. onion, chopped
1 t. garlic, minced
3 (28-oz.) cans Italian plum tomatoes, drained
2 t. fresh basil, chopped
1½ t. red pepper flakes
2 c. chicken broth

1 t. salt
1 t. pepper
16-oz. pkg. penne pasta, uncooked
2½ c. Havarti cheese, grated
½ c. Kalamata olives, sliced
½ c. grated Parmesan cheese
Garnish: ¼ c. fresh basil, chopped

Heat 3 tablespoons oil in a Dutch oven over medium-high heat. Sauté onion and garlic for 5 minutes. Add tomatoes, basil and red pepper flakes; bring to a boil. Mash tomatoes with the back of a spoon, and then add broth. Reduce heat and simmer one hour. Add salt and pepper; set aside. Cook pasta according to package directions; drain. Toss with remaining 3 tablespoons oil and combine with tomato sauce. Stir in Havarti cheese. Pour in an ungreased 13"x9" casserole dish. Top with olives, and then Parmesan cheese. Bake, uncovered, at 375 degrees for 30 minutes. Sprinkle fresh basil on top before serving. Serves 6 to 8.

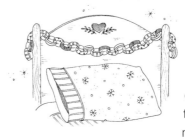

"I KNOW MY LOVE OF CHRISTMAS stems from the many wonderful memories I have of growing up in the small town of Northampton, Pennsylvania. During our childhood, my mom would help my brother and me create a Christmas countdown chain which we could hang on our bedposts and then faithfully remove a link each night until the last magical night. On December 6th, St. Nick always paid us a visit and left apples, oranges, nuts, a gingerbread man and a small toy. Around this time, we would eagerly help Dad in putting up the Christmas decorations, complete with trains, houses, trees and people ice skating on a little lake. It seemed waiting another year was so long until we could once again repeat our ever-anticipated traditions."

Kristen Berke,
Walnutport, PA

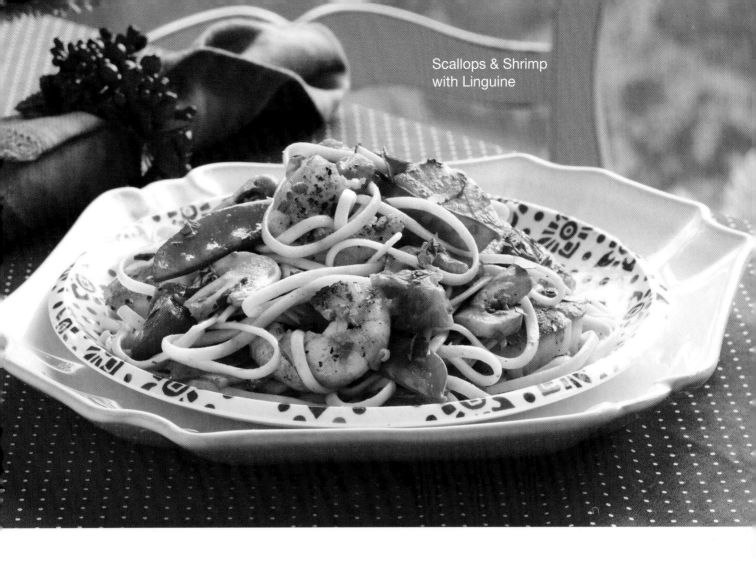

Scallops & Shrimp with Linguine

3 T. butter or margarine, divided
3 T. olive oil, divided
1 lb. uncooked large shrimp, peeled
　　and cleaned
3 cloves garlic, minced and divided
1 lb. uncooked fresh sea scallops
8 oz. pkg. mushrooms, sliced
2 c. snow peas, trimmed

2 tomatoes, chopped
½ c. green onion, chopped
1 t. salt
½ t. red pepper flakes
¼ c. fresh parsley, chopped
2 T. fresh basil, chopped
10 oz. linguine, cooked and kept warm
Parmesan cheese

Everyone will love this!

　　Heat one tablespoon each of butter and olive oil in a large skillet over medium-high heat. Add shrimp and half of garlic; cook 2 to 3 minutes or until shrimp turn pink. Remove shrimp from skillet; keep warm. Repeat procedure with scallops. Heat remaining one tablespoon each of butter and oil in same skillet over medium heat. Add mushrooms, snow peas, tomatoes, green onion, salt, pepper, parsley and basil; cook 4 to 5 minutes. In a large bowl, combine linguine, mushroom mixture, shrimp and scallops; toss well. Serve with Parmesan cheese. Serves 8.

Spicy Tex-Mex Chicken

6 boneless, skinless chicken breasts
2 T. fresh lime juice
½ t. salt
¼ t. cayenne pepper
⅓ c. olive oil, divided
1 red onion, chopped
1 red pepper, chopped

1 yellow pepper, chopped
1 clove garlic, minced
¼ c. plus 2 T. fresh cilantro, chopped
6 to 8 ripe tomatoes, sliced
2 c. shredded Monterey Jack cheese
Garnish: cilantro sprig and lime slices

Place chicken breasts between wax paper, pound until slightly flat. In small bowl, combine lime juice, salt and cayenne pepper. Add chicken to lime mixture; toss to coat. Let stand in marinade for 10 to 12 minutes. In large skillet, heat 2½ tablespoons olive oil over medium heat. Sauté chicken until lightly browned on both sides. Remove from pan. Pour in remaining olive oil; heat. Sauté onion, peppers and garlic until crisp-tender, about 4 to 5 minutes. Remove pan from heat and add cilantro. Mix well. Cover bottom of an ungreased 13"x9" baking pan with half of sliced tomatoes. Layer half of onion-pepper mixture over tomato slices. Sprinkle with one cup of cheese. Place chicken on top of cheese in a single layer. Top with remaining tomato slices and onion-pepper mixture. Bake, uncovered, at 400 degrees for 15 to 25 minutes or until chicken is tender. Sprinkle on remaining cheese and return to oven until cheese is melted. Garnish with cilantro and lime slices. Serves 6.

Speedy Chicken Cordon Bleu

...guiltless gourmet in a flash!

4 boneless, skinless chicken breasts
1 T. butter
¼ lb. cooked ham slices
1 c. shredded Swiss cheese, divided
½ c. white wine or chicken broth

10¾-oz. can cream of chicken soup
¾ c. water
8-oz. pkg. noodles, uncooked
Garnish: flat leaf parsley

In a skillet, cook chicken in butter for 6 to 8 minutes per side, or until done. Set pan aside. Wrap each chicken breast with one ham slice folded in half lengthwise. Transfer chicken to a lightly greased 13"x9" baking pan. Sprinkle with ½ cup cheese. Broil 3 to 5 minutes, or until cheese is melted and lightly golden.

Add wine or broth to skillet; cook over medium heat, using a spoon to scrape up drippings. Add cream of chicken soup, water and ½ cup cheese. Whisk until smooth.

Prepare noodles according to package directions. Serve sauce over chicken and noodles. Garnish with parsley. Serves 4.

Speedy Chicken Cordon Bleu

Chicken Tetrazzini

"This recipe came from one of my mother's best friends, 'Aunt' Cathryn. She always served it for holiday dinners and now my mother makes it for us. I have wonderful memories of 'Aunt' Cathryn; this dish brings her back for a while."

Debbie Musick
Yukon, OK

1 onion, minced
2 T. butter
2 (10¾-oz.) cans cream of mushroom soup
2 (10¾-oz.) cans cream of chicken soup
8-oz. pkg. sharp pasteurized process cheese spread
½ c. milk
½ c. water

1 t. curry powder
¼ t. dried thyme
⅛ t. dried basil
¼ t. dried oregano
2 (7-oz.) pkgs. spaghetti, cooked
5-lb. chicken, cooked and cubed
4-oz. jar pimentos
salt and pepper to taste
½ c. grated Parmesan cheese

Sauté onion in butter in a Dutch oven. Add soups, cheese spread, milk, water and spices. Add spaghetti to soup mixture; fold in chicken and pimentos. Add salt and pepper. Spoon into a lightly greased 13"x9" baking pan. Top with Parmesan cheese. Bake, uncovered, at 350 degrees for 45 minutes. Serves 6 to 8.

Nancy's Turkey Pie

A yummy main course that only needs a salad and a simple dessert for a complete meal.

½ c. butter, softened
1 c. sour cream
1 egg
1 c. all-purpose flour
1 t. salt
1 t. baking powder
½ t. dried sage
⅓ c. carrot, chopped

⅓ c. onion, chopped
⅓ c. green pepper, chopped
⅓ c. red pepper, chopped
⅓ c. celery, chopped
2 c. cooked turkey, chopped
10¾-oz. can cream of chicken soup
½ c. shredded Cheddar cheese

Combine butter, sour cream and egg. Beat with an electric mixer at medium speed until smooth. Add flour, salt, baking powder and sage; blend at low speed, mixing well. Spread batter evenly over the bottom and up the sides of an ungreased 9½" deep-dish pie plate. Mix together vegetables, turkey and soup; place into pie crust and sprinkle with Cheddar cheese. Bake at 375 degrees for one hour. Let stand 15 minutes before serving. Serves 6.

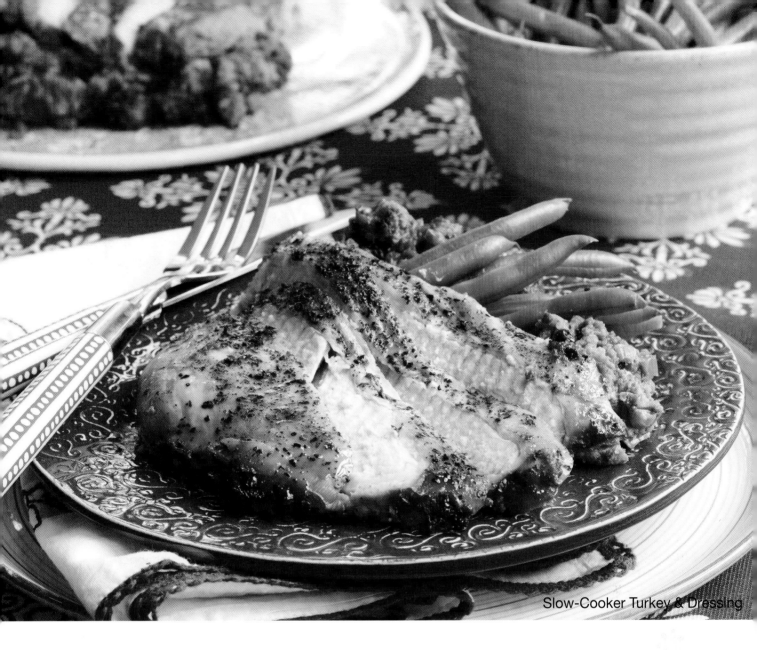

Slow-Cooker Turkey & Dressing

Slow-Cooker Turkey & Dressing

8-oz. pkg. stuffing mix
½ c. hot water
2 T. butter, softened
1 onion, chopped
½ c. celery, chopped

¼ c. sweetened dried cranberries
3-lb. boneless turkey breast, cut in half
¼ t. dried basil
½ t. salt
½ t. pepper

"I like to start this before I leave for work...slice and serve when I get home!"

Geneva Rogers
Gillette, WY

Coat a 4½-quart slow cooker with non-stick vegetable spray; spoon in dry stuffing mix. Add water, butter, onion, celery and cranberries; mix well. Sprinkle turkey breast pieces with basil, salt and pepper and place over stuffing mixture. Cook on high setting, covered, for one hour; reduce to low setting for 5 hours. Remove turkey, slice and set aside. Gently stir the stuffing and allow to sit for 5 minutes. Transfer stuffing to a platter and top with sliced turkey. Serves 4 to 6.

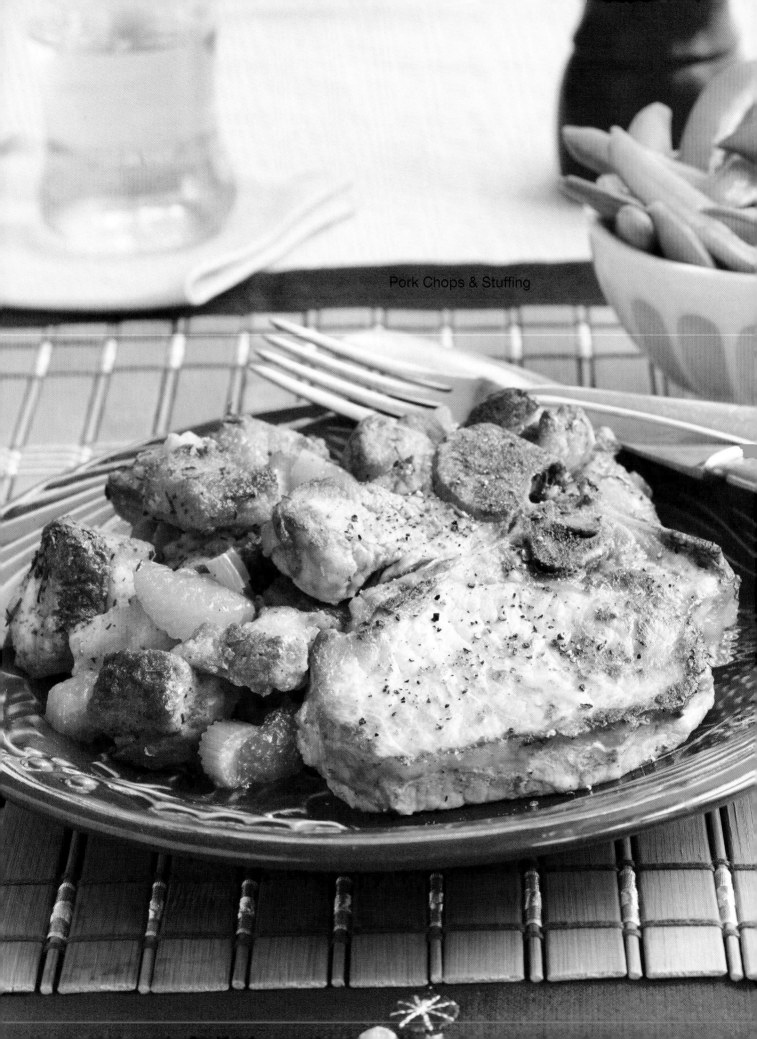

Pork Chops & Stuffing

Pork Chops & Stuffing

6 pork chops
1 T. shortening
1 t. salt, divided
1 c. celery, chopped
¾ c. onion, chopped
¼ c. butter, melted
¼ c. brown sugar, packed

5 c. bread, cubed
1 egg, beaten
1 t. dried sage
½ t. dried thyme
⅛ t. pepper
11-oz. can mandarin oranges, drained

In a skillet, brown pork chops in shortening; remove to a platter and season with ½ teaspoon salt. Lightly brown vegetables in butter in a skillet; stir in brown sugar. Combine bread cubes with egg, sage, thyme, pepper and remaining ½ teaspoon salt; add to vegetables. Stir in oranges and mix gently. Spoon stuffing into the center of an ungreased 3½ quart casserole dish. Place pork chops around the stuffing and cover with foil. Bake at 350 degrees for 30 minutes; uncover and bake 30 more minutes. Serves 6.

"I've been making this recipe for twenty-eight years and it's still one of my favorites! The mandarin oranges and brown sugar make it special."

*Barbara Schmeckpeper
Elwood, IL*

Old-Fashioned Pork Chop Bake

6 pork chops
salt and pepper to taste
1 onion, sliced into 6 thin slices
¾ c. long-cooking rice, uncooked

1 green pepper, sliced into 6 rings
28-oz. can peeled whole tomatoes
15-oz. can tomato sauce

Rinse pork chops and pat dry. Lightly salt and pepper both sides of each pork chop and place in a single layer in a baking pan lightly coated with a non-stick vegetable spray. Place one onion slice and 2 tablespoons of rice on each pork chop. Add one green pepper ring on top of each rice-topped pork chop. In a mixing bowl, combine undrained whole tomatoes and tomato sauce. Pour over the top of pork chops, covering all rice. Cover and bake at 350 degrees for 1½ hours. Serves 4 to 6.

An easy one-dish recipe that can be made ahead of time, refrigerated and put in the oven before taking it to your next potluck.

A QUICK & EASY SEASONING MIX is six parts salt to one part pepper. Keep it handy in a large shaker close to the stove.

Ham Steak with Cider Glaze

This is a tasty, time-saving entrée!

1 to 2-lb. ham steak
1 c. apple cider
¼ c. brown sugar, packed

¼ c. Dijon mustard
¼ c. honey
½ t. liquid smoke

Place ham steak in an ungreased 13"x9" baking pan; set aside. Mix remaining ingredients together; pour over ham steak. Bake, uncovered, at 350 degrees for 30 minutes, basting often. Serves 6.

Reuben Casserole

A favorite sandwich turned into a casserole!

2 (14.4-oz.) cans sauerkraut, drained
2 (12-oz.) cans corned beef, crumbled
2 (8-oz.) pkg. shredded Swiss cheese
1 c. mayonnaise

8-oz. bottle Thousand Island dressing
¼ c. butter, melted
½ c. soft rye bread crumbs
½ t. caraway seeds

Layer sauerkraut, corned beef and half the cheese in a lightly greased 13"×9" baking dish. Mix mayonnaise and dressing together; pour over corned beef mixture. Sprinkle with remaining cheese, mix together butter and bread crumbs; sprinkle over top. Sprinkle with caraway seeds. Bake at 375 degrees for 25 minutes. Serves 8 to 10.

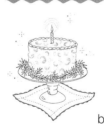

"TEACHING YOUNG CHILDREN THE REAL MEANING of Christmas, when Santa Claus is so prominent, was a goal that my husband and I wanted to accomplish with our two young sons. We began this ritual the Christmas that they were one and three years old. We baked a small cake and placed a candle on it. We sang 'Happy Birthday' to Jesus and blew out the candle before viewing the Christmas tree and the presents. It became an annual tradition until they were young teens…they grew up knowing the true priority of the holiday in our home. Our sons are now 22 and 24 years old and still talk about the 'Baby Jesus birthday cake' when they were small and the meaning that it had to them. I guess we accomplished our goal!"

Debby Rapp
Irmo, SC

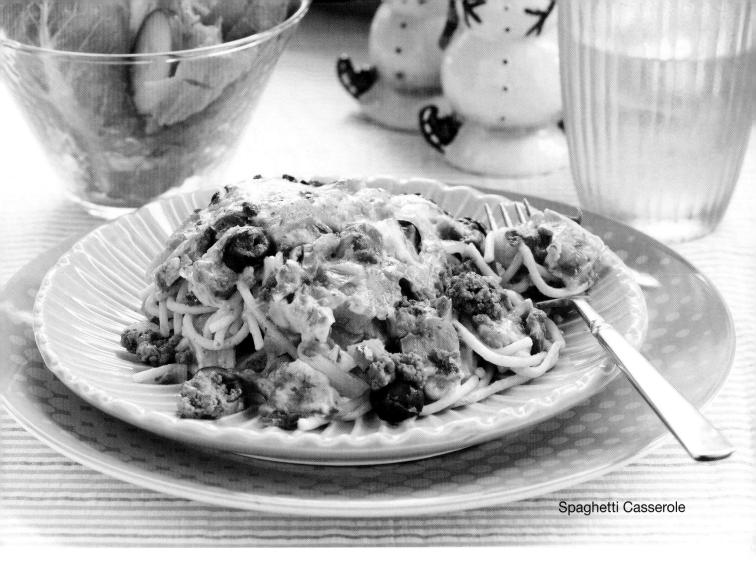

Spaghetti Casserole

Spaghetti Casserole

1 c. onion, chopped
1 c. green pepper, chopped
1 T. butter
28-oz. can tomatoes undrained
4-oz. can mushrooms, drained
2 (2¼-oz.) cans sliced, black olives, drained
2 t. dried oregano
½ t. salt
½ t. pepper
1 lb. ground beef, browned and drained
12 oz. spaghetti, cooked and drained
2 c. shredded Cheddar cheese
10¾-oz. can condensed cream of mushroom soup
¼ c. water
¼ c. grated Parmesan cheese

Feeds a crowd and can be made ahead and refrigerated before baking.

In a large skillet, sauté onion and green pepper in butter until tender. Add undrained tomatoes, mushrooms, olives, oregano, salt and pepper. Add ground beef and simmer, uncovered, for 10 minutes. Place half of the spaghetti in a greased 13"×9" baking dish. Top with half of the vegetable mixture. Sprinkle with one cup of Cheddar cheese. Repeat layers. Combine soup and water; stir until smooth. Pour over casserole. Sprinkle with Parmesan cheese. Bake, uncovered, at 350 degrees for 30 to 55 minutes, or until heated through. Serves 12.

Lasagna Rolls

"When I was little, I remember standing on a chair next to my mom by the stove. I watched her roll these little bundles of noodles, meat and cheese and I would beg her to let me roll up a few. She always let me try some, and even though they were nothing compared to hers, she made me feel like they were perfect."

*Kelli Keeton
Delaware, OH*

1 lb. mild or sage bulk sausage, cooked, crumbled and drained
8-oz. plus 3-oz. pkgs. cream cheese
1 green onion bunch, chopped
1 green pepper, diced
26-oz. jar spaghetti sauce
16 lasagna noodles, uncooked
1½ c. mozzarella cheese, shredded

Combine sausage and cream cheese in the skillet where sausage was browned. Cook over low heat until cream cheese melts. Stir in onion and green pepper; remove from heat. Spread half the spaghetti sauce in the bottom of an ungreased 13"x9" baking pan; set aside. Cook lasagna noodles according to package directions; remove from heat and leave in water. Lay one noodle flat on a cutting board and spoon one to 2 tablespoons of sausage mixture at one end of the noodle. Roll the noodle and place in pan. Repeat with remaining noodles. Pour reserved sauce over top of rolls; top with mozzarella. Bake, uncovered, at 350 degrees for 15 to 20 minutes, or until cheese has melted. Serves 8.

Santa Fe Pie

Just slice and eat!

11-oz. pkg. pie crust mix
2¾ t. chili powder, divided
½ lb. ground beef
½ c. onion, chopped
1 c. water
1½ t. taco sauce
3 T. taco seasoning mix
⅓ c. ripe olives, pitted and chopped
½ c. shredded Monterey Jack cheese
½ c. shredded Cheddar cheese
2 T. chopped green chiles
3 large eggs
1 c. plus 2 T. milk
1 T. all-purpose flour
⅛ t. salt
⅛ t. cayenne pepper

Prepare pie crust according to package directions using entire bag, and adding ¾ teaspoon chili powder to mixture. Roll out dough and place in a pie pan, bake as directed. Brown ground beef and onion in a skillet, draining excess fat. Add water, taco sauce, taco seasoning mix and 1½ teaspoons chili powder to beef mixture; simmer 15 to 20 minutes. Blend in olives; remove from heat. Sprinkle half of each cheese over baked pie crust. On top of cheese, layer beef mixture, remaining cheese and chiles. In a large bowl, beat eggs lightly; add milk. In a separate bowl, combine flour, salt, cayenne pepper and remaining ½ teaspoon of chili powder. Add a small amount of the egg mixture to the flour mixture and whip until smooth. Add flour mixture to remaining egg mixture, blending well. Pour mixture over pie and bake at 375 degrees for 30 to 35 minutes. Serves 8.

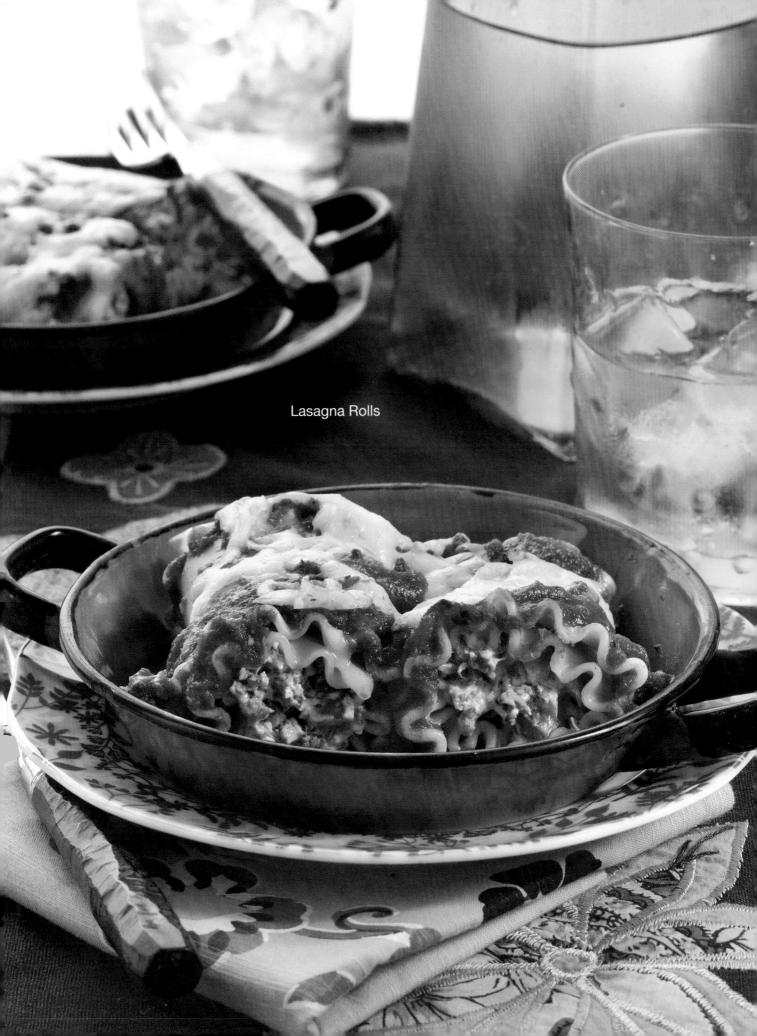

Lasagna Rolls

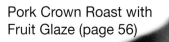
Pork Crown Roast with
Fruit Glaze (page 56)

Fabulous Feast

Turn to these recipes to prepare a meal of classic holiday favorites for your friends and family. Choose from a variety of main dishes, such as Pork Crown Roast with Fruit Glaze and New England Turkey & Stuffing, as well as side dishes like Holiday Sweet Potatoes and Cornbread Dressing. And you can't beat our Old-Fashioned Eggnog!

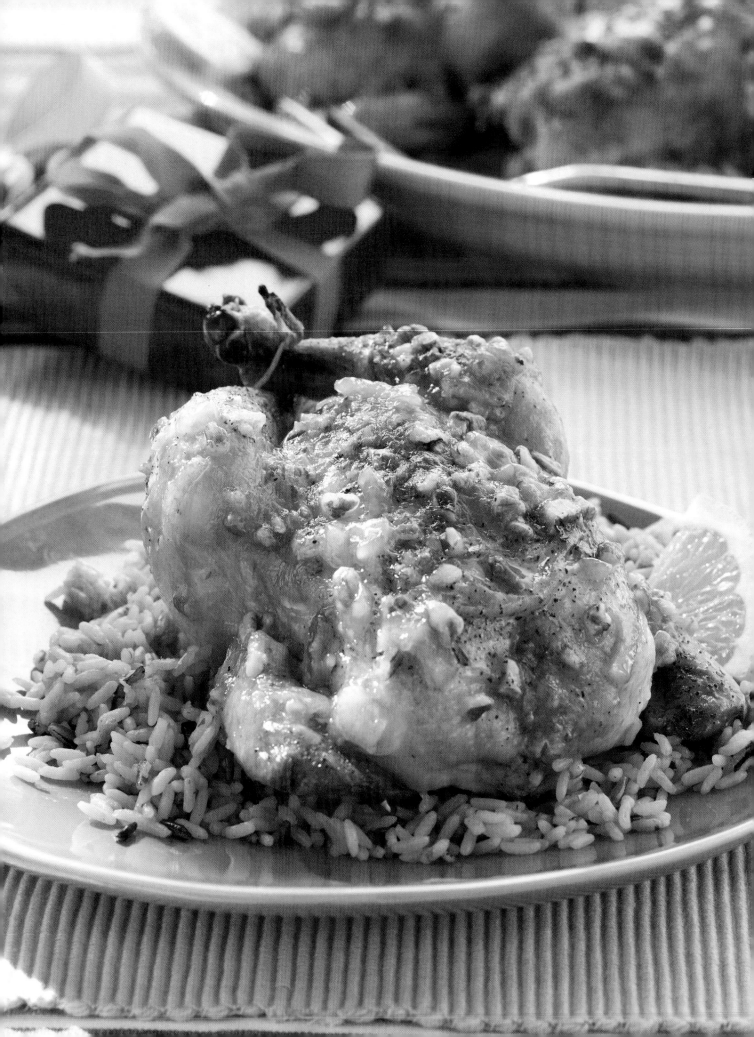

Orange-Pecan Cornish Hens

½ c. butter, melted and divided
4 (1½ lb.) Cornish game hens
1 t. salt
1 t. pepper
½ c. orange marmalade

¼ c. orange juice
1 t. cornstarch
½ c. chopped pecans
Garnish: orange slices

Great to make during the busy holiday season and perfect served with wild rice.

Spread one tablespoon butter equally over hens; season with salt and pepper. Tie ends of legs together, if desired, and place on a lightly greased rack in a roasting pan. Bake at 400 degrees for 1 hour or until a meat thermometer inserted into meaty part of thigh registers 180 degrees. In a saucepan, blend together remaining butter, marmalade and orange juice; bring to a boil. In a bowl, blend together a small amount of cornstarch and water, slowly adding remaining cornstarch until mixture thickens. Slowly add cornstarch mixture to marmalade mixture, stirring constantly; add pecans. Place hens in a greased 15"x10" jelly-roll pan. Pour glaze over chicken and bake for 10 more minutes or until glaze begins to turn golden. Garnish with orange slices. Serves 4.

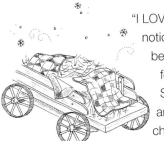

"I LOVE CHRISTMAS! I LOVE EVERYTHING ABOUT IT. But I've noticed in the last few years that a lot of the holiday traditions have been forgotten. So last year I planned a Christmas caroling hayride for my family. Dressed up in his Santa Claus suit, my husband Steve hitched up his wagon to the tractor. We loaded it with hay and cozy quilts and off we went…Steve, myself, our three grown children, our four grandchildren, my sister and her son, and my 70-year-old mother. We sang our hearts out as we rode along. We forgot the words to some of the carols, so we just made them up as we went. It was very cold, but not one person complained…such a wonderful, magical night! At the end of the ride we came back in, gathered around the fireplace and talked about all of our Christmas plans. My children are already calling me asking to do it again this year. I do believe this is going to be one of our very own holiday traditions."

Debra Collins
Gaylesville, AL

New England Turkey & Stuffing

Try using a variety of breads in your stuffing.

2½ loaves day-old bread, torn into
   1-inch pieces
17½ lb. turkey, thawed if frozen
1½ lbs. ground pork sausage,
   browned and drained
2 eggs
2 c. oil
3 c. onion, minced

½ c. celery, diced
3 T. poultry seasoning
1½ T. salt
½ t. pepper
½ c. butter, melted
Garnish: red grapes, pears, fresh
   rosemary sprigs

Place bread in a large bowl; set aside. Remove giblets and neck from thawed turkey; reserve neck for another recipe. Place giblets in a medium saucepan; add water to cover. Simmer gently over medium heat for 1½ hours; drain. Place giblets and remaining ingredients except turkey and butter in a food processor or meat grinder. Process until finely chopped. Pour over bread; mix with hands until bread is coated. Set aside. Rinse turkey and pat dry with paper towels. Stuff turkey with bread mixture; place turkey in a lightly greased roasting pan. Cover turkey with cheesecloth that has been soaked with melted butter. Bake at 450 degrees for 30 minutes. Reduce heat to 350 degrees and bake for 12 to 14 more minutes per pound for remaining time; baste with melted butter every 30 minutes. Remove cheesecloth 30 minutes before turkey is done to allow browning. Garnish with red grapes, pears and fresh rosemary sprigs. Serves 20 to 24.

"THIS STUFFING WAS ALWAYS A THANKSGIVING TRADITION at our home…my dad would grind everything together in a hand-cranked meat grinder. Now I prepare it, and I wouldn't have it any other way!"

Amber Erskine
Hartland, VT

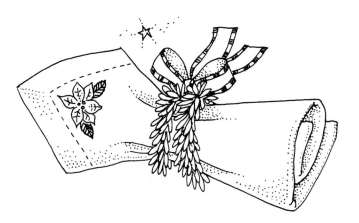

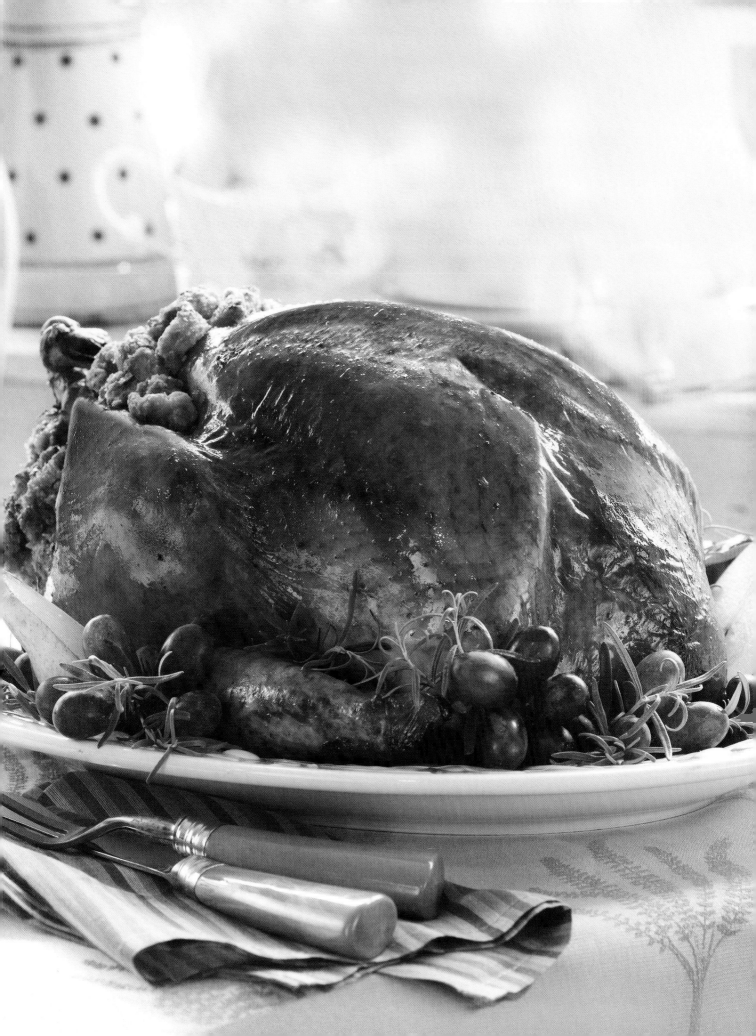

Pork Crown Roast with Fruit Glaze

(pictured on page 50)

The crowning glory of your Christmas table.

1½ t. fennel seed, crushed
1½ t. onion powder
2 t. salt

1 t. pepper
8-lb. pork crown roast
vegetable oil

Combine first 4 ingredients in a small bowl. Rub this mixture on all sides of the roast, cover and refrigerate overnight. Brush the roast lightly with oil and insert a meat thermometer. Cover the bone ends with foil and place roast on a lightly greased rack in a roasting pan. Bake at 425 degrees for 30 minutes; reduce temperature to 325 degrees and bake 1½ hours, or until meat thermometer reads 165 degrees. Allow to stand for 10 minutes before carving. Garnish with Fruit Glaze. Serves 8 to 10.

Fruit Glaze:

½ c. dried apricot halves
½ c. dried peach halves
¾ c. apple juice, divided
¼ t. cardamom or nutmeg

2 t. cornstarch
1 c. seedless green grapes
1 c. seedless red grapes

In a 1½-quart casserole dish, combine fruit, ½ cup of apple juice and cardamom. Cover casserole dish and microwave on high power for 6 minutes or until fruit begins to fill out. In a separate bowl, combine cornstarch and remaining apple juice, stirring well. Add to fruit mixture and microwave on high power for 2 minutes, or until thick. Add grapes and stir gently.

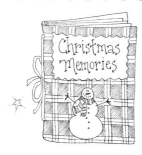

EACH YEAR STARTING DECEMBER 1ST, WE HAVE A MEMORY BOOK that we set out for family and guests who come to our home during the holidays. They write about anything they would like...the weather, births, graduations and family events. We've found it's a great way to keep track of all that's happened throughout the year. Even the little ones add to the book...a chocolate handprint or an outline of their hand or foot is so sweet.

Patty Moyer
Milan, OH

Honey-Roasted Pork Loin and Harvest Dressing (page 62)

Honey-Roasted Pork Loin

2 to 3-lb. boneless pork loin roast
¼ c. honey
2 T. Dijon mustard
2 T. mixed or black peppercorns, crushed

½ t. dried thyme
½ t. salt
Garnish: fresh thyme sprigs

A wonderful, old-fashioned main dish when served with homemade stuffing or noodles.

Place roast on a lightly greased rack in a shallow roasting pan. Combine honey and remaining ingredients; brush half of mixture over roast. Bake at 325 degrees for one hour; brush with remaining honey mixture. Bake 20 more minutes, or until thermometer inserted in thickest portion registers 160 degrees. Garnish with fresh thyme sprigs and serve with Harvest Dressing (recipe on page 62). Serves 8.

Stuffed Beef Tenderloin

Stuffed with spinach and cheese, this roast is so tender you can cut it with a fork!

10-oz. pkg. frozen chopped spinach, thawed and drained
¼ c. dried currants
3 oz. Muenster cheese, grated
1 egg
2 t. balsamic vinegar

1 clove garlic, minced
½ t. salt
½ t. pepper
6-lb. beef tenderloin, butterflied
⅓ c. beef broth

Place spinach in a large mixing bowl and add currants, cheese, egg, vinegar, garlic, salt and pepper; blend well. Open and flatten tenderloin and spoon spinach mixture down the center of the meat. Bring long sides of meat together; cover filling and tie with butcher's twine at one-inch intervals. Place roast in a lightly greased 13"x9" baking pan; pour beef broth over roast. Bake, uncovered, at 425 degrees for 10 minutes. Reduce heat to 350 degrees and bake 25 minutes more for rare or 35 minutes more for medium-rare. Let stand for 15 minutes before carving. Serve with Horseradish Sauce. Serves 8 to 10.

Horseradish Sauce

Low-fat and tasty!

3 T. prepared horseradish
1 c. low-fat mayonnaise

1 t. Dijon mustard

Combine ingredients and refrigerate until needed. Makes about one cup.

Hearty Beef Brisket

Slow-cooking makes the meat tender. Let it roast while you wrap packages or trim the tree!

16-oz. can stewed tomatoes, chopped
8-oz. can sauerkraut
1 c. applesauce

2 T. brown sugar, packed
3½-lb. beef brisket
2 T. cold water
2 T. cornstarch

Combine tomatoes, sauerkraut, applesauce and brown sugar in a Dutch oven. Bring to a boil; then reduce heat. Add brisket, spooning tomato mixture over top; cover and simmer over low heat 2 to 3 hours, or until meat is tender. When brisket is thoroughly cooked, remove from Dutch oven and set aside. In a small bowl, combine cold water and cornstarch, whisking well. Blend into tomato mixture in Dutch oven. Cook until mixture thickens; continue to cook for 2 more minutes. Spread sauce over top of brisket, reserving some as gravy. Serves 6 to 8.

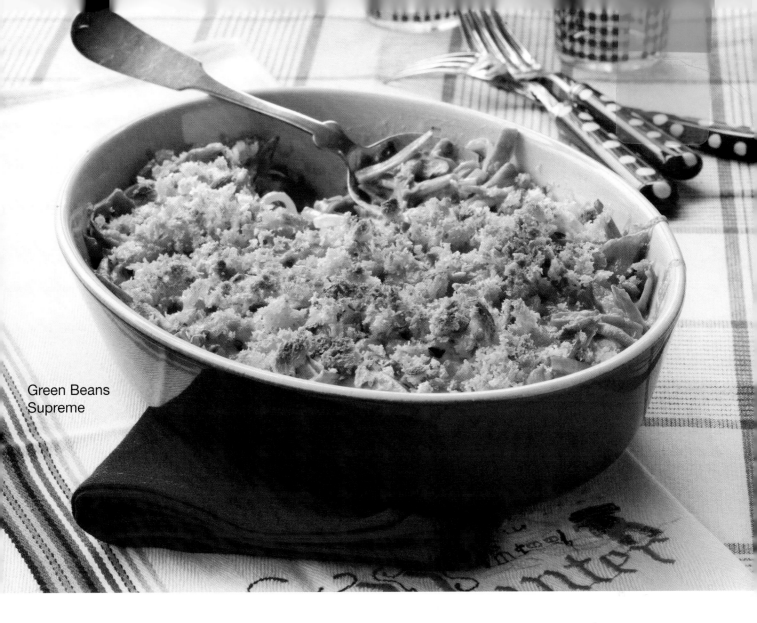

Green Beans
Supreme

Green Beans Supreme

1 onion, sliced
1 T. fresh parsley, snipped
3 T. butter, divided
2 T. all-purpose flour
½ t. lemon zest
½ t. salt
⅛ t. pepper

½ c. milk
8-oz. container sour cream
16-oz. pkg. frozen French-style
   green beans, cooked
½ c. shredded Cheddar cheese
¼ c. fresh bread crumbs

This isn't your usual green bean casserole. Loaded with cheese and sour cream, it will be your new favorite!

Cook onion slices and parsley in 2 tablespoons butter until onion is tender. Blend in flour, lemon zest, salt and pepper. Stir in milk; heat until thick and bubbly. Add sour cream and beans; heat through. Spoon into an ungreased 2-quart baking dish; sprinkle with cheese. Melt remaining butter and toss with bread crumbs; sprinkle on top of beans. Broil 3 to 4 inches from heat source for 3 minutes, or until golden. Serves 4 to 6.

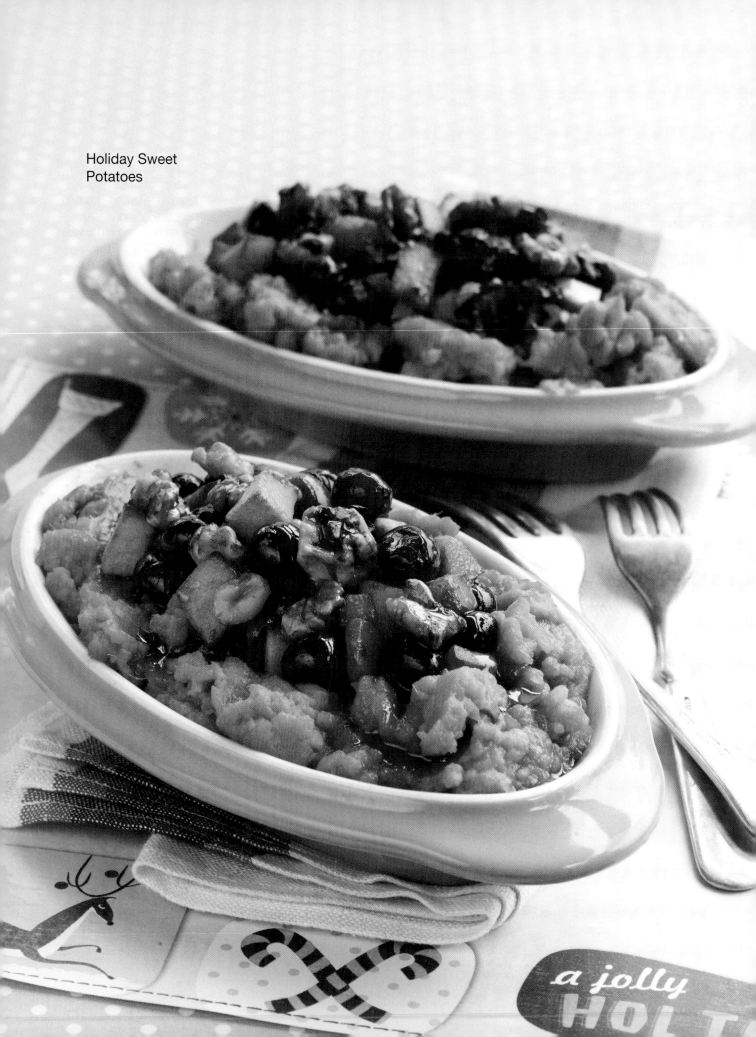

Holiday Sweet
Potatoes

Holiday Sweet Potatoes

2 (29-oz.) cans cut sweet potatoes
   in syrup, drained
⅔ c. brown sugar, packed
¼ t. salt
2 c. fresh cranberries
1 apple, peeled, cored and chopped

⅓ c. sugar
¼ c. plus 2 T. water, divided
1 c. chopped walnuts
½ c. brown sugar, packed
2 T. butter

Combine first 3 ingredients in a bowl. Mash until smooth. Spoon into a lightly greased 11"x7" baking dish.

Stir together cranberries, apple, sugar and ¼ cup water in a saucepan. Cook over medium heat for 8 to 10 minutes, or until cranberries burst. Add walnuts; stir well. Spoon over sweet potatoes in dish.

Combine brown sugar, remaining 2 tablespoons water and butter in a small saucepan. Bring to a boil; boil, stirring constantly, 2 minutes. Pour over cranberries and sweet potatoes. Bake, uncovered, at 350 degrees for 15 minutes, or just until heated through. Serves 8.

This dish combines your sweet potatoes and cranberry sauce into one scoop. For individual casseroles, spoon sweet potato filling into small baking dishes or ramekins. Top evenly with cranberry mixture and brown sugar syrup. Bake at 350 degrees for 10 minutes, or until thoroughly heated.

Creamy Macaroni & Cheese

6 T. butter, divided
3 T. all-purpose flour
2 c. milk
8-oz. pkg. cream cheese, cubed
2 c. shredded Cheddar cheese
2 t. spicy brown mustard

½ t. salt
¼ t. pepper
8-oz. pkg. elbow macaroni,
   cooked
¾ c. bread crumbs
2 T. fresh parsley, minced

The spicy brown mustard gives this a little kick!

Melt 4 tablespoons butter in a large saucepan. Stir in flour until smooth. Gradually add milk; bring to a boil. Cook and stir for 2 minutes. Reduce heat; add cheeses, mustard, salt and pepper. Stir until cheese is melted and sauce is smooth. Add macaroni to cheese sauce; stir to coat. Transfer to a lightly greased 3-quart casserole dish. In a small saucepan, melt the remaining 2 tablespoons butter and toss with bread crumbs and parsley; sprinkle over macaroni. Bake, uncovered, at 400 degrees for 15 to 20 minutes, or until golden. Serves 6 to 8.

SAVE TIME…prepare holiday foods that can be made ahead, and if friends and family volunteer to bring a dish, let them!

Wild Rice Casserole

A warm and hearty side dish.

1 to 1¼ c. wild rice, uncooked
1 t. salt
½ c. butter
1 onion, finely chopped

1 lb. sliced mushrooms
½ c. slivered almonds
1 to 2 c. chicken broth
Garnish: sliced almonds

Place rice in a saucepan, adding enough water to cover; soak overnight. When ready to prepare, add salt to rice and water; simmer for 45 to 50 minutes. Drain rice and sauté in butter with onion and mushrooms until onion is soft, but not brown. Mix cooked rice mixture, almonds and one cup chicken broth in a large casserole dish. Cover tightly and bake at 325 degrees for one hour. If it starts to dry out, add more broth. Garnish with sliced almonds. Serves 8 to 10.

Cornbread Dressing

A snap to prepare, and it's a really tasty change from the more traditional bread stuffing.

4 c. cornbread, cubed
2 c. bread, cubed
½ c. green pepper, chopped
1 c. onion, chopped
½ c. celery, chopped

2 (10-oz.) cans chicken broth
2 eggs, beaten
2 T. dried sage
salt and pepper to taste

Lay cornbread and bread on parchment paper overnight to dry. When ready to prepare dressing, combine cornbread and bread cubes with remaining ingredients; blend well. Spoon into a greased 9"x9" baking pan and bake, uncovered, at 350 degrees for 45 minutes. Serves 6.

Harvest Dressing
(pictured on page 57)

Not your ordinary dressing…delicious with pork or poultry!

2 apples, cored and chopped
½ c. golden raisins
3 T. butter
½ c. walnuts or pecans, coarsely
   chopped

¼ c. brown sugar, packed
2 c. whole-wheat bread, cubed
½ c. apple juice or cider

Sauté apples and raisins in butter; add nuts, brown sugar and bread cubes. Add enough juice to moisten to desired texture. Bake, uncovered, in a 1½-quart casserole dish at 400 degrees for 18 minutes. Serves 4.

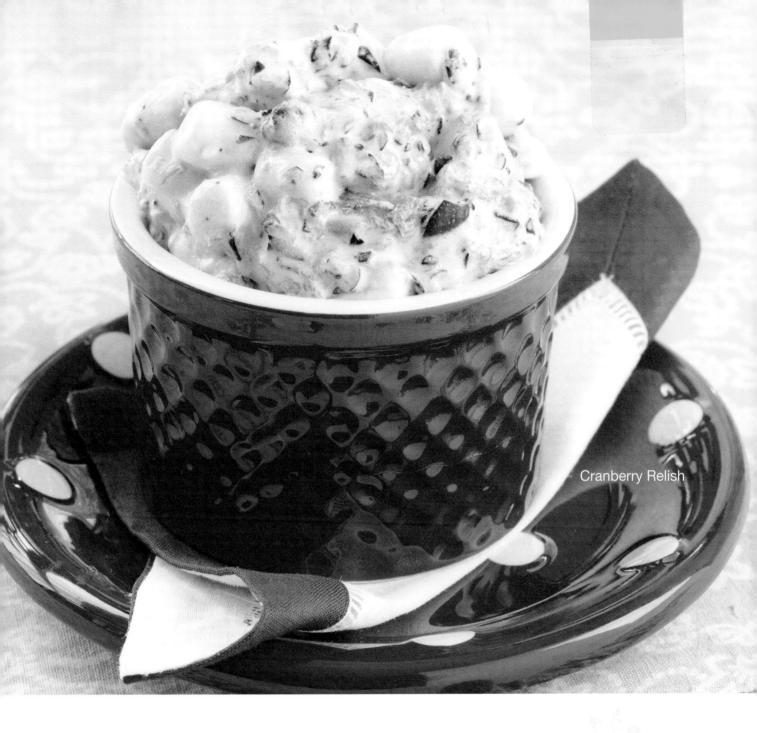

Cranberry Relish

Cranberry Relish

8-oz. can crushed pineapple with juice
4 c. mini marshmallows
2 c. fresh cranberries, ground

1 c. sugar
2 c. whipped cream

An easy make-ahead dish!

Pour crushed pineapple with juice over marshmallows; let stand overnight. Mix cranberries and sugar; let stand overnight. In the morning, combine mixtures and fold in whipped cream. Serves 6.

Old-Fashioned
Fruitcake

Old-Fashioned Fruitcake

1 c. butter, softened
2½ c. sugar
6 eggs
2 t. brandy flavoring
4 c. all-purpose flour
1½ t. cinnamon
1 t. nutmeg
1 t. salt

1½ lbs. ready mix candied fruit
1 lb. seedless raisins
¾ lb. candied pineapple
¾ lb. whole candied cherries
2 c. pecan halves
Garnish: light corn syrup and pecan
  halves

What would Christmas be without a fruitcake? You'll like this one.

In a large bowl, beat butter, sugar and eggs with an electric mixer until fluffy, adding eggs one at a time until yolk disappears. Stir in flavoring. Sift together next 4 ingredients and mix thoroughly with butter and egg mixture. Work the fruit and nuts into batter with hands. Grease and flour a 10" tube pan. Fill pan ⅔ full with batter. Bake at 275 degrees for 3 hours. One-half hour before cake is done, brush top with corn syrup. Decorate with pecan halves and finish baking. Cool. If desired, place cake, wrapped in a wine-soaked cloth, in an airtight container. Store in a cool place for several weeks; this blends and mellows the cake. Serves 16.

Maple-Spice Pecan Pie

9-inch pie crust
3 eggs
¾ c. brown sugar, packed
1 c. maple syrup
3 T. butter, melted

1 T. lemon juice
1 t. vanilla extract
¾ t. nutmeg
¼ t. salt
1½ c. chopped pecans

The sweet maple flavor makes this pie special.

Place pie crust in a pie pan; set aside. In a large bowl, whisk eggs and brown sugar. Add maple syrup, butter, lemon juice, vanilla, nutmeg and salt; whisk to blend. Add nuts and pour into pie crust. Bake at 450 degrees for 10 minutes. Lower temperature to 350 degrees and bake an additional 30 to 35 minutes. Serves 8.

Christmas Plum Pudding

Prepare two weeks before Christmas Day.

½ c. dates, chopped
½ c. golden raisins
¾ c. brandy or apple juice, divided
2 c. all-purpose flour
1 t. baking soda
1 t. cinnamon
½ t. nutmeg
½ t. salt

1 c. butter, softened
1 c. dark brown sugar, packed
½ c. molasses
3 eggs
¼ c. milk
1 c. almonds, slivered
⅔ c. sweetened flaked coconut
1 c. bread crumbs

Soak dates and raisins in half cup brandy or apple juice overnight. Sift together next 5 ingredients. In a separate bowl, beat together butter and brown sugar. Add molasses and eggs to butter mixture; beat in flour mixture and milk alternately. Add ¼ cup brandy or apple juice. Stir in dates, raisins, almonds, coconut and bread crumbs. Pour into a greased 6-cup mold. Cover with buttered wax paper, tie with string and cover again with foil. Place on rack in a large pot. Add water to just below rack. Cover and steam 3 hours. Keep adding water to pan so it does not dry out . Cool and store at room temperature until Christmas Day. To serve, steam 2 hours, remove and cool 10 minutes. Loosen edges and invert onto plate. Serve with Brandy Butter. Serves 6 to 8.

Brandy Butter:

1 c. powdered sugar
½ c. butter, softened
1 T. brandy or apple juice

1 T. rum or 1 t. rum extract plus
2 t. water

Beat sugar and butter. Beat in remaining ingredients and chill.

Old-Fashioned Eggnog

When was the last time you had real eggnog?

6 eggs
1 c. sugar
½ t. salt
1 qt. light cream, divided

1 c. golden rum or 1 T. rum extract plus
1 c. water
Garnish: nutmeg, cinnamon sticks

Beat eggs until light and foamy. Add sugar and salt, beating until thick. Combine egg mixture and 2 cups light cream in a large saucepan. Stirring constantly, cook over low heat until mixture coats the back of a metal spoon and reaches 160 degrees on a candy thermometer. Remove from heat. Stir in remaining light cream; add rum or extract and water. Chill several hours. Sprinkle with nutmeg before serving. Garnish with cinnamon sticks. Makes 6 cups.

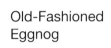

Old-Fashioned
Eggnog

Butternut Squash Soup
(page 70)

Soup's On

Ease the chill of winter with comforting soups, stews and chowders. To round out a meal, try Parmesan-Onion Soup or Red Pepper Soup. If it's a main dish you're looking for, you can't go wrong with Burgundy Beef Stew or Sausage-Potato Chowder. Stay in and warm up with one of these delicious recipes!

Butternut Squash Soup

(pictured on page 68)

2½ lbs. butternut squash, halved,
    seeded, peeled and cubed
2 c. leeks, chopped
2 Granny Smith apples, peeled, cored
    and diced

2 (14½-oz.) cans chicken broth
1 c. water
seasoned salt and white pepper to taste
Garnish: freshly ground nutmeg and
    sour cream

Combine squash, leeks, apples, broth and water in a 4-quart slow cooker.
Cover and cook on high setting for 4 hours, or until squash and leeks are tender.
Carefully purée the hot soup, in 3 or 4 batches, in a food processor or blender
until smooth. Add seasoned salt and white pepper. Garnish with nutmeg and sour
cream. Serves 8.

Red Pepper Soup

*Spicy, but not too hot,
it's a nice change from
traditional rice soups.*

6 red peppers, chopped
2 carrots, chopped
2 onions, chopped
1 celery stalk, chopped
4 cloves garlic, minced
1 T. olive oil
2 (32-oz.) cartons chicken broth

½ c. long grain rice, uncooked
2 t. dried thyme
1½ t. salt
¼ t. pepper
⅛ to ¼ t. cayenne pepper
⅛ to ¼ t. crushed red pepper flakes
Garnish: croutons

In a large Dutch oven, sauté red peppers, carrots, onions, celery and garlic
in olive oil until tender. Stir in broth, rice, thyme, salt, pepper and cayenne pepper; bring to a boil. Reduce heat; cover and simmer for 20 to 25 minutes, or until
vegetables and rice are tender. Cool for 30 minutes. Purée in small batches in a
food processor or blender, return to pan and add red pepper flakes. Heat through.
Garnish with croutons. Serves 12 to 14.

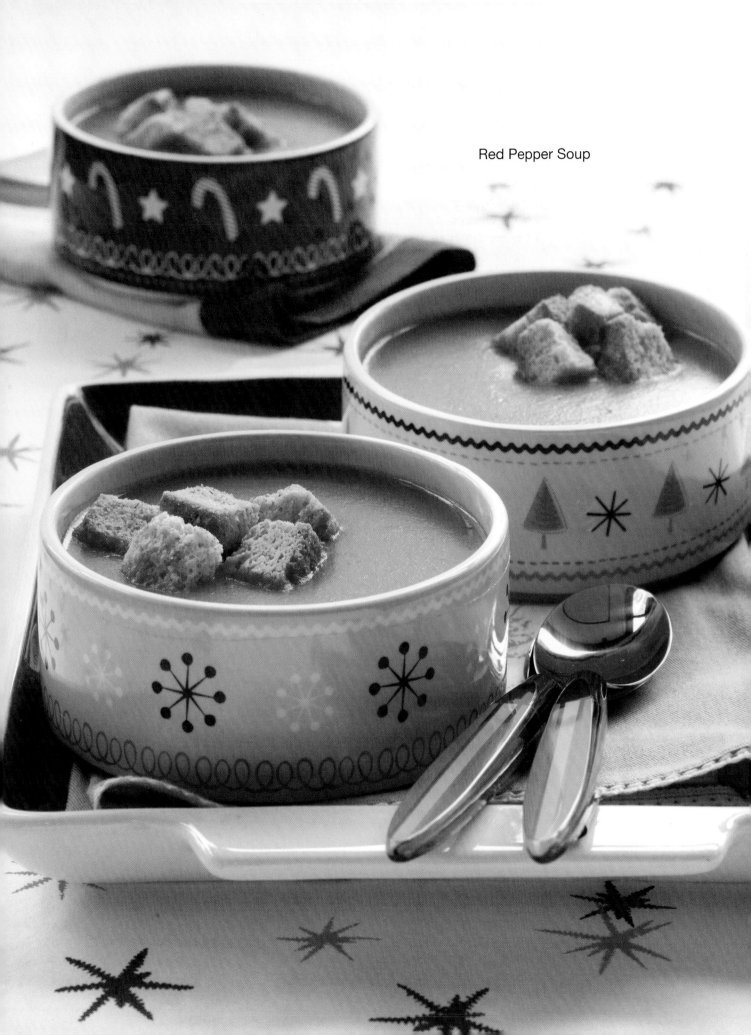

Red Pepper Soup

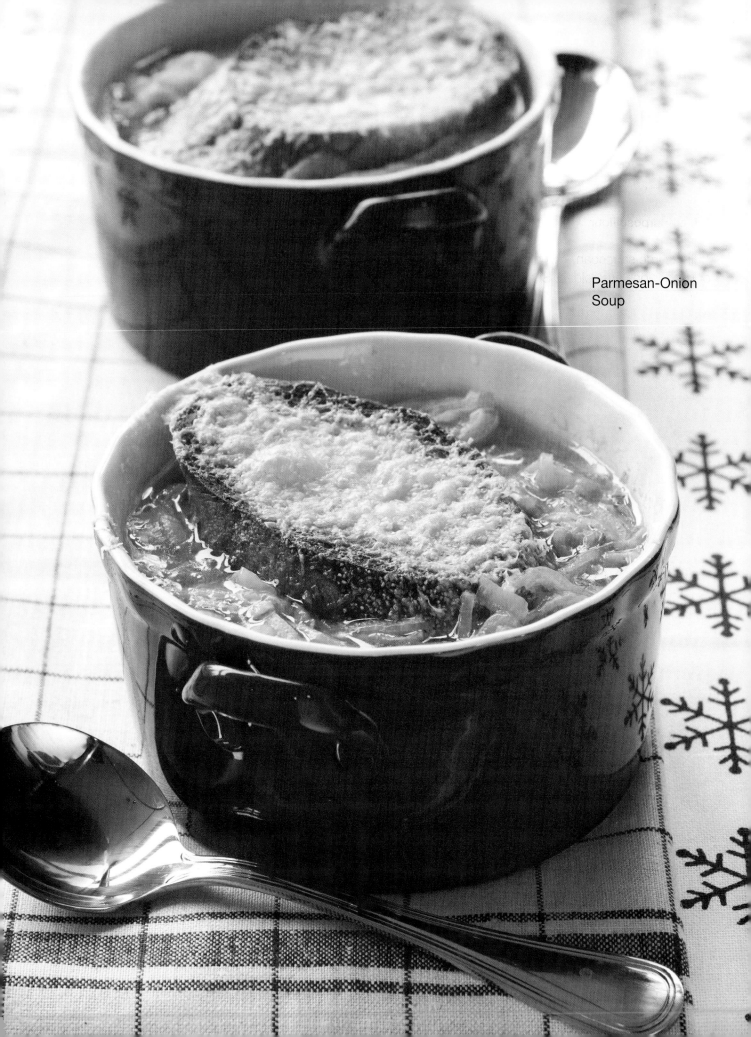

Parmesan-Onion
Soup

Parmesan-Onion Soup

3 T. butter, melted
4 c. onions, thinly sliced
½ t. sugar
1 T. all-purpose flour

4 c. water
salt and pepper to taste
4 French bread slices, toasted
½ c. freshly grated Parmesan cheese

A rich and flavorful soup that'll warm you to your toes!

In a large saucepan, combine butter, onions and sugar; sauté 20 to 25 minutes or until onions are golden. Stir in flour; continue to cook for 3 to 5 minutes. Add water and simmer, partially covered, for 30 minutes. Add salt and pepper, blending well. Fill 4 oven-proof bowls with soup; top each with a bread slice and sprinkle generously with Parmesan cheese. Bake at 400 degrees until cheese melts. Serves 4.

Spinach-Tortellini Soup

2 cloves garlic, pressed
1 T. butter
3¼ c. chicken broth
8-oz. pkg. cheese tortellini, uncooked
⅛ t. cayenne pepper

¼ t. pepper
10-oz. pkg. frozen chopped spinach, thawed
16-oz. can stewed tomatoes, chopped and juice reserved
Garnish: grated Parmesan cheese

Tasty served with warm homemade bread.

In a large saucepan, sauté garlic in butter over medium heat for 3 to 5 minutes. Add chicken broth and tortellini; heat to boiling. Reduce heat, add peppers and simmer for 10 minutes. Stir in spinach and tomatoes with juice; continue to simmer 5 more minutes. Serve topped with Parmesan cheese to taste. Serves 6 to 8.

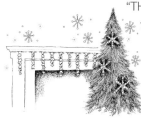

"THERE WASN'T A CHRISTMAS THAT GRANDPA JUNE, my dad, didn't take a picture of the grandkids under the tree. It all started with their first Christmas in the infant seat on the floor. As the years passed, the kids grew and the tree looked smaller and smaller. It's been such fun to look back and see how the kids have changed over the years. I now have a granddaughter and I follow Dad's tradition...Ava had her picture taken in her car seat in front of the tree!"

Cheri Stees
Lena, IL

Black-Eyed Pea Soup

Add bacon, garlic and chiles to a classic soup recipe and you get this delicious variation!

6 slices bacon, crisply cooked and crumbled, drippings reserved
1 onion, finely chopped
1 clove garlic, minced
½ t. salt
½ t. pepper

4-oz. can chopped green chiles, drained
4 (15½-oz.) cans black-eyed peas
2 (14½-oz.) cans beef broth
10-oz. can diced tomatoes and green chiles

Add onion, garlic, salt, pepper and chiles to bacon drippings in a Dutch oven; sauté until onion is golden. Add bacon, undrained peas and remaining ingredients. Increase heat to medium-high and bring to a boil; remove from heat. Serve with cornbread. Serves 12 to 14.

Wild Rice Soup

For a special touch, top with crispy homemade croutons and crumbled bacon.

1⅓ c. chicken broth
1½ c. quick-cooking wild rice, uncooked
1 lb. sliced bacon, cooked and crumbled, drippings reserved
1 onion, chopped
2 (4½ oz.) jars sliced mushrooms

2 (10¾-oz.) cans cream of potato soup
2 (4½-oz.) jars sliced mushrooms, undrained
2 c. half-and-half
⅔ c. sharp pasteurized process cheese spread
Garnish: croutons

In a saucepan, bring chicken broth to a boil; add rice. Cover, reduce heat and simmer 5 minutes or until liquid is absorbed. Spoon bacon drippings into another saucepan and sauté onion. Reserve ⅓ cup crumbled bacon for topping. Stir in undrained mushrooms, remaining ingredients and rice. Heat, but don't boil. Sprinkle each serving with croutons and reserved bacon. Serves 6.

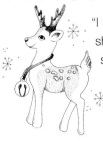

"I HAVE A VERY SPECIAL BOND WITH MY GREAT-NIECE, and ever since she was two years old we've been making a big batch of reindeer food. We simply pour oats into a container, add chopped nuts and a pinch of glitter; shake and sprinkle on the lawn for Santa's reindeer. My niece looks forward to this ritual every year. It's been a great way to show children that we believe in things we can't always see, and to have faith and hope in everything that we do."

Michelle Eva Papp
Rutherford, NJ

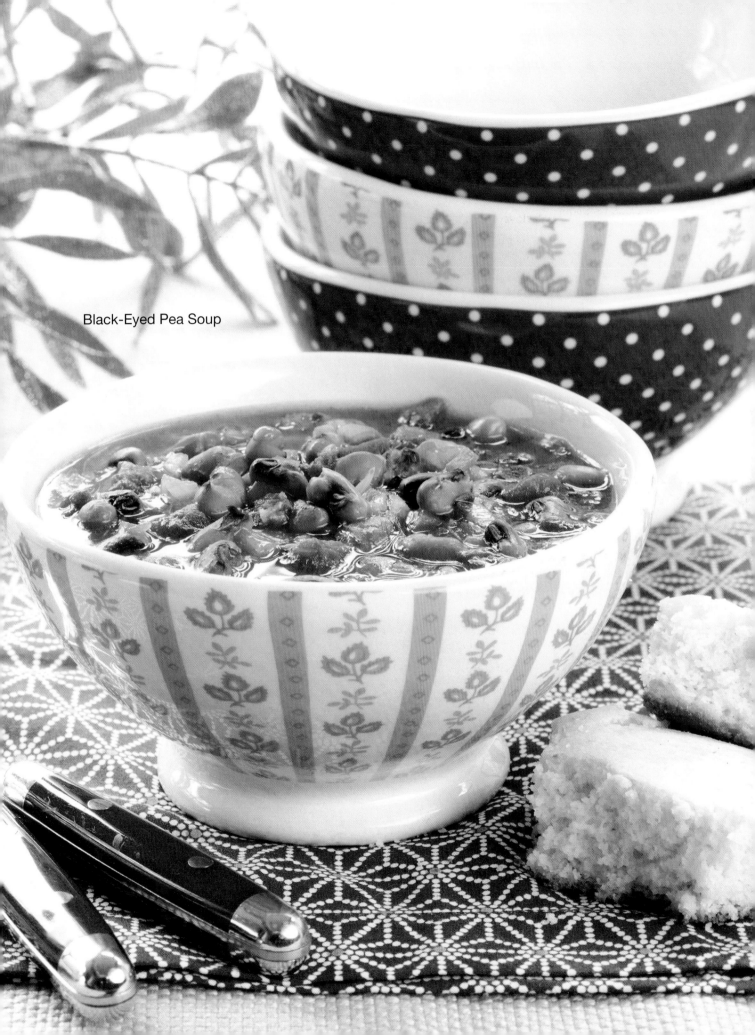

Black-Eyed Pea Soup

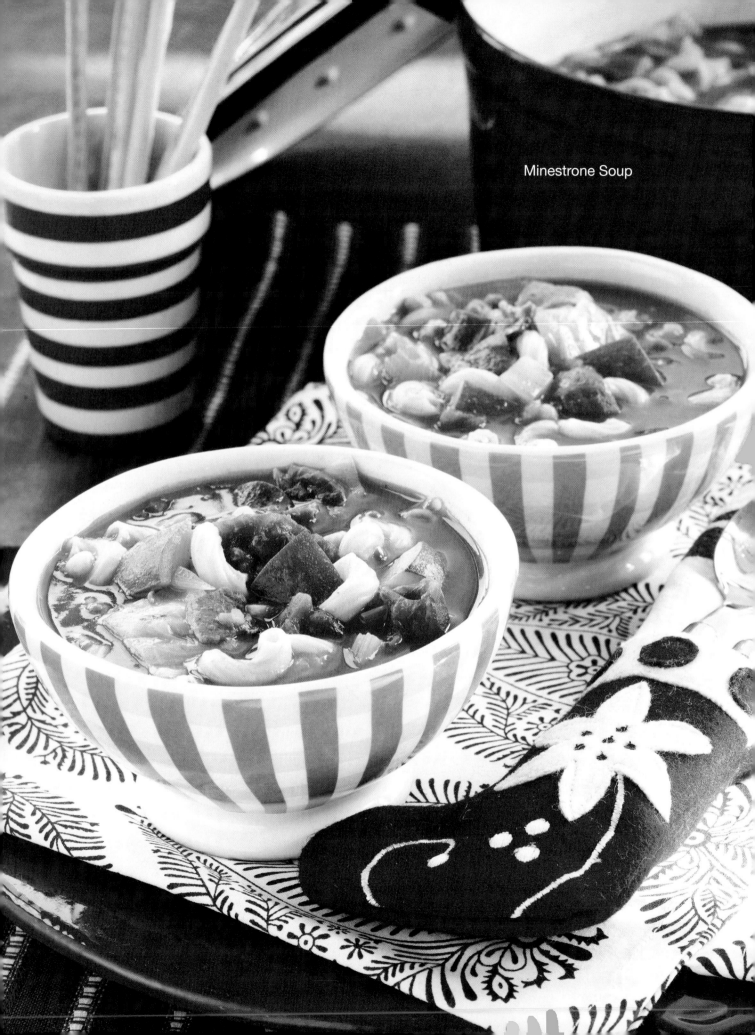

Minestrone Soup

Minestrone Soup

6 slices bacon, chopped
1 onion, chopped
1 c. celery, chopped
2 cloves garlic, minced
2 t. fresh basil, chopped
½ t. salt
3½ c. water

2 (10¾-oz.) cans bean & bacon soup
2 (14½-oz.) cans beef broth
2 (14½-oz.) cans stewed tomatoes,
    chopped and juice reserved
2 c. zucchini, peeled and chopped
2 c. cabbage, chopped
1 c. elbow macaroni, uncooked

"My aunt gave this recipe to me about 20 years ago. It's a wonderful main dish soup and it is very easy to prepare."

*Linda Newkirk
Central Point, OR*

In a large stockpot, brown bacon, onion, celery and garlic; drain drippings. Add basil, salt, water, soup, broth, tomatoes and juice, zucchini, cabbage and macaroni. Boil until macaroni is tender. Serves 6 to 8.

Beef, Vegetable & Macaroni Soup

1 lb. stew beef, cubed
1 t. salt
½ t. pepper
1 t. oil
1 onion, diced
2 stalks celery, chopped

14½-oz. can stewed tomatoes,
    undrained
1 bay leaf
2 qts. water
4 carrots, peeled and sliced
14½-oz. can green beans, drained
1 c. elbow macaroni, uncooked

"My mother and grand-mother made this soup on cold, snowy days. Serve with homemade bread!"

*Pam Vienneau
Derby, CT*

Sprinkle beef with salt and pepper; brown in oil in a large stockpot. Add onions and celery; cook until tender. Blend in stewed tomatoes, bay leaf, water and carrots. Simmer, covered, for at least 2 hours. Stir in green beans and uncooked macaroni. Bring to a boil and cook for 20 minutes. Add more water if mixture begins to boil dry. Serves 6 to 8.

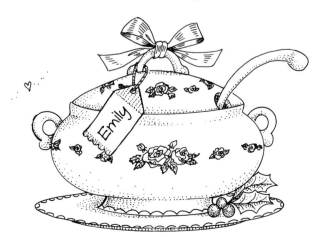

Corn Chowder

Spoon this yummy soup into individual bread bowls for a tasty change!

10-oz. pkg. frozen corn
½ c. potato, peeled and cubed
½ c. onion, chopped
⅓ c. water
1 t. instant chicken bouillon granules
⅛ t. white pepper

1¾ c. milk, divided
2 T. powdered milk
2 T. all-purpose flour
Garnish: 1 T. bacon, crisply cooked
   and crumbled

In a large saucepan, combine corn, potato, onion, water, bouillon granules and pepper. Bring to a boil and reduce heat. Cover and simmer about 10 minutes, or until potatoes are tender, stirring occasionally. Stir in 1½ cups milk. In a small bowl, stir together powdered milk and flour. Gradually stir in the remaining ¼ cup milk until smooth. Stir the flour mixture into the corn mixture. Stirring constantly, cook until mixture is thick and bubbly. Cook and stir for one minute longer. Garnish with bacon pieces before serving. Serves 4.

Sausage-Potato Chowder

"We start making this soup when the first hint of frost is in the air."

Carol Wakefield
Indianapolis, IN

2 T. butter
1 onion, chopped
½ c. celery, sliced
3 c. potatoes, cubed
3 c. chicken broth

1 lb. smoked sausage, chopped
½ c. sour cream
10¾-oz. can cream of mushroom soup
1 c. milk

Melt butter in a Dutch oven; sauté onion and celery until onion is translucent. Add potatoes and chicken broth; bring to a boil. Cover, reduce heat, add sausage and simmer until potatoes are tender, about 15 to 20 minutes. In a small bowl, combine sour cream and mushroom soup; add to chowder, then stir in milk. Heat, but do not boil. Serves 6 to 8.

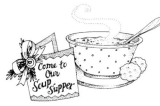

INVITE FRIENDS OVER FOR A SOUP SUPPER on a frosty winter evening. Everyone can bring their favorite soup or bread to share...you provide the bowls, spoons, and a crackling fire!

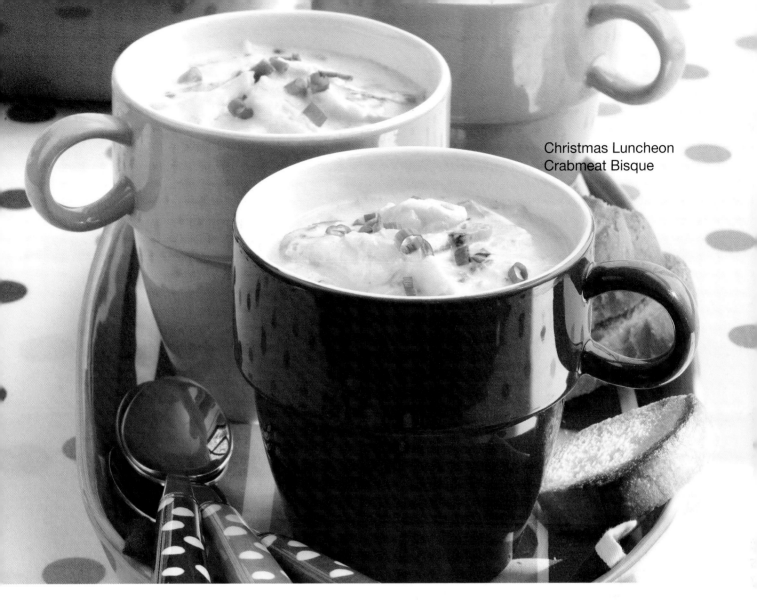

Christmas Luncheon
Crabmeat Bisque

Christmas Luncheon Crabmeat Bisque

6 T. butter, divided
¼ c. green pepper, finely chopped
¼ c. onion, finely chopped
1 green onion, chopped
2 T. fresh parsley, chopped
1½ c. sliced mushrooms
2 T. all-purpose flour
1 c. milk

1 t. salt
⅛ t. white pepper
⅛ t. hot pepper sauce
2 c. half-and-half
1½ c. cooked crabmeat
Optional: 3 T. dry sherry
Garnish: additional chopped green
  onion

*For a shrimp bisque,
replace crab with 1½
cups cooked, peeled
and cleaned shrimp.*

Heat 4 tablespoons butter in a skillet over medium heat. Add next 5 ingredients
and sauté until soft. In a saucepan, heat remaining 2 tablespoons butter and stir in
flour. Add milk and cook, stirring until thickened and smooth. Stir in salt, pepper and
hot pepper sauce. Add sautéed vegetables and half-and-half. Bring to a boil, stirring;
reduce heat. Add crabmeat, simmer uncovered for 5 minutes. If desired, stir in
sherry just prior to serving. Top with additional green onion. Serves 4.

Chicken Stew

Let the slow cooker do all the work for you!

2 sweet potatoes, peeled and cubed
1 onion, sliced
6 boneless, skinless chicken breasts
½ t. dried thyme
¼ t. pepper

2 bay leaves
3½ c. water, divided
2 (3-oz.) pkgs. chicken ramen noodles
   with seasoning packets

In a 5-quart slow cooker, layer potatoes, onion and chicken. Sprinkle with thyme and pepper. Add bay leaves. Combine one cup water and seasoning packets from noodle soup, reserving noodles. Pour seasoning mixture over chicken; add remaining 2½ cups water to slow cooker. Cover and cook on high for one hour and low for 3 hours. Shred chicken. Stir in reserved noodles; increase heat to high setting and cook 10 minutes. Remove bay leaves before serving. Serves 8 to 10.

Red Bandanna Stew

A slow cooker makes this dish a low-fuss meal for families on the go.

1 lb. ground beef, browned
2 (15-oz.) cans new potatoes, drained
   and chopped
8¼-oz. can sliced carrots, drained

1¼-oz. pkg. taco seasoning mix
½ c. water
1 c. picante sauce
1 c. shredded Cheddar cheese

Place browned beef in a slow cooker; add potatoes and carrots. In a separate mixing bowl, combine taco seasoning with water; pour into slow cooker. Cook on high setting for about 30 minutes to one hour; garnish with picante sauce and cheese. Serves 4 to 6.

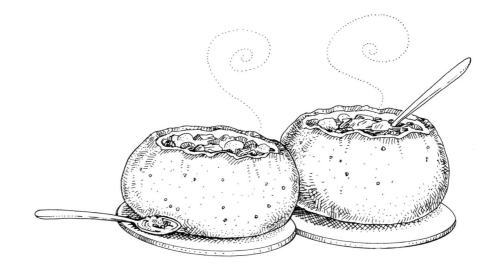

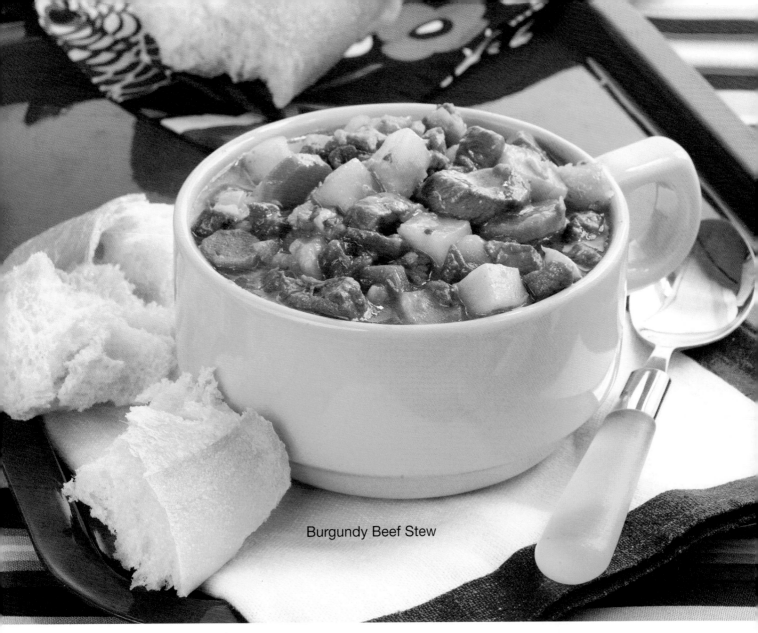

Burgundy Beef Stew

Burgundy Beef Stew

1½ lbs. boneless chuck, cubed

2 T. oil

2 baking potatoes, chopped into
   ½-inch cubes

2 onions, peeled and chopped

4 carrots, chopped

1 turnip, chopped

3 T. all-purpose flour

1 c. beef broth

1 c. Burgundy wine or beef broth

3 bay leaves

1 t. fresh basil, chopped

14½-oz. can chopped tomatoes

Fork-tender and richly flavored.

Brown beef in oil in a large stew pot. Add all vegetables, except tomatoes, and sauté over medium-low heat for 5 minutes. Sprinkle flour over meat and vegetables and stir to coat. Add broth, wine or broth, seasonings and tomatoes. Bring to a boil; reduce heat to low and simmer, covered, for 1½ hours, or until meat is very tender, stirring occasionally. Serves 4 to 6.

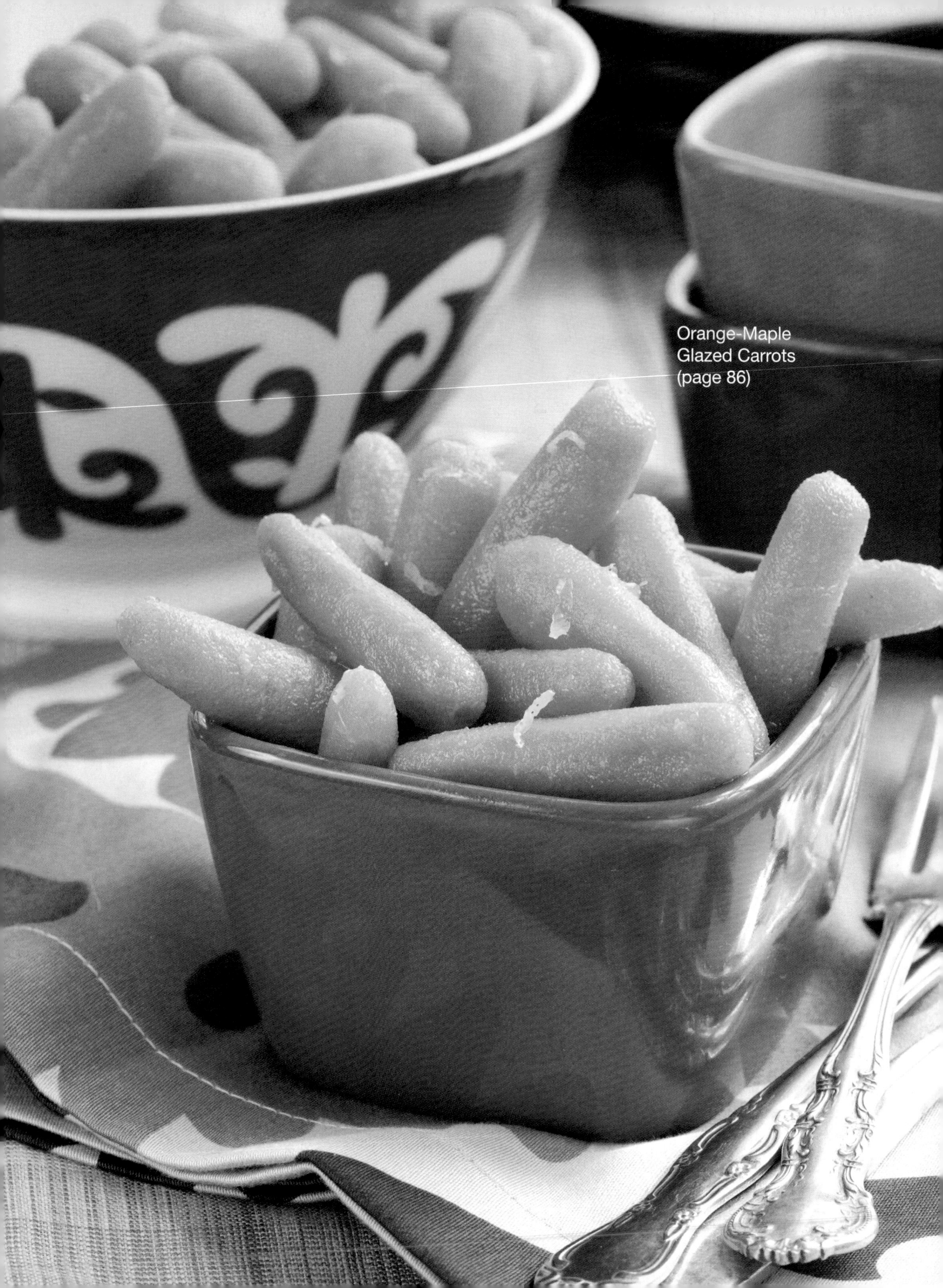

Orange-Maple
Glazed Carrots
(page 86)

Holiday Sideboard

Complete your Christmas meal with one of these irresistible sides and salads. From tasty Broccoli-Cheddar Casserole to tempting Savory Mashed Potatoes, Wild Rice Stuffing and Three Layer Ruby Red Salad, you're sure to find a recipe to please even the pickiest of eaters. Enjoy!

Squash Casserole

For a spicier dish, use hot sausage.

8 oz. ground pork sausage
3 zucchini, sliced
1 onion, finely chopped
2 T. butter
2 (8¾-oz.) cans cream-style corn

2 c. shredded Monterey Jack cheese
¾ c. cornbread stuffing
4½-oz. can chopped green chiles, drained

Brown sausage in a skillet, stirring until it crumbles; drain well and set aside. In a large skillet over medium heat, sauté zucchini and onion in butter until tender. Combine zucchini mixture, sausage, corn, cheese, stuffing and chiles; stir well. Spoon into a lightly greased 2-quart casserole dish. Bake, uncovered, at 350 degrees for 40 minutes, or until golden and bubbly. Serves 8.

Broccoli-Cheddar Casserole

A side dish that everyone can agree on!

8 c. broccoli, chopped
1 c. onion, finely chopped
2 T. butter
12 eggs

2 c. whipping cream
2 c. shredded Cheddar cheese, divided
2 t. salt
1 t. pepper

In a skillet over medium heat, sauté broccoli and onion in butter for about 5 minutes or until crisp-tender; set aside. In a large bowl, beat eggs. Add whipping cream and 1¾ cups cheese; mix well. Stir in the broccoli mixture, salt and pepper. Pour into a greased 3-quart casserole dish; set into a larger pan filled with one inch of hot water. Bake, uncovered, at 350 degrees for 45 to 50 minutes or until knife inserted in center comes out clean. Sprinkle with remaining cheese; let stand for 10 minutes before serving. Serves 12 to 16.

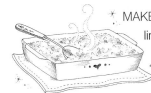

MAKE AND STORE CASSEROLES AHEAD for quick, easy meals! Simply line a casserole dish with foil, fill with your favorite casserole, then freeze. Once the ingredients are completely frozen, lift the foil and casserole from the dish, wrap tightly in freezer wrap and return to the freezer. When you need a quick meal, pop the frozen casserole back in a dish and bake!

Squash Casserole

Aunt Tillie's Green Beans

"This recipe is one that has been a favorite in our family for years. Even though most of my family doesn't care for vegetables, they always ask for seconds of this dish!"

Barbara Czachowski
Dallas, TX

1 lb. pkg. frozen French-style green
   beans, thawed
2 T. plus 1 t. butter, divided
2 T. all-purpose flour
½ t. salt
1 t. sugar

¼ t. pepper
¼ c. onion, finely chopped
1 c. sour cream
1 c. shredded Swiss cheese
1 c. corn flake cereal, crushed

Drain beans; set aside. Melt 2 tablespoons butter over low heat; blend in flour. Stir in salt, sugar, pepper and onion. Add sour cream; stir until smooth. Remove from heat and fold in green beans. Spoon mixture into a greased 1½-quart casserole dish. Sprinkle cheese over top. Layer cereal over cheese. Melt remaining butter and drizzle over cereal. Bake, uncovered, at 350 degrees for 30 minutes. Serves 4 to 6.

Baked Creamed Corn

A well-loved addition to any meal!

2 eggs, beaten
1 c. milk
1 T. sugar
1 t. salt

2 T. butter
⅛ t. pepper
1 c. cream-style corn
¼ c. shredded Cheddar cheese

In a large bowl, combine eggs, milk, sugar, salt, butter, pepper and corn. Pour into a greased 2-quart casserole dish. Sprinkle cheese over top. Bake at 350 degrees for 30 minutes. Serves 3.

Orange-Maple Glazed Carrots

(pictured on page 82)

This dish always impresses guests...don't let them know you did it in the microwave.

⅔ c. orange juice
16-oz. pkg. peeled baby carrots
2 T. orange zest

⅓ c. maple syrup
1 t. fresh nutmeg, grated
⅓ c. butter

Heat orange juice in a microwave-safe casserole dish in the microwave on high for 1½ minutes. Add carrots and orange zest; stir to coat. Cover dish and microwave on high for 7 minutes. Stir in the remaining ingredients and microwave, uncovered, for 2 minutes. Carrots should be crisp-tender; if not, microwave 2 more minutes. Serves 3 to 4.

Broccoli Bake

3 eggs, beaten
1 c. all-purpose flour
1 c. milk
1 onion, chopped

3 c. shredded Cheddar cheese
10-oz. pkg. frozen, chopped broccoli, thawed
1 t. baking powder

A speedy side dish to make for a progressive dinner.

In a large mixing bowl, combine all ingredients. Place in a greased 13"x9" baking pan. Bake, uncovered, at 350 degrees for 35 minutes. Serves 2 to 4.

Fruited Yams

2 yams, peeled and sliced
1 c. pineapple, chopped
1 banana, sliced
¾ c. apple, peeled and chopped
¼ c. raisins
⅓ c. apple juice

1 T. brown sugar, packed
1 t. lemon zest, grated
1 t. cinnamon
½ t. ground ginger
¼ t. nutmeg

This is a good side dish any time of year, but especially on blustery winter days!

Spray a 13"x9" baking pan with non-stick vegetable spray. Layer half of the yams in pan. Mix pineapple, banana, apple and raisins. Spread half of the fruit mixture over yams. Repeat with remaining yams and fruit mixture. Mix remaining ingredients. Pour evenly over yams and fruit mixture. Cover and bake at 350 degrees for 50 to 60 minutes, or until yams are tender. Serves 6.

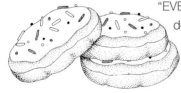

"EVERY YEAR AT CHRISTMASTIME, the children and I bake dozens of cookies from recipes we pick out of one of our many Gooseberry Patch cookbooks. We make a special little craft that we have selected from one of the craft books, pack them together in special bags and deliver them via wagon throughout the neighborhood. When we started, we had just moved here and didn't know many people at all. Now our list is up to nineteen and is growing every year. It's a great way for the children to recognize the importance of giving and reaching out to others...we've made a lot of friends along the way too!"

Mary Therese Onoshko
Brick, NJ

Savory Mashed Potatoes

Sweet Potato Pudding

10 sweet potatoes, baked, peeled
  and mashed
¾ c. brown sugar, packed
½ c. butter

4 eggs, beaten
¾ to 1 c. half-and-half
1 t. cinnamon

"This recipe has been in my family as long as I can remember! Every holiday, I get requests to bring this pudding."

Carolyn Celeste
Brick, NJ

Place potatoes in a large bowl, beat in brown sugar and butter; mix well. Blend in eggs, half-and-half and cinnamon. Whip until well blended; pour into an ungreased 13"x9" baking pan. Bake, uncovered, at 350 degrees for 30 to 40 minutes, or until heated through. Serves 10 to 12.

Savory Mashed Potatoes

5 potatoes, peeled and diced
¼ c. milk
½ t. seasoned salt
3 T. butter, divided
1 c. sour cream

3-oz. package cream cheese, softened
2 t. dried chives
½ c. round buttery crackers, crushed
⅔ c. shredded Cheddar cheese

This recipe can be pre-pared a day in advance if you wish.

Cook potatoes in salted water until tender; drain. Beat potatoes, milk, seasoned salt and 2 tablespoons butter in a mixing bowl until fluffy. Mix in sour cream, cream cheese and chives. Pour into greased 13"x9" baking pan. Combine remaining one tablespoon of butter with crushed cracker crumbs; sprinkle on top of potato mixture. Bake, uncovered, at 350 degrees for 30 minutes. Top with shredded cheese during last 10 minutes of baking time. Serves 5.

Quick Smackeroni

1 c. milk, divided
16-oz. pkg. elbow macaroni, cooked
1 c. onions, minced
¼ t. hot pepper sauce

2 (8-oz.) pkgs. shredded sharp Cheddar
  cheese
salt and pepper to taste

In a bowl, mix ½ cup milk, macaroni, onions, hot sauce, half of cheese, salt and pepper. Spread in a lightly greased 13"x9" baking dish. Sprinkle with remaining cheese and ½ cup milk. Bake, covered, at 325 degrees for 30 minutes, or until cheese is melted. Serves 8 to 10.

Wild Rice Stuffing

Dates and crunchy almonds make this stuffing recipe special!

1⅓ c. wild rice, uncooked
2 T. butter
2 c. onion, chopped
1 c. carrots, grated
1 c. green pepper, chopped
6 c. herb-seasoned stuffing mix
1 c. slivered almonds

½ c. fresh parsley, chopped
10-oz. pkg. pitted dates, chopped
1½ t. dried rosemary
1½ t. dried thyme
1½ t. dried sage
3 c. chicken broth

Prepare rice according to package directions; set aside. Combine butter, onion, carrots and pepper in a medium skillet over medium-high heat and sauté until onion is transparent; remove from heat. Blend in remaining ingredients; stir in rice. Spoon stuffing into a greased 13"x9" baking pan. Bake, covered, at 325 degrees for 45 minutes. Uncover and bake 15 more minutes. Serves 10 to 12.

Simple Spoon Bread

A perfect recipe for the beginning baker!

1 c. cornmeal
3 c. milk, divided
3 eggs, beaten

1 t. salt
3 T. butter, melted
1 T. baking powder

Bring cornmeal and 2 cups milk to a boil in a saucepan over medium heat; stir often. Remove from heat and add remaining milk, eggs and salt; mix well. Add butter and baking powder; mix well. Place in a greased 9"x5" loaf pan. Bake at 350 degrees for 45 minutes. Serves 4 to 6.

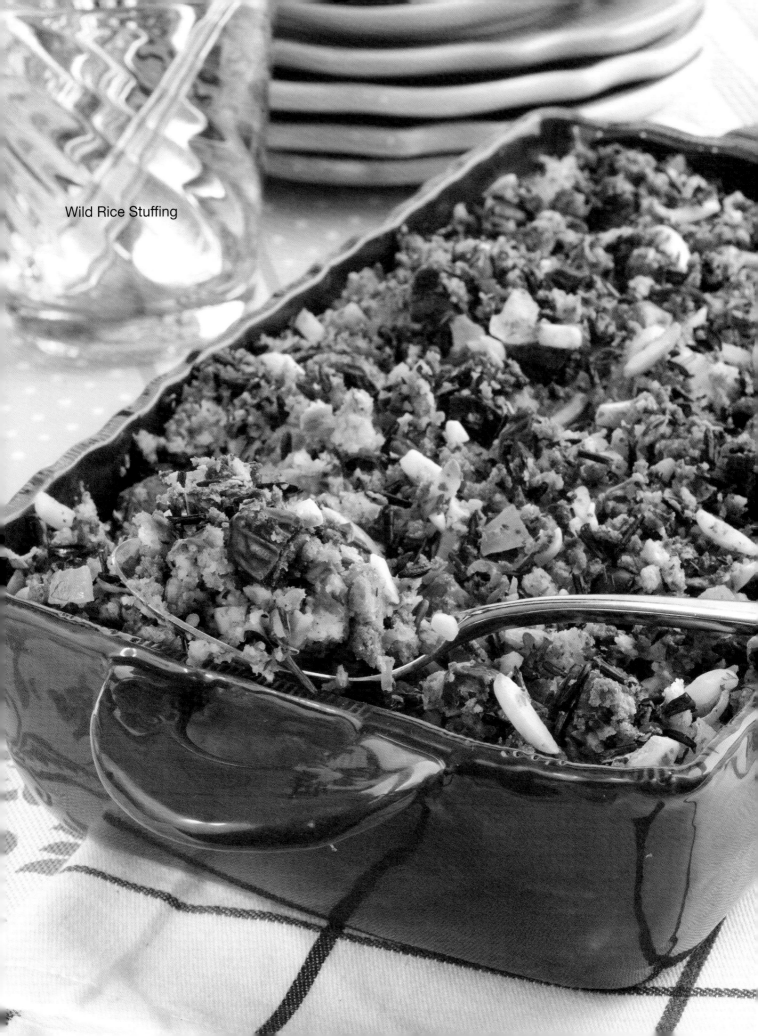

Wild Rice Stuffing

Asparagus & Tomato Salad

This salad has a tasty combination of flavors.

16 stalks asparagus
1 lb. Roma tomatoes, diced
1½ T. fresh basil, chopped
1 t. salt

½ t. pepper
8-oz. pkg. Feta cheese, crumbled
⅓ c. balsamic vinegar

Cut the stems from asparagus stalks; discard. Slice asparagus on the diagonal and blanch in boiling water for 5 minutes. Remove from boiling water and immediately immerse in cold water to stop the cooking. In a large serving bowl, combine asparagus and tomatoes. Add basil, salt and pepper. Stir in Feta cheese; toss and refrigerate. Before serving, toss with balsamic vinegar. Serves 8.

Mandarin Orange Salad

Quick and easy to prepare, this salad is best topped with fresh dressing like Raspberry Vinaigrette.

4 c. green or red loose leaf lettuce,
  torn into bite-size pieces
2 (15-oz.) cans mandarin oranges,
  drained

½ c. walnut pieces, toasted
½ red onion, sliced

Combine all ingredients together. Toss with desired amount of Raspberry Vinaigrette and serve. Serves 4.

Raspberry Vinaigrette:

⅓ c. raspberry vinegar
⅓ c. seedless raspberry jam
1 t. dried ground coriander or cumin

½ t. salt
¼ t. pepper
¾ c. olive oil

Combine first 5 ingredients in blender. Turn blender on high, gradually adding oil. Chill.

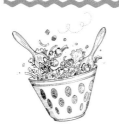

FOR AN EASY SIDE, WHIP UP A MARINATED SALAD to keep in the fridge…cut up crunchy veggies and toss with Zesty Italian salad dressing.

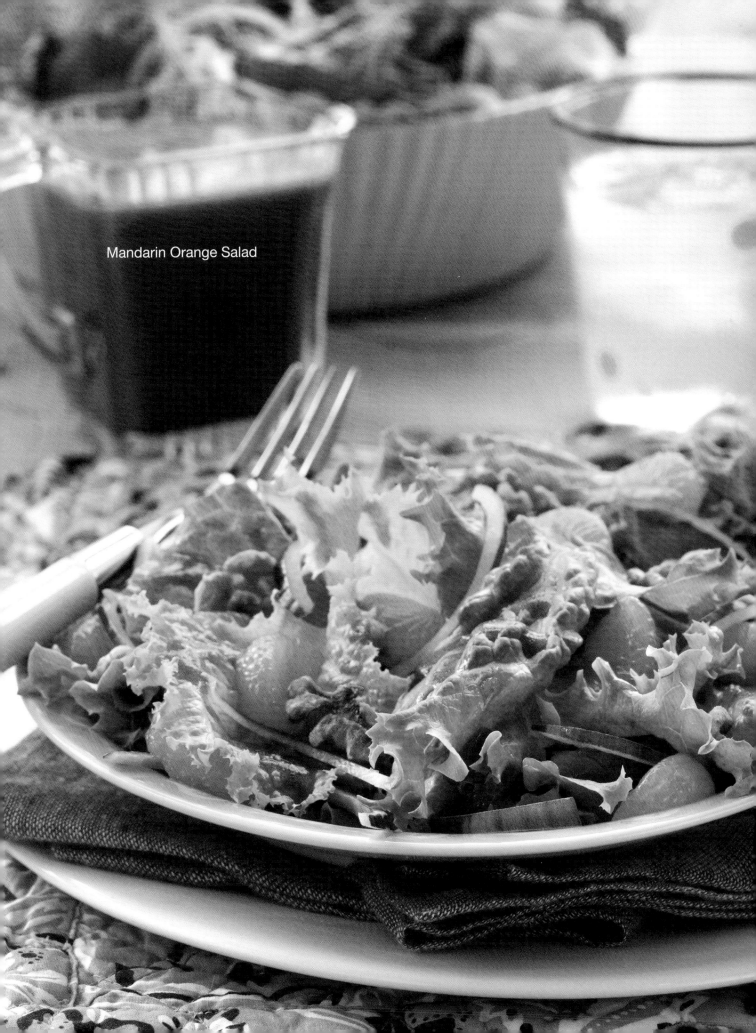
Mandarin Orange Salad

Crunchy Granny Smith Salad

Crisp Granny Smith apples make this salad especially refreshing.

1 head red leaf lettuce, torn, washed and pat dry
2 Granny Smith apples, cored, sliced and cut in half
1 c. shredded Swiss cheese
1 c. cashews, chopped

1 c. oil
1 T. onion, minced
1 t. dry mustard
½ c. sugar
⅓ c. cider vinegar
2 t. poppy seed

Layer the first 4 ingredients in a bowl. Combine the next 5 ingredients in a blender; process until smooth. Add poppy seed; pulse two times. Pour desired amount of dressing over salad. Serves 10 to 12.

Fruit Salad with Orange Dressing

Add any fruits in season to this special creamy dressing.

2 (8¼-oz.) cans mandarin oranges, drained
2 (15-oz.) cans sliced peaches, drained
2 (20-oz.) cans pineapple chunks, drained
1 apple, cored and diced

1½ c. milk
3.4-oz. pkg. instant vanilla pudding mix
¾ c. sour cream
6-oz. frozen orange juice concentrate, thawed

Mix all fruits together in a large bowl. Gradually whisk milk into pudding mix. Stir in sour cream and orange juice concentrate. Serves 10.

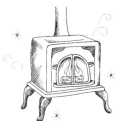

"DURING THE HOLIDAYS, I remember the excitement of Christmas shopping at the 5 & dime store and of our family gathered around the piano. We weren't the best singers, but it gave us all that special feeling of family. Getting up on Christmas morning with the wood stove roaring, the smell of popcorn balls and of course the tree and presents…Mom really made Christmas special."

Brenda Degreenia
Barre, VT

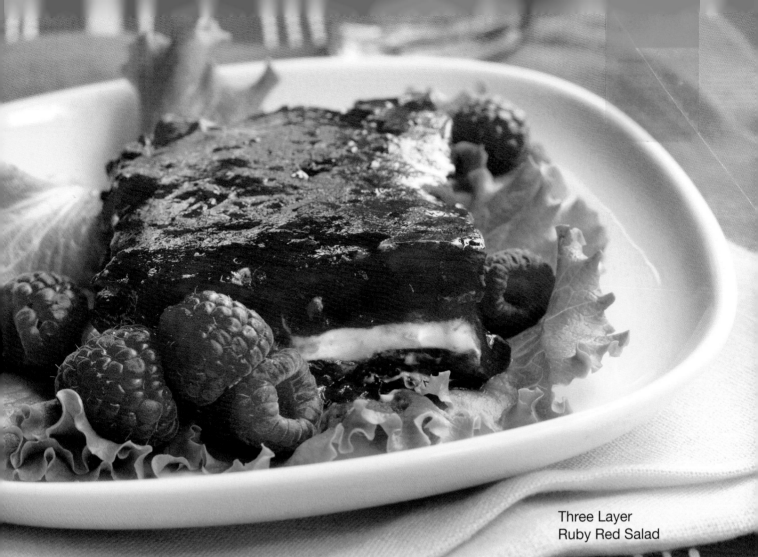

Three Layer
Ruby Red Salad

Three Layer Ruby Red Salad

3.4-oz. pkg. raspberry gelatin mix
2 c. boiling water, divided
12-oz. pkg. frozen raspberries
  in syrup
1 c. sour cream
3-oz. pkg. cream cheese, softened
2 T. sugar

½ c. pecans, chopped
3.4-oz. pkg. cherry gelatin mix
8-oz. can crushed pineapple, drained
16-oz. can whole-berry cranberry sauce
spinach or lettuce leaves
Garnish: fresh raspberries

This bright red salad is perfect for the holidays!

    For bottom layer, dissolve raspberry gelatin in one cup boiling water. Add frozen raspberries and stir until thawed and separated. Pour into a greased 9" square pan. Place in refrigerator for gelatin to thicken. For middle layer, combine sour cream, cream cheese, sugar, and pecans; carefully spread on top of thickened raspberry gelatin. Chill. For top layer, dissolve cherry gelatin in one cup boiling water. Stir in pineapple and cranberry sauce. Let thicken slightly at room temperature. Carefully spoon over sour cream mixture. Chill until firm. Cut into squares and serve on spinach or lettuce leaves. Garnish with fresh raspberries. Serves 9.

Orange Biscuits
(page 98)

Bountiful Breads

Sweet breads, savory breads, quick breads, and yeast breads...we've got them all! If you're looking for that perfect roll to accompany your Christmas dinner, try our Make-Ahead Dinner Rolls or Golden Butter Rolls. Satisfy sweet cravings by baking up Orange Biscuits or Damascus Brick Sweet Rolls.

Orange Biscuits

(pictured on page 96)

"My grandmother kept a journal and always included lots of recipes alongside her memories. I remember her always serving these with ham… oh, the aroma from the kitchen was wonderful!"

Peg Baker
La Rue, OH

½ c. orange juice
¾ c. sugar, divided
½ c. butter, divided
2 t. orange zest
2 c. all-purpose flour

1 t. baking powder
½ t. salt
⅓ c. shortening
¾ c. milk
½ t. cinnamon

Combine orange juice, ½ cup sugar, ¼ cup butter and orange zest in a medium saucepan. Cook and stir over medium heat for 2 minutes. Fill 12 ungreased muffin cups each with 1¼ tablespoon of mixture; set aside. Sift together flour, baking powder and salt; cut in shortening until mixture resembles coarse crumbs. Stir in milk and mix with a fork until mixture forms a ball. On a heavily floured surface, knead dough for one minute. Roll into a 9-inch square about ½-inch thick; spread with ¼ cup softened butter. Combine cinnamon and remaining ¼ cup sugar; sprinkle over dough. Roll up dough and cut into 12 slices about ¾-inch thick. Place slices, cut side down, in muffin cups. Bake at 450 degrees for 14 to 17 minutes. Cool for 2 to 3 minutes; remove from pan. Makes one dozen.

"MY HUSBAND, TWO CHILDREN AND I ALWAYS GET OUR CHRISTMAS TREE from a tree farm. It may take us a while, but we walk around until we find just the right tree. Once we find it, we always stop for hot cocoa on the way home. Then, when Christmas vacation starts for the kids, we take one night and camp out on the floor in front of the tree. We have our hot cocoa and read to them from a Christmas story book my mother used to read to my sisters and brother and me when we were small. When Christmas Eve arrives, my parents come and spend the night with us. The best thing of all is that when I think I'm not doing enough as a mom to make their holidays memorable, they tell me that they don't ever want any of it to change, no matter how old they get."

Nikki Canterbury
Cross Lanes, WV

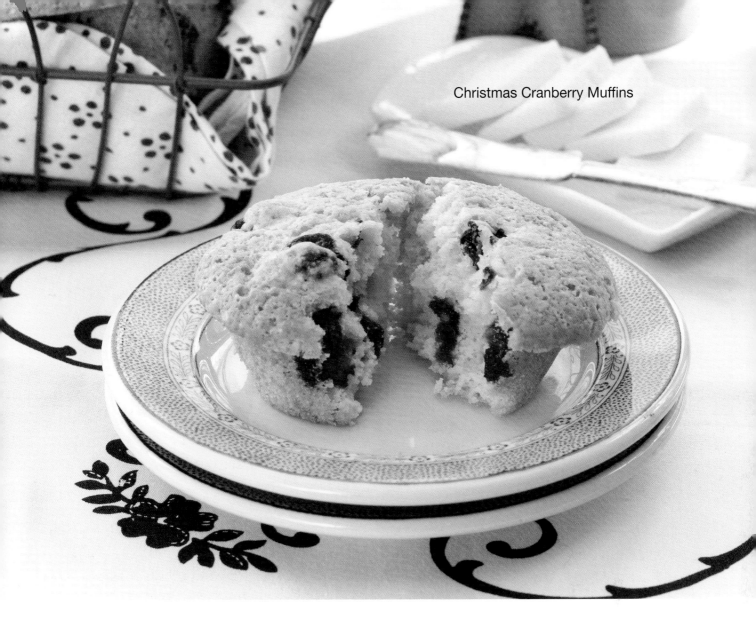

Christmas Cranberry Muffins

2 c. all-purpose flour
1 c. sugar
1½ t. baking powder
½ t. baking soda
½ t. salt

2 T. shortening
juice and zest of one orange
water
1 egg, beaten
1 c. cranberries, halved

These muffins create a wonderful aroma while baking and they are so colorful, too!

In a large bowl, combine first 5 ingredients; blend in shortening. Add orange zest. Place juice from orange in a measuring cup and add enough water to bring liquid equal to ¾ cup. Blend into flour mixture. Add egg and fold in cranberries. Pour into greased muffin cups, filling ⅔ full. Bake at 350 degrees for 15 to 18 minutes. Remove from pan and cool on a rack. Makes approximately 1½ dozen. This can also be made into quick bread by pouring batter into a greased 9"x5" loaf pan and baking at 350 degrees for 50 to 60 minutes.

Buttery Scones

Buttery Scones

1 c. buttermilk
1 egg
2 to 3 T. sugar
3½ c. unbleached white flour, divided
2 t. baking powder

1 t. baking soda
½ t. salt
½ c. butter, melted
½ c. raisins

Serve warm with butter, honey, jam and, of course, your favorite tea!

Beat buttermilk, egg and sugar together with an electric mixer at medium speed. Sift 3 cups of flour with baking powder, soda and salt. Add ⅔ of the flour mixture to the buttermilk mixture and stir well. Gradually add melted butter, stirring well; add remaining flour mixture. Add raisins and a bit more flour if needed. Knead dough on a floured surface 2 to 3 times. Cut dough into 3 parts. Form each into a 1½-inch thick circle and cut into 4 equal quarters. Place on a greased baking sheet. Bake at 400 degrees for 15 minutes, or until tops are golden. Makes one dozen.

Eggnog Quick Bread

2 eggs
1 c. sugar
1 c. dairy eggnog
½ c. butter, melted
2 t. rum extract

1 t. vanilla extract
2¼ c. all-purpose flour
2 t. baking powder
¼ t. nutmeg

Mix up this quick & tasty treat for drop-in company!

Beat eggs in a large bowl, then add next 5 ingredients, blending well. Add remaining ingredients and stir until just moist. Pour into a greased 9"x5" loaf pan and bake at 350 degrees for 45 to 50 minutes. Makes one loaf.

FOR A NICE CHANGE OF PACE, try a progressive dinner! Bundle everyone up and travel from house-to-house for each course, enjoying the holiday sights along the way. At the last house, serve desserts and coffee while exchanging little Christmas gifts!

Dilly Onion Bread

An easy-to-make quick bread that's full of flavor!

3 c. all-purpose flour
½ c. plus 2 T. sugar
1½ T. baking powder
⅔ c. butter

1 c. milk
4 eggs
1 T. plus 2 t. dill seed
2 t. dried, minced onion

In a large bowl, combine flour, sugar and baking powder and mix well; cut in butter. In a separate bowl, blend milk, eggs, dill seed and onion. Add to flour mixture and stir. Pour equal amounts into 4 greased 6" loaf pans. Bake at 350 degrees for 30 minutes, or until a knife inserted in the center comes out clean. Cool on a rack and serve warm. Makes 4 loaves.

Zesty Salsa & Cheese Bread

"This is one of my favorite family recipes… enjoy!"

Cheryl Wilson
Coshocton, OH

10-oz. tube refrigerated pizza dough
8-oz. jar salsa
garlic salt to taste

8-oz. pkg. shredded Cheddar cheese
8-oz. pkg. shredded mozzarella cheese

Spread pizza crust on a lightly greased baking sheet. Spread salsa down the middle of the pizza crust. Sprinkle salsa with garlic salt and cheeses. Bring edges of pizza crust to middle, leaving approximately one inch open. Bake at 375 degrees for 15 to 20 minutes or until cheese is melted and crust is golden. Slice and serve warm. Serves 4.

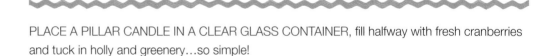

PLACE A PILLAR CANDLE IN A CLEAR GLASS CONTAINER, fill halfway with fresh cranberries and tuck in holly and greenery…so simple!

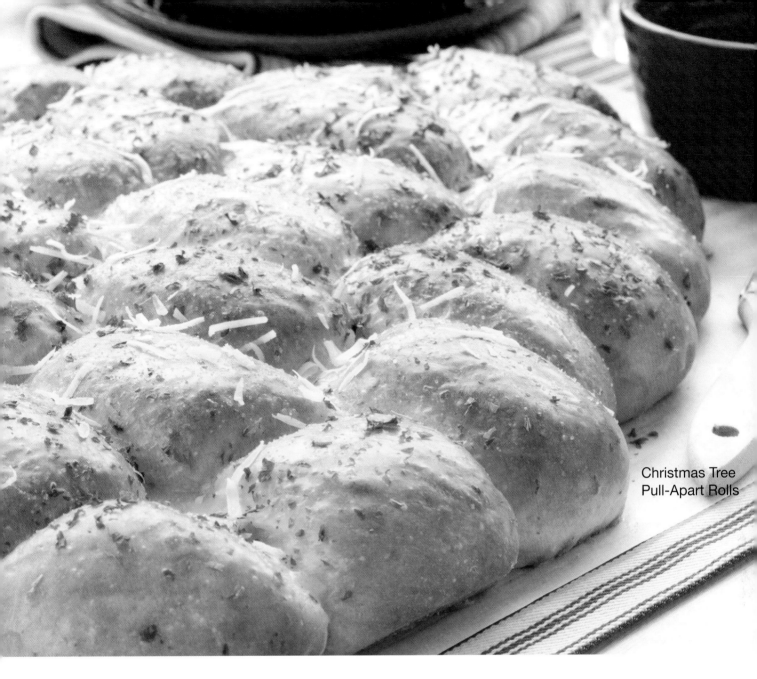

Christmas Tree
Pull-Apart Rolls

Christmas Tree Pull-Apart Rolls

48-oz. pkg. (36 count) frozen rolls
2 T. butter, melted
2 t. dried parsley, crumbled

garlic salt to taste
¼ c. Romano cheese, grated
additional dried parsley

*Very yummy…so festive
with dinner!*

Arrange rolls on a baking sheet in a Christmas tree pattern. (As they rise, the "balls" come together.) Bake according to package directions. When you remove them from the oven, they will be formed into a single piece. Transfer to a platter. Combine butter, parsley and garlic salt; brush onto rolls. Sprinkle with cheese and dried parsley. Serve immediately. Makes 3 dozen.

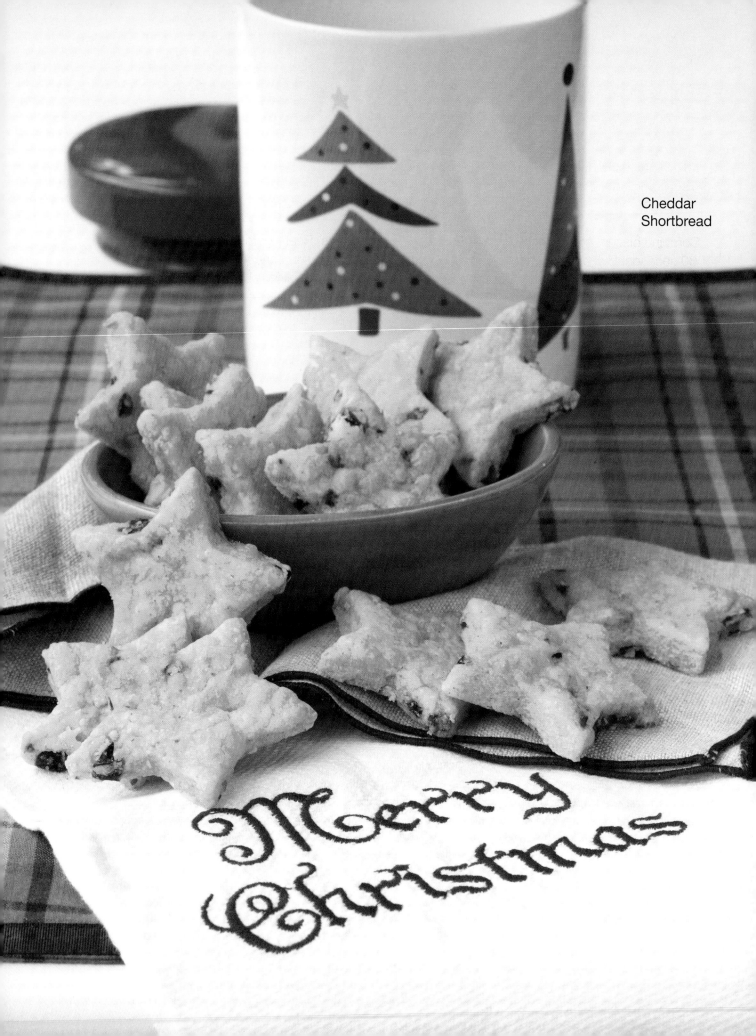

Cheddar
Shortbread

Savory Herb Biscuits

2 c. biscuit baking mix
½ c. shredded Cheddar cheese
⅔ c. milk

½ t. dried basil leaves
½ t. garlic powder
¼ c. butter or margarine, melted

Delicious and very easy!

Combine biscuit mix, cheese and milk until a soft dough forms. Beat vigorously for 30 seconds. Roll out dough to ½-inch thickness and cut with a star-shaped cookie cutter or drop by heaping tablespoonfuls onto an ungreased baking sheet. Bake at 450 degrees for 10 to 12 minutes, or until golden. Combine basil and garlic powder with melted butter and brush over hot biscuits after removing from oven. Makes one dozen.

Cheddar Shortbread

2 c. shredded sharp Cheddar cheese
1½ c. all-purpose flour
¾ t. dry mustard
¼ t. salt
¼ t. cayenne pepper

¼ c. sun-dried tomatoes, chopped
2 cloves garlic, minced
½ c. butter, melted
Optional: 1 to 2 T. water

Toss first 7 ingredients together; mix in butter. Mix with your hands to form a dough. Add water if dough feels too dry. On a floured surface, roll out half the dough to ¼-inch thickness. Cut with a 2½-inch star-shaped cookie cutter and place on an ungreased baking sheet. Reroll scraps and repeat with the remaining dough. Bake at 375 degrees for 10 to 12 minutes. Remove to a rack to cool. Makes 2½ dozen.

"OUR FAMILY BEGAN A FUN TRADITION ABOUT 10 YEARS AGO. My great-aunt had moved into a new condo, and she needed new Christmas ornaments. So she purchased plain glass ornaments in red, green and blue. After Thanksgiving dinner, each of us…men, women and children…painted Christmas scenes on them with acrylic paints. The fun and easy craft kept everyone from falling asleep after that turkey dinner. The following year, no one asked what was on the menu for Thanksgiving dinner, but everyone wanted to know about the Christmas craft. So, from that year forward, we have continued to begin the Christmas season with family & friends on Thanksgiving afternoon. The ornaments, bowls, sock snowmen and T-shirts bring us laughter and memories, but most importantly, bring us even closer as a family."

Laura Hartman
Oswego, IL

Sour Cream Cornbread

Easy to make!

1 c. self-rising cornmeal
8-oz. container sour cream

3 eggs, lightly beaten
¼ c. oil

Heat a lightly greased 8-inch cast-iron skillet or deep-dish pie pan in a 400-degree oven for 5 minutes. Combine all ingredients, stirring just until moistened. Remove prepared skillet from oven and spoon batter into skillet. Bake at 400 degrees for 30 minutes, or until golden. Serves 4 to 6.

Make-Ahead Dinner Rolls

A county fair blue ribbon winner...so easy for busy days!

1 pkg. active yeast
½ c. sugar
1 c. warm milk
2 eggs, beaten

½ c. butter, melted
1 t. salt
4 c. all-purpose flour

Mix together first 3 ingredients and let stand for 30 minutes. Add next 3 ingredients, then mix in flour, 2 cups at a time. Cover and chill until ready to bake. Divide the dough in half, rolling each half into a 9-inch circle. Cut each circle into 12 equal pie-shaped wedges, and roll up beginning at wide end. Place on a greased baking sheet and let rise in a warm place (85 degrees), away from drafts, until doubled in size. Bake at 375 degrees for 12 to 15 minutes. Makes 2 dozen.

WHEN TIME'S SHORT, make a warm loaf of Crostini to serve with dinner...it's easy! Slice a loaf of French bread into one-inch diagonal slices. Melt together ½ cup olive oil with ½ cup butter and coat one side of each slice of bread. Bake at 300 degrees for 30 minutes, or until toasty.

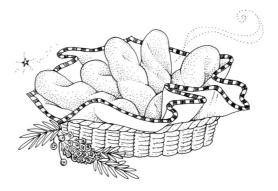

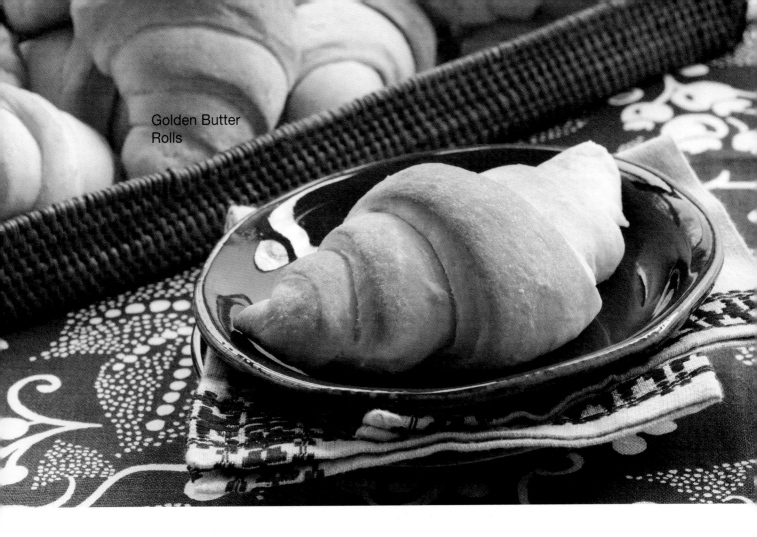

Golden Butter Rolls

Golden Butter Rolls

1 c. milk
1¼ c. butter, divided
1 pkg. active dry yeast
½ c. plus 1 t. sugar, divided
½ c. warm water

1 t. salt
3 eggs, beaten
1 c. whole-wheat flour
3½ to 4 cups all-purpose flour

In a heavy saucepan, heat milk and ½ cup butter. Remove from heat and cool. In a small bowl, dissolve yeast and one teaspoon sugar in warm water (110 to 115 degrees). When mixture foams, add to a large mixing bowl with remaining sugar, salt, eggs, whole-wheat and all-purpose flours. Add the cooled milk mixture and blend until smooth. Knead on a lightly floured surface until smooth and elastic, and then place in a large greased bowl; brush top of dough with ¼ cup softened butter. Cover and let rise in a warm place (85 degrees), away from drafts, until doubled in size. Divide dough into 3 portions. Roll each portion into a ½-inch-thick circle. Cut each circle into 10 or 12 pie-shaped wedges. Roll up each wedge beginning at wide end and place one inch apart on a greased baking sheet. Brush tops of each roll with ¼ cup softened butter; let rise until doubled. Bake at 375 degrees for 15 to 20 minutes, or until golden. Remove and brush with ¼ cup butter while rolls are still warm. Makes 2½ to 3 dozen.

"I'm very blessed to have a wonderful mom, and doubly blessed that she's also a great cook. This recipe may seem like a lot of work, but it's well worth the effort. Our entire family loves these delicious rolls!"

*Susan Ingersoll
Cleveland, OH*

Twisty Rolls

"I have been making these for years…but my dear Aunt Betty will always be the undisputed world champion Twisty Roll maker!"

*Debi Gilpin
Bluefield, WV*

1 pkg. active yeast
¼ c. warm water
3 T. sugar, divided
1½ t. salt
4¼ c. all-purpose flour, divided
¼ c. butter, melted and cooled

¾ c. milk
1 egg, lightly beaten
1 T. water
1 egg, beaten
1 c. powdered sugar
2 T. milk

Dissolve yeast and 1 teaspoon sugar in warm water (110 to 115 degrees); set aside. Mix remaining sugar, salt and 2 cups flour. Add yeast mixture, melted butter and milk. Stir until smooth. Beat in egg. Add enough flour to make a soft dough. Knead in remaining flour until dough is smooth and elastic (about 5 minutes). Place in greased bowl, cover and let rise in a warm place (85 degrees), away from drafts, until doubled, about 40 minutes. Punch down and roll out to a ¼-inch thickness on a floured surface. Cut into ½"x 6" strips, and braid 3 strips together to form a roll. Combine 1 tablespoon water and remaining egg. Place braids on a baking sheet and brush with egg mixture. Let rise 15 to 20 more minutes. Bake at 375 degrees for 10 to 12 minutes. Let cool. Blend together powdered sugar and milk; drizzle over cooled rolls. Makes 14.

Damascus Brick Sweet Rolls

There's nothing like the aroma of fresh bread baking to welcome guests. The memories and smells of their childhood soon warm their hearts.

1 c. plus 2 T. milk, divided
1 c. butter, divided
2 t. salt
½ c. plus 1 t. sugar, divided
2 pkgs. active dry yeast
1 c. warm water

1 egg, beaten
6 to 7 c. bread flour
Cinnamon-sugar to taste
2 c. powdered sugar
½ t. vanilla extract

In a large saucepan, combine one cup milk, ½ cup butter, salt and ½ cup sugar; heat until just warm. In a small mixing bowl, combine yeast and warm water (110 to 115 degrees) until yeast is dissolved; add remaining sugar. When yeast mixture begins to foam, add to milk mixture; mix well. Fold in egg. Add flour and knead just until smooth. Roll dough out on a floured surface to a 16"×12" rectangle. Sprinkle with cinnamon-sugar mixture to taste; dot with remaining butter. Roll up dough lengthwise and cut into one-inch slices. Place on a lightly greased baking sheet; cover and let rise in a warm place (85 degrees), away from drafts, for 25 minutes or until doubled. Bake at 375 degrees for 12 to 15 minutes. Combine powdered sugar, remaining milk and vanilla; drizzle over rolls. Makes 1½ dozen.

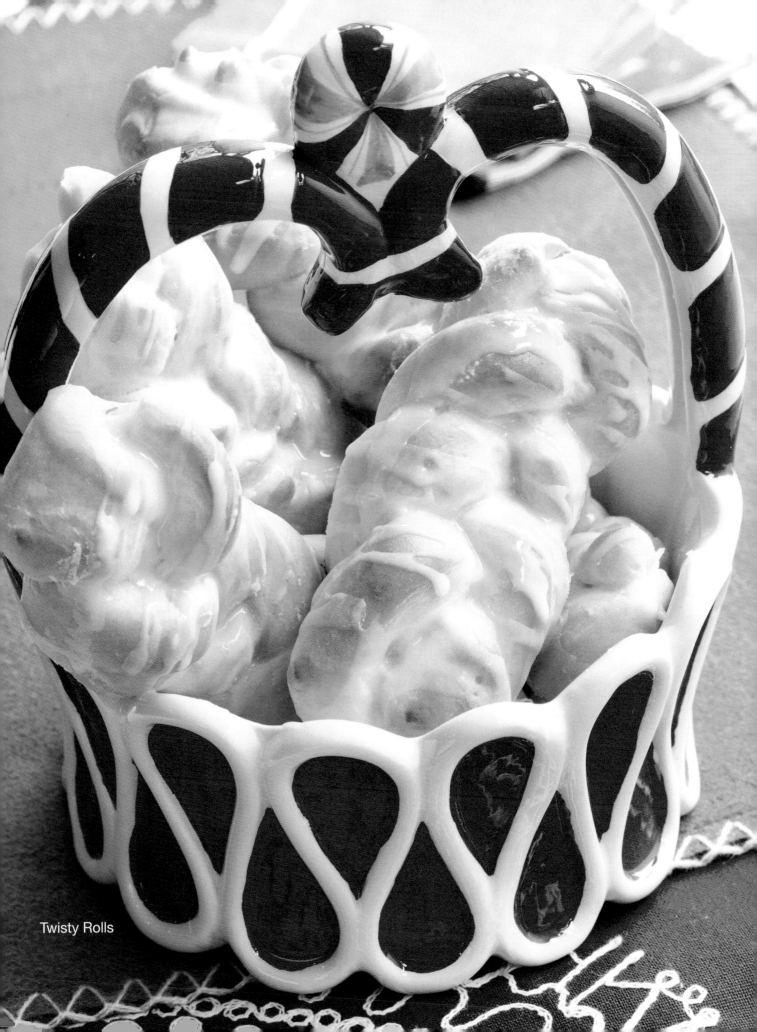

Twisty Rolls

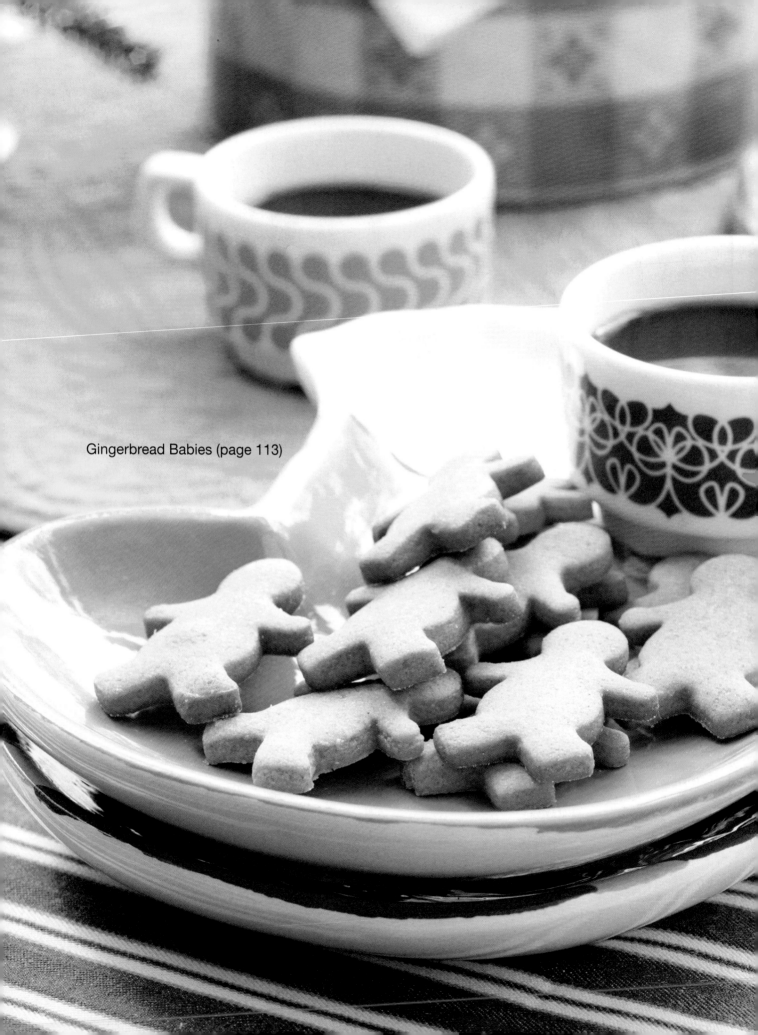

Gingerbread Babies (page 113)

Cookie Swap

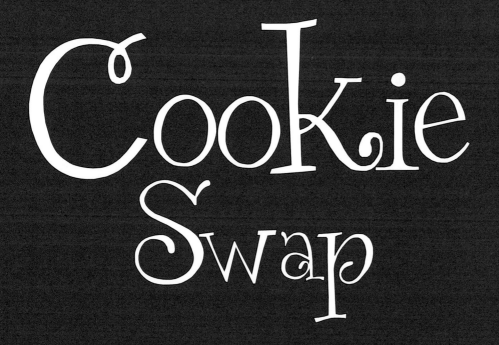

Cookies, bars, brownies and homemade candies...there's nothing like a little something sweet to get you in the spirit of Christmas! Children young and old won't be able to resist Old-Fashioned Iced Sugar Cookies topped with Royal Icing. Let the little ones do the decorating! If chocolate is your weakness, look no further than the Chocolate Cappuccino Brownies. Bet you can't eat just one!

Old-Fashioned Iced Sugar Cookies

These cookies will make memories for years to come.

2 c. shortening
2½ c. sugar
1½ t. orange zest
1½ t. vanilla extract
3 eggs

¼ c. orange juice
6 c. all-purpose flour
4½ t. baking powder
¾ t. salt

In a large bowl, blend together shortening, sugar, orange zest and vanilla. Add eggs to shortening mixture; mix well. Add orange juice and mix. In a separate bowl, sift together flour, baking powder and salt; add to shortening mixture and blend. Divide dough in half; flatten into two disks. Cover with wax paper and chill for 1 hour. Roll out dough ⅛ to ¼-inch thick on lightly floured surface. Cut out with favorite cutters. Use floured spatula to place cookies on ungreased baking sheet. Bake at 375 degrees for 9 to 10 minutes. Cool before removing from baking sheet. Ice cooled cookies with Royal Icing. Once dry, layer cookies in boxes or tins with wax paper between each layer. Makes about 4 dozen.

Royal Icing:

3¼ c. powdered sugar
½ c. water

2½ T. meringue powder

Beat powdered sugar, water and meringue powder in a medium bowl at high speed of an electric mixer 7 to 10 minutes, or until stiff.

Orange Teacake Cookies

"I grew up on these Orange Teacake Cookies. This recipe and my cookie jar are all I have of my grandma...but oh, what a legacy!"

Joy Torkelson

1 c. butter, softened
1 c. sugar
1 T. orange zest
1 T. orange juice
2 t. orange extract

2 eggs
3 c. all-purpose flour
1 t. baking powder
Garnish: sugar

In a large bowl, blend together butter and sugar. Add orange zest, orange juice and orange extract. Add the eggs, beating well. In a separate bowl, sift together flour and baking powder; add to butter mixture. Cover and chill dough for 30 minutes. Divide dough in half. Roll out half of dough at a time between two sheets of wax paper. Roll out to ⅛-inch thickess, cut with cookie cutters and place on greased baking sheets. Sprinkle with sugar. Bake at 350 degrees for 8 minutes. Makes about 2 dozen.

Gingerbread Babies

(pictured on page 110)

¾ c. butter, softened
¾ c. brown sugar, packed
1 egg
½ c. dark molasses
2⅔ c. all-purpose flour

2 t. ground ginger
½ t. nutmeg
½ t. cinnamon
½ t. ground allspice
¼ t. salt

In a large bowl, blend together butter and brown sugar until fluffy. Add egg and molasses. In a separate bowl, combine remaining ingredients; gradually stir into butter mixture. Turn dough out onto well-floured surface; roll out to ⅛-inch thickness. Cut dough with a 2-inch gingerbread man cookie cutter. Place on a greased baking sheet. Bake at 350 degrees for 9 to 10 minutes, or until firm. Makes 12 dozen.

Tuck them into a little box and leave them on someone's doorstep… surely you know someone who will give them a good home at Christmas!

Gramma's Snappiest Ever Ginger Snap Cookies

¾ c. shortening
1½ c. sugar, divided
¼ c. molasses
1 egg
2 c. all-purpose flour

2 t. baking soda
1 t. ground ginger
1 t. ground cloves
1 t. cinnamon

In a large bowl, beat shortening. Add one cup sugar, molasses and egg; beat well. Sift together flour, baking soda and spices; add to shortening mixture. Beat until smooth. Mixture will be very stiff. Shape a teaspoonful of mixture into a ball; then roll ball in remaining sugar. Place on a greased baking sheet. Bake at 350 degrees for 10 to 12 minutes. Makes about 4 dozen.

The smell of these spicy cookies baking will bring back memories.

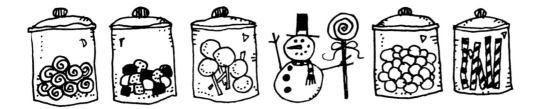

Simple Scottish Shortbread

A favorite cookie from Scotland that will melt in your mouth. Delicious with tea!

1 c. butter, softened
½ c. powdered sugar

½ t. vanilla
2¼ c. all-purpose flour

Beat together butter, powdered sugar and vanilla until well blended. Add flour, one cup at a time, to butter mixture. On a floured surface, roll out dough to ¼ to ½-inch thickness. With a sharp knife, cut dough into 2-inch squares or cut into 1¾-inch rounds with a cookie cutter. Place on ungreased baking sheet and prick top of cookies with a fork. Bake at 325 degrees for 20 minutes, or until bottoms are golden and tops are light in color. Cool on wire racks. Store in airtight containers. Makes about 4 dozen.

The Peanut Butter Bars

"Many years ago when I was in elementary school, our 'Lunch Lady,' Mrs. Hopkins, made these for us once a week. The aroma filled the school as they were baking and we knew we were in store for the best possible treat. I've never had anything that tasted so good! Now I make these for my own family and they agree… they are THE Peanut Butter Bars."

Carol Bull
Delaware, OH

1½ c. plus 2 T. butter, softened
¾ c. creamy peanut butter
¾ c. corn syrup
1 c. sugar

1¾ c. all-purpose flour
2 eggs
1 t. salt

In a large bowl, blend together butter and peanut butter; add corn syrup, sugar, flour, eggs and salt. Mix about 5 minutes. Spread in greased a 13"×9" baking pan. Bake at 350 degrees for 25 minutes, watching carefully. Let cool. Frost with Chocolate Icing and cut into squares. Makes 1½ to 2 dozen.

Chocolate Icing:

¼ c. shortening, melted and cooled
½ c. baking cocoa
¼ t. salt

⅓ c. milk
1½ t. vanilla extract
3½ c. powdered sugar

Combine shortening, cocoa and salt. Add milk and vanilla. Stir in powdered sugar in three parts; beat well.

Simple Scottish
Shortbread

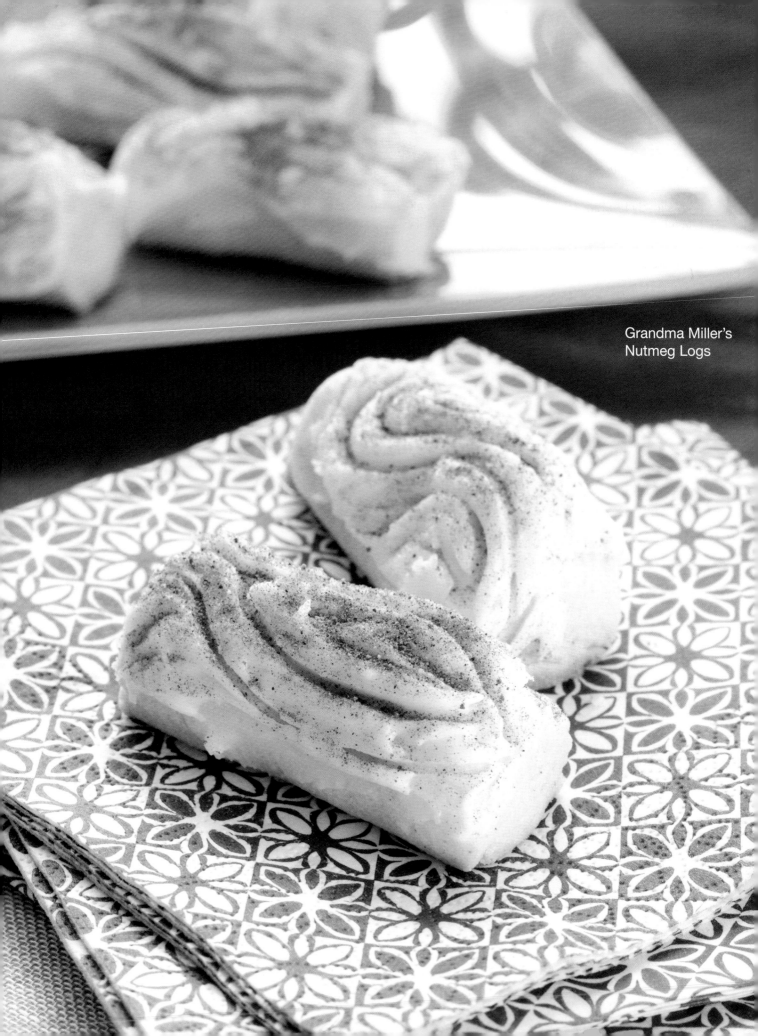

Grandma Miller's
Nutmeg Logs

Grandma Miller's Nutmeg Logs

1 c. butter, softened
¾ c. sugar
1 egg, slightly beaten
2 t. vanilla extract

2 t. rum extract
1 t. nutmeg
3 c. all-purpose flour
Garnish: ¼ t. nutmeg

You'll want more than just one!

In a large bowl, blend together butter and sugar; add egg. Stir in vanilla and rum extract. Mix nutmeg and flour into butter mixture. Divide dough into 52 portions. Roll each portion into 1-inch wide logs and cut into a 1½-inch lengths. Place on ungreased baking sheets. (Since cookies don't spread, they can be placed close together.) Bake at 350 degrees for 10 to 15 minutes. Let cool. Spread Frosting on cookies. Run the tines of a fork across frosting to resemble a log. Sprinkle with ¼ teaspoon nutmeg. Makes 52.

Frosting:

3 T. butter, softened
½ t. vanilla extract
1 t. rum extract

2½ c. powdered sugar
3 T. milk

Mix first 4 ingredients together; add milk until desired consistency.

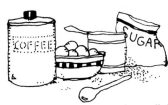

"I REMEMBER THE CHRISTMAS SEASON, with its blustery nights, when I would find my precious mother in the kitchen making fudge and hear the sound of dancing popcorn on the stove. My two sisters and I would linger at Mom's side to see which one of us would get the privilege of licking the chocolate off the old wooden spoon…the chocolate aroma in the air, mixed with the scent of popcorn, just made our tiny mouths water for the tasty treats! Our evenings together were magical as we tasted the delights of tempting snacks, and it gave Mom and Dad time to hear the three of us tell them our Christmas wishes and dreams. Time is such a fleeting thing. Grab every wonderful moment and each loving memory, then hold them in your heart."

Thais Menges
Three Rivers, MI

Chocolate Cappuccino Brownies

Chewy and chocolatey together...delicious!

½ c. butter, melted
1 c. brown sugar, packed
2 T. instant coffee granules
3 eggs, slightly beaten
1 t. vanilla extract
½ c. brewed coffee, cooled
1 t. baking powder

½ t. salt
1¼ c. unbleached white flour, sifted
⅓ c. plus 1 T. baking cocoa
1 c. walnuts, chopped
1 c. semi-sweet chocolate chips
Garnish: powdered sugar

In a bowl, combine butter, brown sugar and coffee granules; blend well. Add eggs, vanilla and cooled coffee; stir. In a separate bowl, combine baking powder, salt, flour and cocoa; add to butter mixture. Stir in walnuts and chocolate chips. Pour batter into a greased 13"x9" pan and bake at 350 degrees for 25 to 30 minutes. Allow to cool and cut into squares. Dust with powdered sugar before serving. Makes 1½ to 2 dozen.

Cream Cheese Brownies

"I have made these brownies so many times I could bake them with my eyes closed!"

Jean Landolfi
Northford, CT

8-oz. pkg. cream cheese, softened
2⅓ c. sugar, divided
3 eggs, divided
⅔ c. baking cocoa
½ c. butter
¾ c. water

2 c. all-purpose flour
1 t. baking soda
½ t. salt
1 t. vanilla extract
½ c. sour cream
1 c. chocolate chips

Combine cream cheese, ⅓ cup sugar and one egg; set aside. Mix cocoa, butter and water in a saucepan and heat until butter is melted. In a bowl, mix together flour, remaining sugar, baking soda, salt, vanilla, 2 eggs and sour cream. Beat cocoa mixture into flour mixture. Spread into a greased and floured 17½"x11" pan. Spoon cream cheese mixture over chocolate mixture; pull a knife through the layers to marble. Sprinkle chocolate chips on top. Bake at 375 degrees for 20 to 25 minutes. Let cool and cut into squares. Makes about 2 dozen.

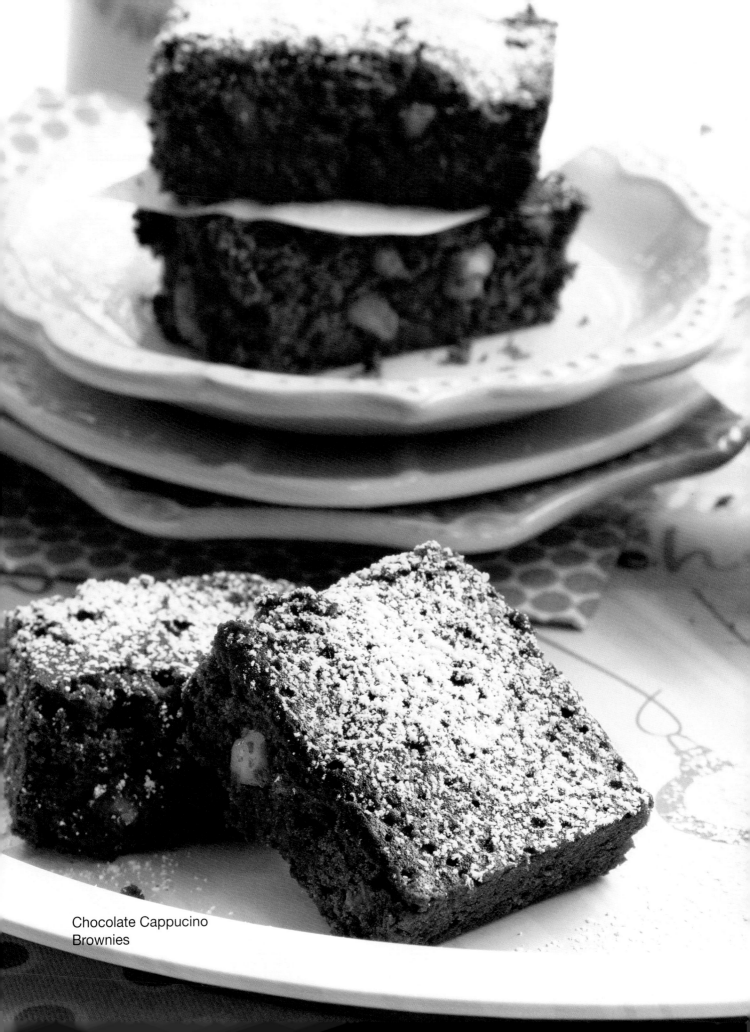

Chocolate Cappucino
Brownies

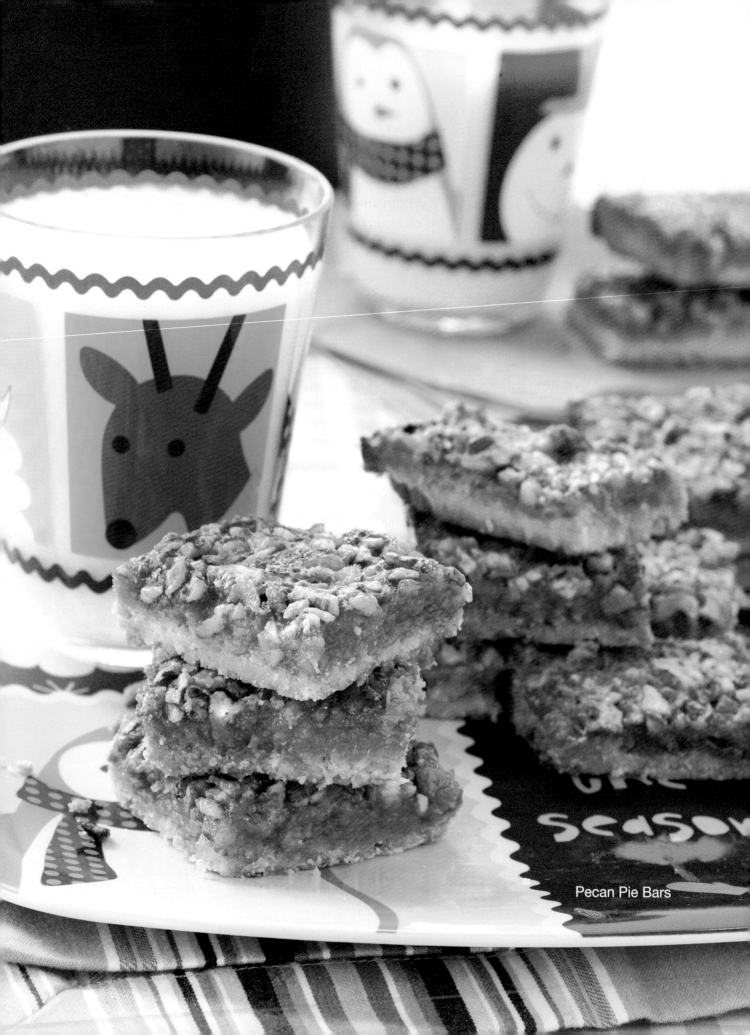

Pecan Pie Bars

Pecan Pie Bars

1¼ c. all-purpose flour
½ c. plus 3 T. brown sugar, packed
    and divided
½ c. plus 2 T. butter, divided

2 eggs
½ c. light corn syrup
1 t. vanilla extract
½ c. chopped pecans

Wonderful little pecan pie bars you can't stop eating! Great for a church social or holiday cookie exchange.

Combine flour with 3 tablespoons brown sugar; cut in ½ cup butter until coarse crumbs form. Press into a lightly greased 11"x7" baking pan. Bake at 375 degrees for 20 minutes. While crust is baking, beat eggs in a large bowl and add remaining brown sugar, 2 tablespoons melted butter, corn syrup and vanilla. Blend in pecans and pour mixture into hot crust. Bake for 15 to 20 minutes. Cool and cut into bars. Makes 2 dozen.

Southern Pecan Pralines

1½ c. brown sugar, packed
1½ c. sugar
3 T. corn syrup

1 c. milk
1 t. vanilla extract
1½ c. chopped pecans

"While touring plantations in Georgia and South Carolina, I found a wonderful book that shared Christmas traditions of the old South. These wonderful pralines are reminiscent of that simpler time."

Juanita Williams
Jacksonville, OR

Combine sugars, corn syrup and milk in a heavy 3-quart saucepan. Cook over medium heat, stirring constantly, until the mixture comes to a boil. Turn the heat to low and continue stirring until a little of the mixture dropped into cold water forms a soft ball or mixture reaches 234 to 240 degrees on a candy thermometer. Remove from heat and let stand for 10 minutes. Stir in the vanilla and beat for 2 minutes, using a wooden spoon. Add pecans and stir until creamy. Drop by tablespoonfuls onto wax paper to make patties about 2½ inches in diameter. Let pralines stand until firm, and then peel from the wax paper. Makes 2½ dozen.

"I HAVE SUCH FOND CHRISTMAS MEMORIES of my sisters, brothers and myself lining up at the kitchen table for cookie decorating. Mom and my older sister would frost the cut-outs and pass them down the 'assembly line,' where each of us had our own container of candy sprinkles or red cinnamon candies to apply. We were quite creative, but even more so when we turned the frosted cookies upside-down to gather up all the scattered sugars and sprinkles. What a mess, but what fun we had! It still makes me smile."

Lori Krigbaum
Stoughton, WI

Divinity

"Our family loved making divinity every Christmas. I feel so blessed to have such fond memories of the holidays and I hope, with Mom's help, to carry on the family tradition for years to come."

Tina Kutchman
Johnstown, PA

2 egg whites, stiffly beaten
1 t. vanilla extract
3 c. sugar
1 c. corn syrup

1 c. water
Optional: 2 drops food coloring
Optional: ¼ c. chopped walnuts

Blend egg whites and vanilla; set aside. Combine sugar, corn syrup and water in a saucepan. Stir to dissolve sugar, then bring to a boil. Continue to boil until mixture reaches the hard-ball stage or 260 degrees on a candy thermometer. Remove from heat and pour in a thin stream over egg whites. Continue to beat until mixture stands in peaks; add food coloring, if desired. Beat with a wooden spoon until candy is dull in color and holds its shape when dropped onto wax paper. Working very quickly, drop candy onto wax paper by tablespoonfuls and top with nuts, if desired. Makes 2 pounds.

Coconut Joys

"My daughter and I love these...we can't get enough of them!"

Flo Burtnett
Gage, OK

½ c. butter
2 c. powdered sugar
3 c. sweetened flaked coconut

2 (1-oz.) sqs. milk baking chocolate, melted
Garnish: finely chopped nuts

In a large saucepan, melt butter; remove from heat. Add powdered sugar and coconut; mix well. Shape rounded teaspoonfuls into balls. Place balls on a parchment-lined baking sheet, and then make indentations in the center of each. Fill indentations on each ball with chocolate; sprinkle nuts over chocolate. Chill 3 hours or until firm. Makes 3 dozen.

Chocolate-Peanut Candy

Candy made in a slow cooker...so easy!

1 T. oil
3 T. baking cocoa
24 oz. white melting chocolate
12-oz. pkg. chocolate chips

16-oz. container unsalted, dry roasted peanuts
16-oz. container salted, dry roasted peanuts

Combine oil, cocoa, white melting chocolate and chocolate chips in a 5-quart slow cooker. Cook on high setting until chocolate is melted and smooth. Turn off slow cooker and add peanuts; stir well. Drop by teaspoonfuls onto wax paper; cool. Makes about 8 dozen.

Easy Cream Cheese
Truffles

Easy Cream Cheese Truffles

8-oz. pkg. cream cheese, softened
4¼ c. powdered sugar, divided
5 (1-oz.) sqs. unsweetened baking
    chocolate, melted and cooled

¼ c. baking cocoa
¼ c. almonds, toasted and finely
    chopped
¼ c. sweetened flaked coconut, toasted

It's fun rolling these in the different coatings.

    Beat cream cheese until fluffy. Slowly add 4 cups powdered sugar. Beat until smooth. Add melted chocolate and beat until blended. Chill for approximately one hour. Shape chilled mixture into one-inch balls. Roll some in ¼ cup powdered sugar, some in cocoa, some in nuts and some in coconut. Store in an airtight container in the refrigerator for up to 2 weeks. Makes 6½ dozen.

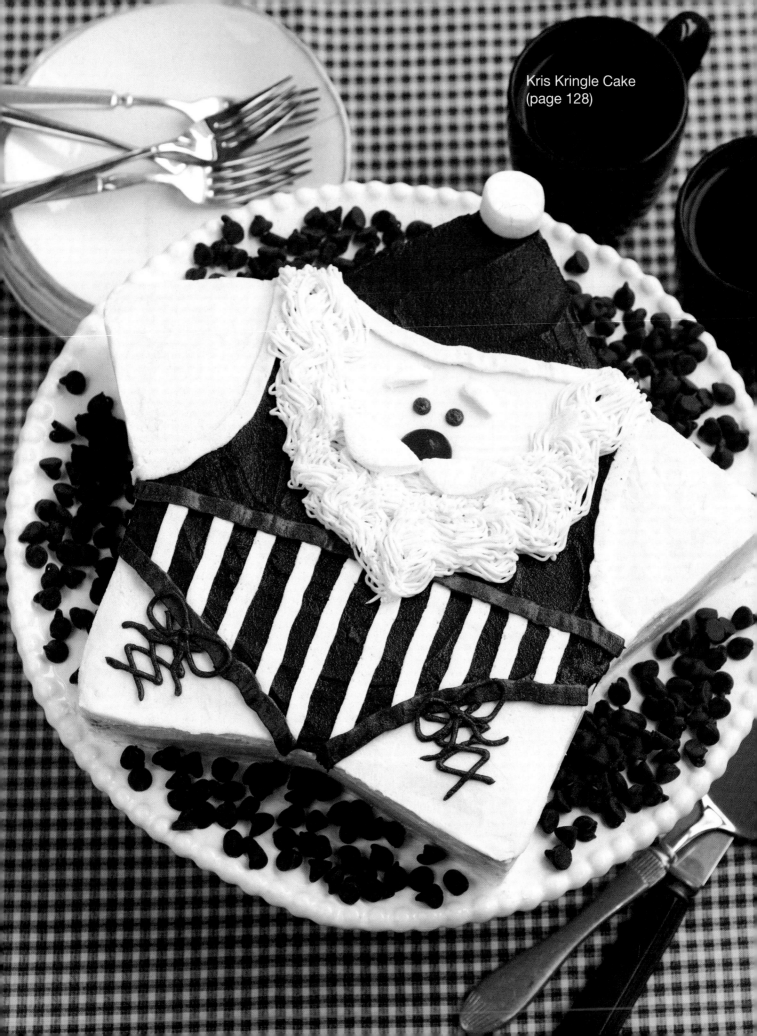

Kris Kringle Cake
(page 128)

Yuletide Sweets

Make the holiday season that much sweeter with these decadent cakes, pies and other mouth-watering desserts. Impress your guests with the beautifully layered Old-Fashioned Jam Cake. And you'll have them begging for more with the Chocolate Chip Cookie Dough Pie or the Holiday Hot Fudge Dessert!

German Chocolate Cake

18¼-oz. white cake mix
5.9-oz. pkg. instant chocolate
  pudding mix

1 c. milk
1 c. water
3 egg whites

Combine all ingredients in a large bowl and beat with an electric mixer at medium speed for 2 minutes. Pour into 2 greased and floured round cake pans. Bake at 350 degrees for 25 to 35 minutes. Cool 10 minutes in pans and remove. Cool completely. Frost with Coconut-Pecan Frosting. Serves 6 to 8.

Coconut-Pecan Frosting:

1⅓ c. evaporated milk
1⅓ c. sugar
4 egg yolks, beaten
⅔ c. butter

1½ t. vanilla extract
1⅓ c. sweetened flaked coconut
1⅓ c. chopped pecans

Combine milk, sugar, egg yolks and butter in a heavy saucepan; bring to a boil and cook over medium heat 12 minutes, stirring constantly. Add vanilla, coconut and pecans; stir until frosting is cool and spreadable.

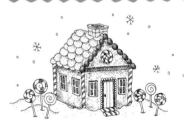

"EACH YEAR AT CHRISTMAS, SINCE MY SONS WERE YOUNG, I have baked a gingerbread house. The decorating part is a family event and so we set aside one night to assemble and decorate the house. The kitchen table is loaded down with a variety of candy, chocolates, sugar cubes and decorations. We've learned that the more icing we use, the sturdier the house is and so far it has never collapsed!

My sons are now 18 and 13 years old and around Thanksgiving they began asking what night is set aside for decorating our gingerbread house. I'm not sure which I enjoy more…the family fun building the house, or the sight of all the neighborhood children coming in for the demolition and eating. Both are precious memories that I hope will carry on to the next generation."

*Elaine Pettit
Clearwater, FL*

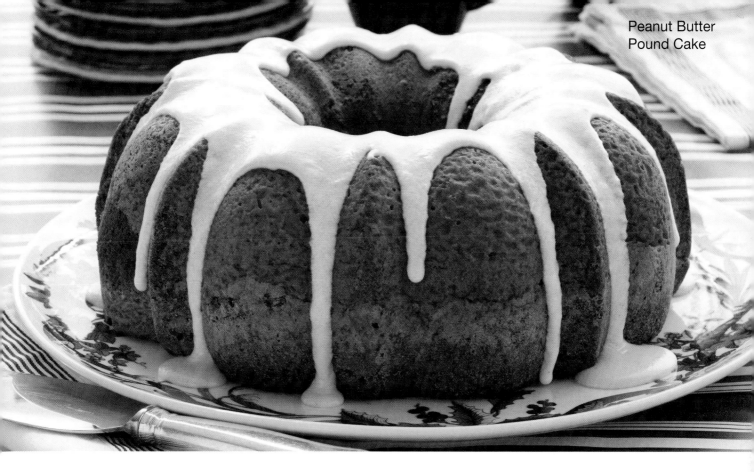

Peanut Butter Pound Cake

1 c. butter, softened
2 c. sugar
1 c. light brown sugar, packed
½ c. creamy peanut butter
5 eggs
1 T. vanilla extract

3 c. cake flour
½ t. baking powder
½ t. salt
¼ t. baking soda
1 c. whipping cream or whole milk

Delicious without the frosting, too!

In a bowl, beat butter and sugar until fluffy. Add brown sugar and peanut butter; beat thoroughly. Add eggs, one at a time, beating well after each addition; stir in vanilla. Sift together the dry ingredients and add alternately with whipping cream. Pour into a lightly greased and floured 10" tube pan. Bake at 325 degrees for one hour, or until it tests done. Frost, if desired, with Peanut Butter Frosting. Serves 10 to 12.

Peanut Butter Frosting:

¼ c. butter, softened
⅛ t. salt
5 to 6 T. milk

⅓ c. creamy peanut butter
16-oz. pkg. powdered sugar

Combine all ingredients and beat until smooth.

Kris Kringle Cake

(pictured on page 124)

A special cake for a special time of year.

1¼ c. butter or margarine, softened and divided
1½ c. brown sugar, packed
3 eggs
1 c. sour cream
½ c. plus 3 T. milk, divided
2 c. all-purpose flour
2 t. cinnamon
1½ t. baking soda
1 t. baking powder

½ t. cloves
½ t. nutmeg
½ t. salt
6 c. powdered sugar
¾ c. shortening
1 T. vanilla extract
brown and red paste food coloring
red candied cherry, halved
4 large marshmallows

For cake, beat ½ cup butter and brown sugar in a large bowl until fluffy. Add eggs, one at a time, beating well after each addition. Add sour cream and ½ cup milk; stir until well blended. In a medium bowl, sift together flour, cinnamon, baking soda, baking powder, cloves, nutmeg and salt. Add dry ingredients to butter mixture, stirring until well blended. Spoon batter into a greased and floured 12½-inch-wide star-shaped baking pan. Bake at 350 degrees for 35 to 40 minutes or until a toothpick inserted in the center tests done. Cool in pan 10 minutes. Remove cake from pan and cool completely on a wire rack.

For frosting, combine powdered sugar, shortening, ¾ cup butter, 3 tablespoons milk and vanilla in a large bowl; beat until smooth. Spoon 1½ cups frosting into a pastry bag; cover end of bag with plastic wrap and set aside. Spoon ¼ cup frosting into small bowl; tint brown. Spoon brown frosting into a pastry bag; cover end of bag with plastic wrap and set aside. Spoon one cup frosting into another small bowl; tint red.

Spread remaining white frosting on sides of cake, on top of four tips of cake for hands and feet and on top of cake for face. Spread red frosting on top of cake for hat and suit. Use table knife or small metal spatula dipped in water to smooth frosting.

Using white frosting and a basketweave tip with smooth side of tip facing up, pipe stripes on pants and trim on shirt and hat. Using brown frosting and a basketweave tip with smooth side of tip facing up, pipe belt and trim on top of boots. Using brown frosting and a small round tip, pipe eyes and laces on boots. Using white frosting and a grass tip, pipe beard.

Place one cherry half on cake for nose. Cut one marshmallow in half crosswise. Place one marshmallow half on top of hat for pom-pom. Draw and cut out patterns for mustache and eyebrows. Use a rolling pin to roll out remaining marshmallows to ⅛-inch thickness. Place patterns on marshmallow pieces and use small sharp knife to cut out 2 mustache pieces and 2 eyebrows; place on cake. Store in an airtight container in refrigerator. Serves 16.

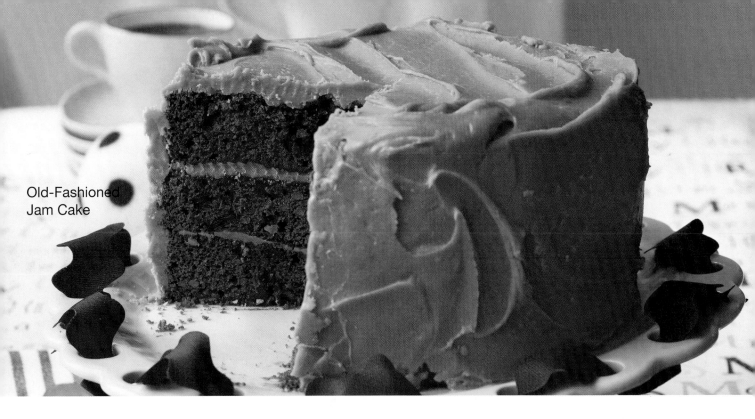

Old-Fashioned
Jam Cake

Old-Fashioned Jam Cake

1 c. plus 6 T. shortening, divided
5¾ c. sugar, divided
½ c. water
½ c. applesauce
1 c. seedless blackberry jam
2 eggs
3 c. all-purpose flour
½ c. baking cocoa
1 t. baking powder
1 t. baking soda

½ t. salt
1 t. each ground cinnamon, ground
    allspice and ground nutmeg
1 c. buttermilk
1 c. raisins
1 c. chopped pecans
6 T. butter
1½ c. milk
1½ t. vanilla extract

*For neat slices, cut with
an electric knife.*

Beat one cup shortening until creamy; gradually beat in 2 cups sugar. Add water; beat until fluffy. Beat in applesauce and jam; add eggs, one at a time. Combine flour, cocoa, baking powder, baking soda, salt and spices; add to shortening mixture alternately with buttermilk. Stir in raisins and pecans. Pour into 3 lightly greased 9" round pans. Bake at 350 degrees for 24 minutes, or until toothpick tests clean. Cool in pans 10 minutes; remove from pans and cool completely on wire racks.

Combine 3 cups sugar, remaining shortening, butter and milk in heavy saucepan. Bring to a boil; remove from heat. Heat ¾ cup sugar in a separate saucepan over medium heat until sugar melts and is golden. Stirring rapidly, pour into icing in saucepan; bring to a boil over medium heat. Cook, stirring for about 15 minutes, until icing reaches soft ball stage (234 to 243 degrees on a candy thermometer). Remove from heat; stir in vanilla. Let stand 10 minutes, then beat icing with wooden spoon until thick and creamy but still hot. Ice between layers, on sides and top of cake; smooth with spatula dipped in hot water if necessary. Serves 12.

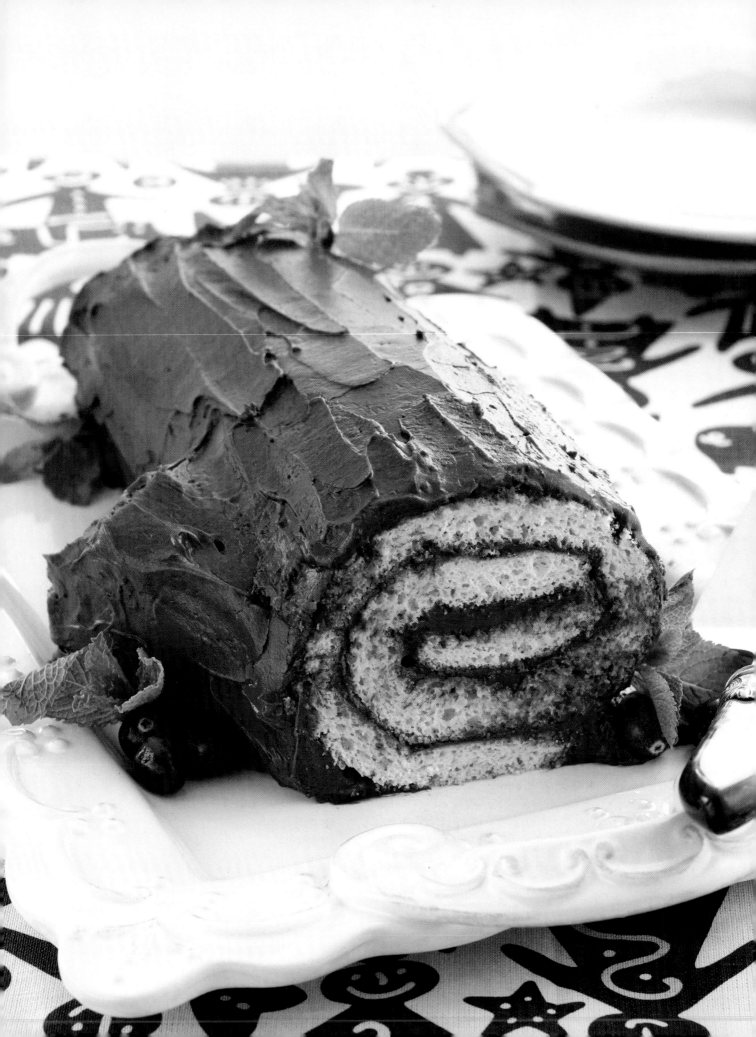

Bûche de Noël

1 c. all-purpose flour
1 t. baking powder
¼ t. salt
4 eggs, separated
¾ c. sugar, divided

⅓ cup water
1 t. vanilla extract
3 T. powdered sugar
Garnish: fresh mint and fresh
   cranberries

This traditional French cake resembles the Yule logs of long ago.

Combine flour, baking powder and salt; set aside. Beat egg whites with an electric mixer at high speed until foamy. Gradually add ¼ cup sugar, 1 tablespoon at a time, beating until stiff peaks form and sugar dissolves, about 2 to 4 minutes; set aside. Beat egg yolks in a large mixing bowl with an electric mixer at high speed, gradually adding ½ cup sugar; beat 5 minutes, or until thick and pale. Add water and vanilla extract; beat well. Add flour mixture; beat just until blended. Fold in about ⅓ of egg white mixture. Gently fold in remaining egg white mixture. Grease bottom and sides of a 15"x10" jelly-roll pan. Line with wax paper; grease and flour. Spread batter evenly into pan. Bake at 375 degrees for 10 minutes, or until top springs back when lightly touched. Sift powdered sugar in a 15"x10" rectangle on a cloth. When cake is done, immediately loosen from sides of pan; turn out onto cloth. Peel off wax paper. Starting at narrow end, roll up cake and cloth together; cool completely on a wire rack, seam side down.

Unroll cake and remove towel. Spread half Chocolate Frosting onto cake; carefully reroll. Cut a 1-inch-thick diagonal slice from one end of cake roll. Place cake roll on a serving plate, seam side down. Position slice against side of cake roll to resemble knot; use frosting to "glue" in place. Spread remaining frosting over cake and knot. If frosting is soft, chill cake before serving. Garnish with fresh mint and fresh cranberries. Serves 8 to 10.

Chocolate Frosting:

3¾ c. sifted powdered sugar
½ c. baking cocoa

6 T. milk
6 T. butter, softened

In a large bowl, combine powdered sugar and cocoa. Add milk and butter to sugar mixture; beat with an electric mixer at medium speed until smooth.

Pumpkin-Dutch Apple Pie

Two favorite flavors in one wonderful pie.

2 Granny Smith apples, peeled, cored and thinly sliced
1 c. plus 1 T. sugar, divided
½ c. plus 2 t. all-purpose flour, divided
1 t. lemon juice
1 t. cinnamon, divided
9-inch deep-dish pie crust

2 eggs, lightly beaten
1½ c. canned pumpkin
1 c. evaporated milk
5 T. butter, divided
⅛ t. nutmeg
¼ t. salt
⅓ c. walnuts, chopped

For apple layer, toss apples with ¼ cup sugar, 2 teaspoons flour, lemon juice and ¼ teaspoon cinnamon. Place in pie crust.

For pumpkin layer, combine eggs, pumpkin, evaporated milk, ½ cup sugar, 2 tablespoons melted butter, ¾ teaspoon cinnamon, nutmeg and salt. Pour over apple layer. Bake at 375 degrees for 30 minutes. While pie is baking, mix together ½ cup flour, ⅓ cup sugar, 3 tablespoons softened butter and walnuts; sprinkle over pie. Return to oven and bake 20 more minutes, or until filling is set. Cool. Serves 8.

Nutty Maple Pie

Rich and flavorful; a twist on traditional pecan pie.

⅔ c. sugar
6 T. butter, melted and cooled
4 eggs

1 c. maple syrup
1 c. whole hazelnuts, chopped
9-inch pie crust

Combine sugar, butter, eggs, maple syrup and hazelnuts. Pour into pie crust and bake at 400 degrees for 10 minutes; reduce heat to 325 degrees and bake 25 more minutes. Cool. Serves 8.

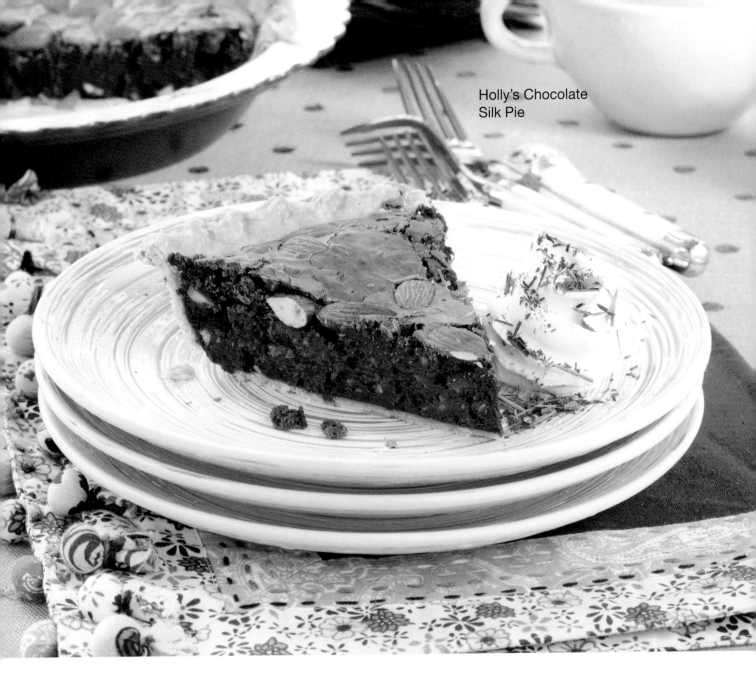

Holly's Chocolate
Silk Pie

Holly's Chocolate Silk Pie

¾ c. brown sugar, packed
¼ c. butter, softened
3 eggs
1¼ c. semi-sweet chocolate chips,
  melted
1½ t. instant coffee granules

½ t. almond extract
1 c. almonds, toasted and chopped
¼ c. all-purpose flour
9-inch pie crust
½ c. whole almonds

The rich filling is as smooth as silk!

In a mixing bowl, beat brown sugar and butter until fluffy. Beat in eggs, one at a time. Mix in chocolate chips, coffee and almond extract. Add chopped nuts and flour; mix well. Pour filling into pie crust. Decorate top with whole almonds. Bake at 375 degrees for 30 minutes on lower rack in oven. Cool. Serves 6 to 8.

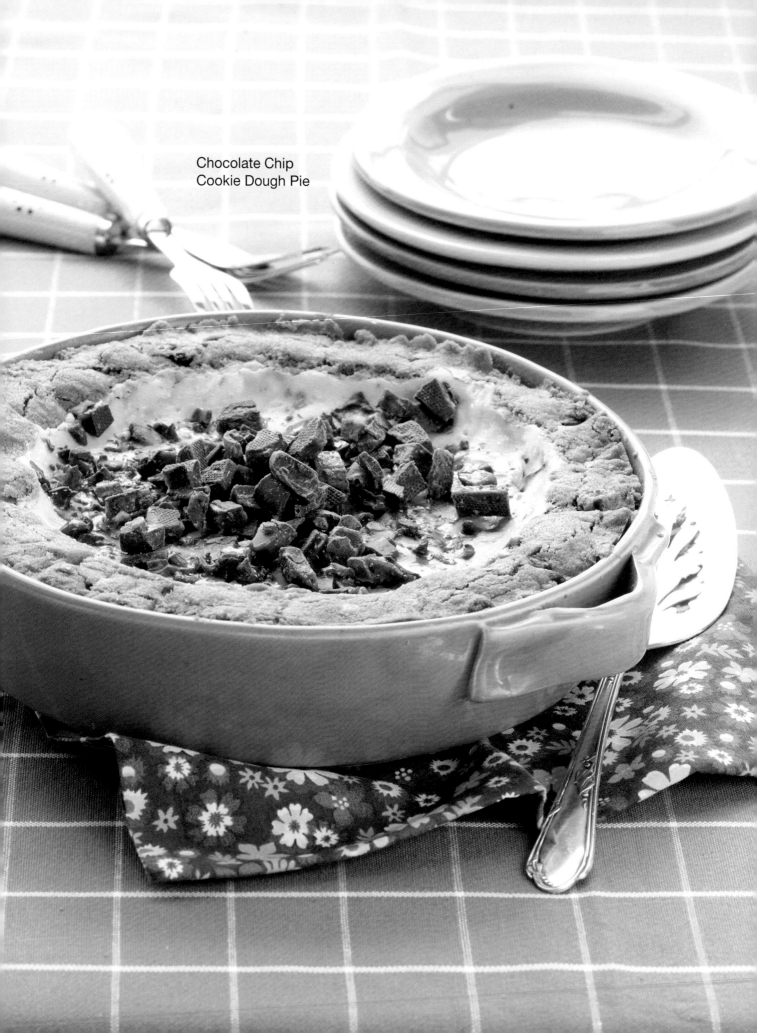

Chocolate Chip
Cookie Dough Pie

Chocolate Chip Cookie Dough Pie

16½-oz. tube refrigerated chocolate
   chip cookie dough
2 (8-oz.) pkgs. cream cheese, softened
2 eggs

½ c. sugar
5 (1.4-oz.) bars chocolate covered
   toffee candy, divided

There is nothing better than chocolate chip cookie dough!

Press cookie dough into an ungreased 9" pie plate to make crust. In a large mixing bowl, combine cream cheese, eggs, sugar and 3 crumbled candy bars; pour into cookie dough crust. Bake, uncovered, at 325 degrees for 30 to 35 minutes. Cool completely. Sprinkle top with remaining 2 crumbled candy bars. Chill until ready to serve. Serves 8.

White Chocolate-Macadamia Brownie Pie

½ c. butter, softened
1 c. sugar
2 eggs
½ c. all-purpose flour

¼ c. baking cocoa
1 t. vanilla extract
½ c. macadamia nuts, chopped
½ c. white chocolate chips

The crunchy macadamia nuts combine with the creamy white chocolate to create a fabulous taste sensation.

Cream butter and sugar together and beat in the eggs. Add flour, cocoa and vanilla. Fold in the nuts and chips. Pour into a greased 9" pie plate. Bake at 325 degrees for 35 minutes. Pie should be moist; toothpick will not come out completely clean. Let cool, but serve slightly warm. Serves 8.

IT'S OH-SO- EASY TO MAKE VANILLA SUGAR for flavoring cookies, pastries or even a cup of coffee! Simply put a vanilla bean in a jar of sugar and seal tightly…the longer it sits, the stronger the flavor.

Marbled Pumpkin Cheesecake

This looks so pretty on a holiday buffet table.

¾ c. gingersnaps, crushed
¾ c. graham crackers, crushed
1¼ c. sugar, divided
¼ c. butter, melted
2 (8-oz.) pkgs. cream cheese, softened
4 eggs

15-oz. can pumpkin
½ t. cinnamon
¼ t. ginger
¼ t. nutmeg
Garnish: whipped cream, additional nutmeg

In a bowl, combine gingersnaps and graham crumbs with ¼ cup sugar and butter. Press into the bottom of a 9" springform pan. Bake at 350 degrees for 8 to 10 minutes. In a mixing bowl, beat cream cheese until smooth. Gradually add one cup sugar; beat until light. Add eggs, one at a time, beating well after each. Transfer 1½ cups of cream cheese mixture to a separate bowl and blend in pumpkin and spices. Pour half of pumpkin mixture into prepared pie crust. Top with half of cream cheese mixture. Repeat layers using remaining pumpkin and cream cheese mixtures. Using a table knife, cut through layers with uplifting motion in 4 to 5 places to create marbled effect. Bake at 325 degrees for 45 minutes without opening oven door. Turn off oven and let cake stand in oven for one hour. Remove from oven and run knife around sides of pan to remove sides. Cool and store in refrigerator. Top each serving with a dollop of whipped cream and additional nutmeg. Serves 10 to 12.

Raspberry Crunch Cheesecake

Make this the night before; it's a great time-saver!

1½ c. quick-cooking oats, uncooked
1½ c. brown sugar, packed
1½ c. all-purpose flour
1 c. butter
¾ c. nuts, chopped
5 (8-oz.) pkgs. cream cheese

1 c. sugar
¼ c. cornstarch
½ c. whipping cream
4 eggs
10-oz. jar seedless raspberry jam

In a bowl, mix together oats, brown sugar and flour. Cut in the butter to make crumbs; add nuts. Press 5½ cups of mixture into the bottom and halfway up the sides of a greased 10" springform pan. Save the remaining ¾ cup crumbs for the top of cake. Bake at 350 degrees for 15 to 18 minutes to set crust. In a large bowl, beat cream cheese, sugar, cornstarch and cream with an electric mixer at medium speed. Add eggs, one at a time, beating well after each addition. Pour into crust. Heat jam in microwave 30 seconds. Spoon jam over batter and swirl into batter.

Bake at 325 degrees for 1 hour and 15 minutes. Top hot cake with reserved crumbs. Return to oven and bake for 15 to 20 more minutes, or until crust is golden. Turn off oven and let cake stand in oven for one hour. Chill overnight. Serves 12.

Marbled Pumpkin
Cheesecake

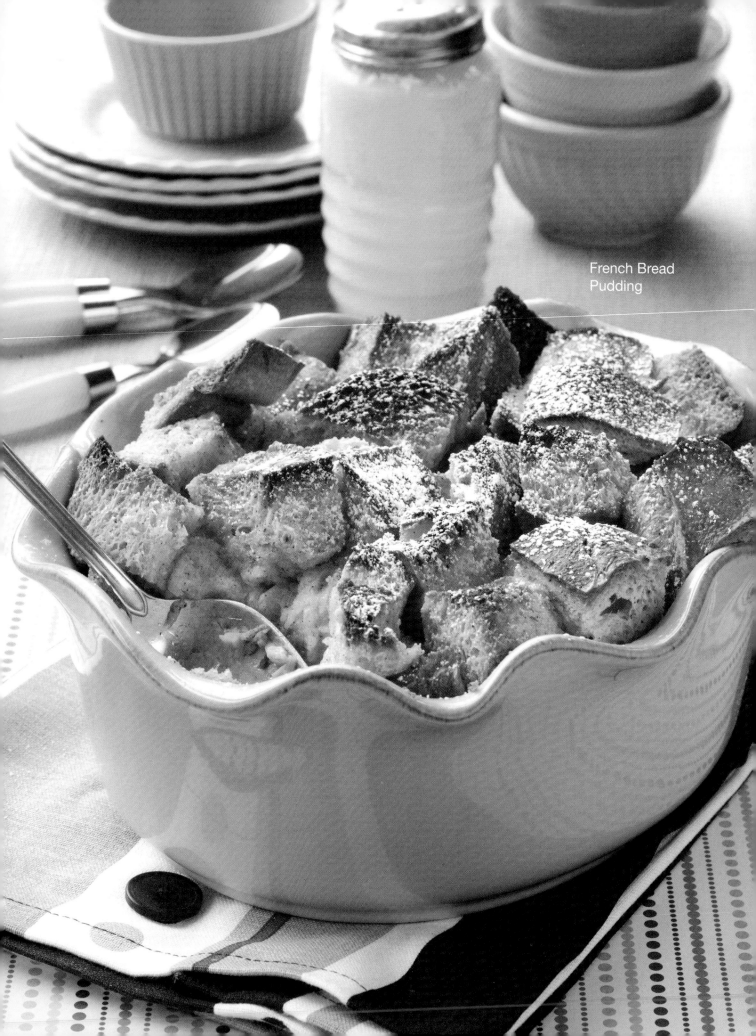

French Bread
Pudding

French Bread Pudding

2½ c. milk
½ c. whipping cream
4 eggs
½ c. sugar
1½ t. vanilla extract
½ t. cinnamon, or to taste if using
    plain bread

½ t. nutmeg
Optional: 1 t. orange zest, finely grated
⅛ t. salt
7 c. cinnamon, French or rich egg bread,
    crusts trimmed and cut into cubes
3 T. butter, melted
Garnish: powdered sugar

A soul-satisfying treat the whole family will love!

Whisk together milk, cream, eggs, sugar, vanilla, cinnamon, nutmeg, orange zest, if desired, and salt in a medium mixing bowl until well blended. Toss with bread in a bowl to coat. Spoon into greased 2 quart casserole dish; drizzle with melted butter. Bake at 325 degrees for 1 hour or until knife inserted in center comes out clean. Before serving, sprinkle with powdered sugar. Serve warm or chilled. Serves 6.

Holiday Hot Fudge Dessert

1 c. all-purpose flour
2 t. baking powder
¾ c. sugar
¼ t. salt
6 T. baking cocoa, divided
½ c. chopped nuts
½ c. milk

2 t. oil
1 t. vanilla extract
1 c. brown sugar, packed
1½ c. hot water
Garnish: whipped cream and
    peppermint candies, crushed

Serve with vanilla ice cream or whipped cream.

Combine flour, baking powder, sugar, salt, 2 tablespoons cocoa and nuts. Add milk, oil and vanilla. Spread into a lightly greased 8"×8" baking pan. Combine brown sugar and remaining cocoa and sprinkle on top of mixture in pan. Pour hot water over entire batter. Do not stir. Bake at 350 degrees for 45 to 50 minutes. Garnish with whipped cream and peppermint candies. Serves 6 to 8.

IT'S AN OLD ENGLISH CUSTOM to wrap tiny treasures in paper and bake them inside the Christmas cake. A bell means a wedding soon, a thimble blesses its owner, a wishbone grants any wish and a horseshoe means good luck. Be sure to let your guests know about the surprises before they dig in!

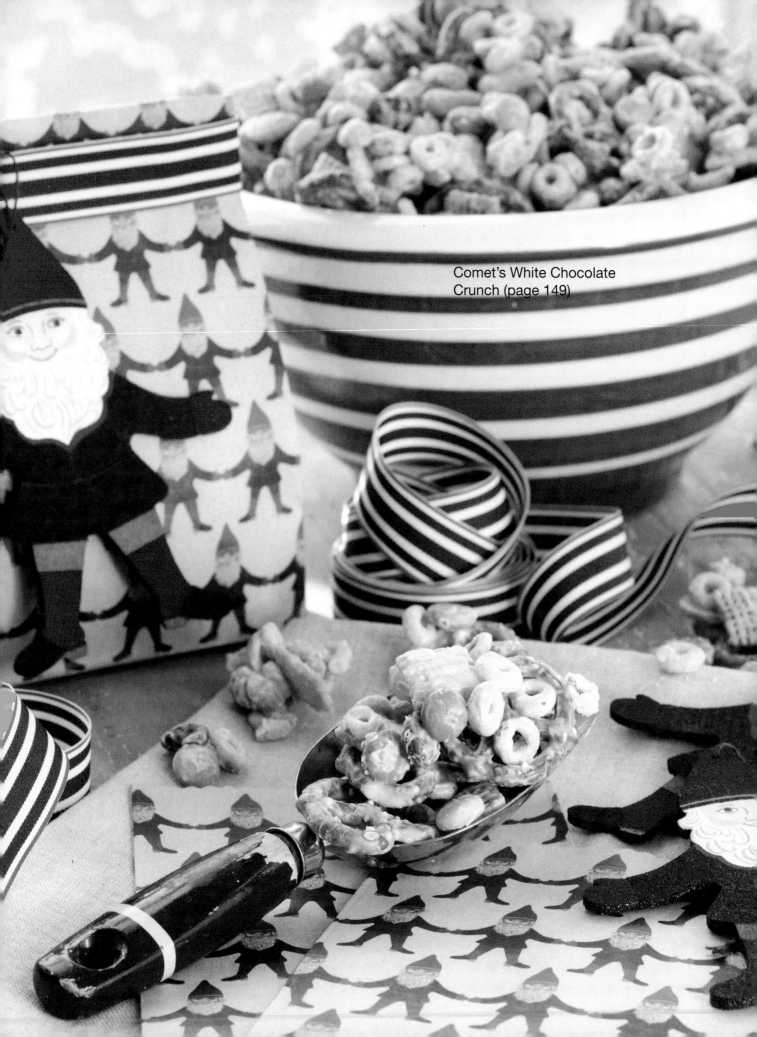

Comet's White Chocolate
Crunch (page 149)

Goodies for Giving

A heartfelt gift from your kitchen will mean the world to your friend or family member this Christmas. Whether you choose to give Patchwork Bean Soup Mix, Holiday Gift Cakes or even the adorable Santa Claus Cookie Pops, your gift...and the thought that went into making it...will be remembered for years to come.

Patchwork Bean Soup Mix

This colorful soup mix would be great paired with crazy quilt potholders or oven mitts!

½ c. dried kidney beans
½ c. dried black-eyed peas
½ c. dried black beans
½ c. dried red beans
½ c. dried split green pas
½ c. dried Great Northern beans
½ c. dried kidney beans
½ c. dried lima beans

3 T. chicken bouillon
1 T. dried, minced onion
salt and pepper to taste
½ t. garlic powder
1 T. dried parsley flakes
1 t. celery seeds
¼ c. brown sugar, packed

Layer beans in a one-quart jar. In a plastic zipping bag, blend together seasonings. For gift-giving, attach the bag of seasonings and the following instructions: Add beans to a large stockpot; cover with hot water and soak overnight. Drain and add 2 quarts water. Bring to a boil; reduce heat and simmer, covered, 1 to 2 hours or until beans are almost tender. Stir in two 14½-ounce cans stewed tomatoes and seasoning mix. Simmer, uncovered, 1 to 1½ hours, or until beans are tender. Makes 12 cups.

Chill-Chaser Chili

½ c. dried pinto beans
½ c. dried kidney beans
2 T. dried minced onion

1 T. dried pepper flakes
½ t. dried minced garlic

Rinse and sort through beans; discard any that are shriveled. Spread on a paper towel to dry overnight. Combine beans and remaining ingredients. Package in a gift bag or glass jar along with Seasoning Packet. For gift-giving, attach the following instructions: Cover bean mix with water in a saucepan. Bring to a boil; boil 10 minutes. Cover pan and turn off heat. Let stand one hour; drain. Cover beans with fresh water; simmer 60 to 90 minutes or until tender. Drain and set aside. Brown 1 pound ground beef with ¼ cup chopped onion and ¼ cup chopped green pepper. Drain. Add one 28-oz. can stewed tomatoes, Seasoning Packet and 1 to 2 cups water. Simmer 1 to 1½ hours. Add beans and simmer 30 to 60 more minutes. Serves 6.

Seasoning Packet:

1½ t. paprika
1 t. cumin
1 t. chili powder
1 t. oregano

½ t. turmeric
½ t. pepper
½ t. red pepper flakes
⅛ t. cayenne pepper

Combine all ingredients in a plastic zipping bag.

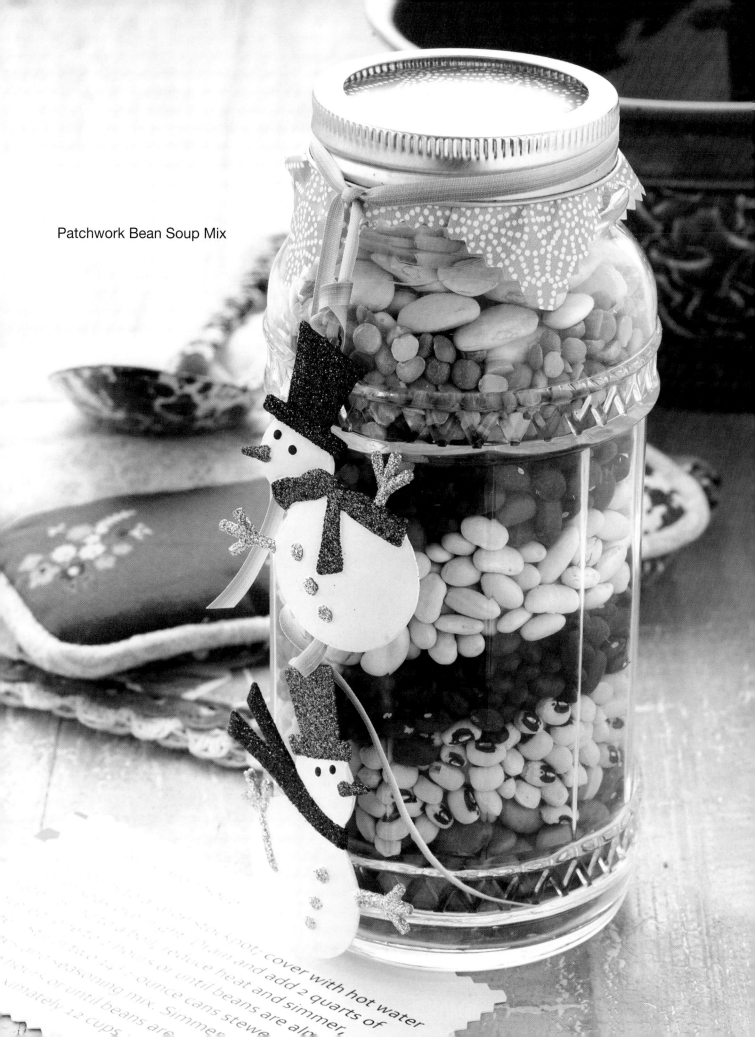

Patchwork Bean Soup Mix

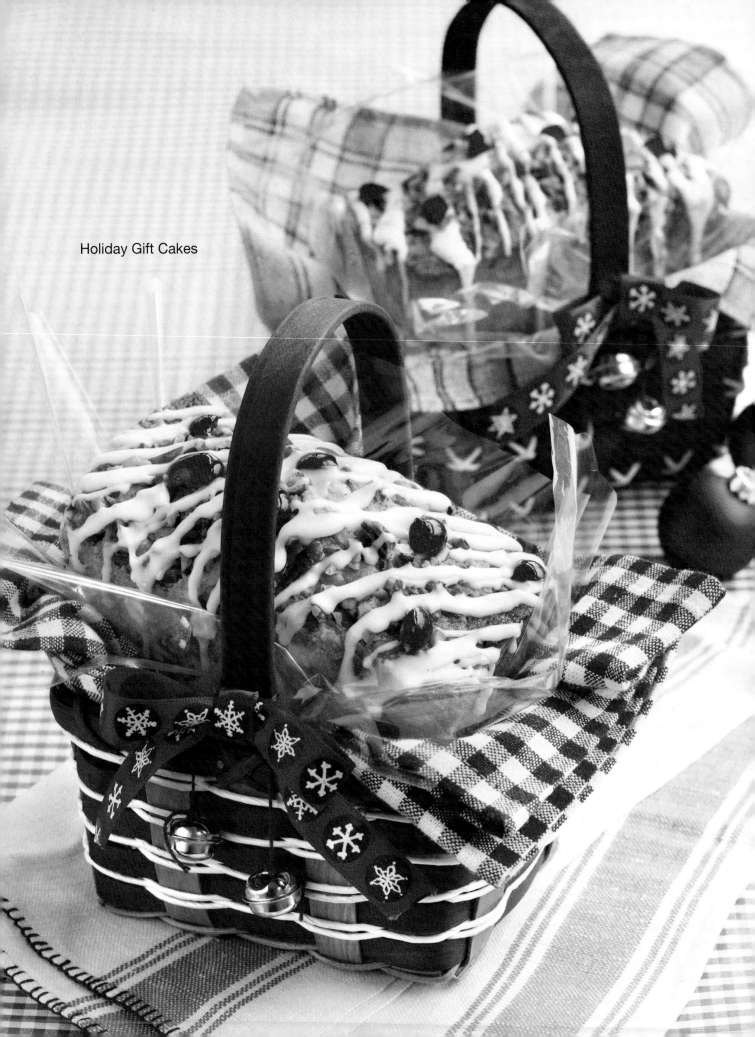

Holiday Gift Cakes

Holiday Gift Cakes

8-oz. pkg. cream cheese, softened
1 c. butter, softened
1½ c. sugar
1½ t. vanilla extract
4 eggs
2¼ c. cake flour, sifted and divided
1½ t. baking powder

8-oz. jar maraschino cherries, well-
  drained and chopped
1 c. pecans, finely chopped and divided
1½ c. powdered sugar, sifted
2 T. milk
Garnishes: red or green maraschino
  cherry and pecan halves

Thoroughly blend cream cheese, butter, sugar and vanilla. Add eggs, one at a time, mixing well after each addition. Sift together 2 cups flour and baking powder. Gradually add sifted flour mixture to batter. Dredge cherries and ½ cup pecans with remaining ¼ cup flour; fold into batter. Grease 4 (3"x5½") loaf pans; sprinkle with remaining ½ cup pecans. Pour batter into pans. Bake at 325 degrees for 45 minutes, or until toothpick tests clean. Cool 5 minutes; remove from pans. To prepare glaze, combine powdered sugar and milk. Add more milk, if needed, for drizzling consistency. Drizzle glaze over top and sides of cake. Garnish with cherry and pecan halves, as desired. Makes 4 small loaves.

Friendship Scone Mix

1¾ c. all-purpose flour
1 T. baking powder
½ t. salt

1 c. quick-cooking oats, uncooked
½ c. chopped walnuts
⅓ c. mini semi-sweet chocolate chips

Substitute ½ cup sweetened, dried cranberries or ½ teaspoon orange zest in place of the mini chocolate chips for variety.

Sift together first 3 ingredients in a large mixing bowl; stir in remaining ingredients. Mix well. Store in an airtight container in a cool, dry place. Makes 3½ cups mix. For gift-giving, attach the following instructions: Place scone mix in a large mixing bowl; cut in ½ cup butter until mixture resembles coarse crumbs. In a separate bowl, whisk ¼ cup milk with one egg. Add to crumb mixture; stir just until moistened. Knead gently on a lightly floured surface 8 to 10 times; pat dough into an 8-inch circle on a lightly greased baking sheet. Cut into 8 wedges; do not separate. Bake at 375 degrees for 10 to 12 minutes, or until golden. Cut wedges again and serve warm. Makes 8.

Santa Claus Cookie Pops

Put one at each place setting.

1 c. sugar
½ c. shortening
2 T. milk
1 egg
1½ t. vanilla extract, divided
2 c. all-purpose flour
1 t. baking powder
½ t. baking soda
½ t. salt

sugar
16 wooden ice-cream sticks
1½ c. powdered sugar
2 to 3 T. water
¼ c. red decorating sugar
1 c. shredded coconut
16 miniature marshmallows
32 raisins
16 red cinnamon candies

Beat together sugar and shortening. Beat in milk, egg and one teaspoon vanilla. Stir in flour, baking powder, baking soda and salt. Shape dough into 1¼-inch balls. Place balls 2 inches apart on a baking sheet. Insert a stick into the side of each dough ball, and flatten with the bottom of a glass dipped in sugar. Bake at 350 degrees for 8 to 10 minutes, or until cookies are golden. Let cool on baking sheet 2 minutes. Remove from baking sheet and cool on a wire rack.

In a small bowl, combine powdered sugar and remaining ½ teaspoon vanilla; add water, one teaspoon at a time, until spreadable. Spread frosting on top ⅓ for a hat and on bottom ⅓ for a beard, one cookie at a time. Sprinkle red sugar for a hat and coconut on beard. Press on a marshmallow for tassel of hat, raisins for eyes and a cinnamon candy for nose. Makes 16 cookies.

Pignoli (Italian cookies)

This crunchy little cookie is perfect alongside a dish of spumoni ice cream or a cup of cappuccino.

1 lb. almond paste
1¼ c. sugar

4 egg whites
3½ c. pine nuts or slivered almonds

Break almond paste into pieces and place in a mixing bowl with sugar. Beat with an electric mixer to crumble paste and sugar until evenly combined. In a separate bowl, beat egg whites to soft peaks. Gradually fold egg whites into the almond mixture. Place nuts in a shallow bowl. Roll the dough into one-inch balls and press each ball into the nuts, gently turning to coat evenly. Place one-inch apart on a greased baking sheet. Bake at 350 degrees for 15 minutes, or until light golden in color. Cool 5 minutes on the pan before transferring to a rack. Store in an airtight container. Makes about 3 dozen.

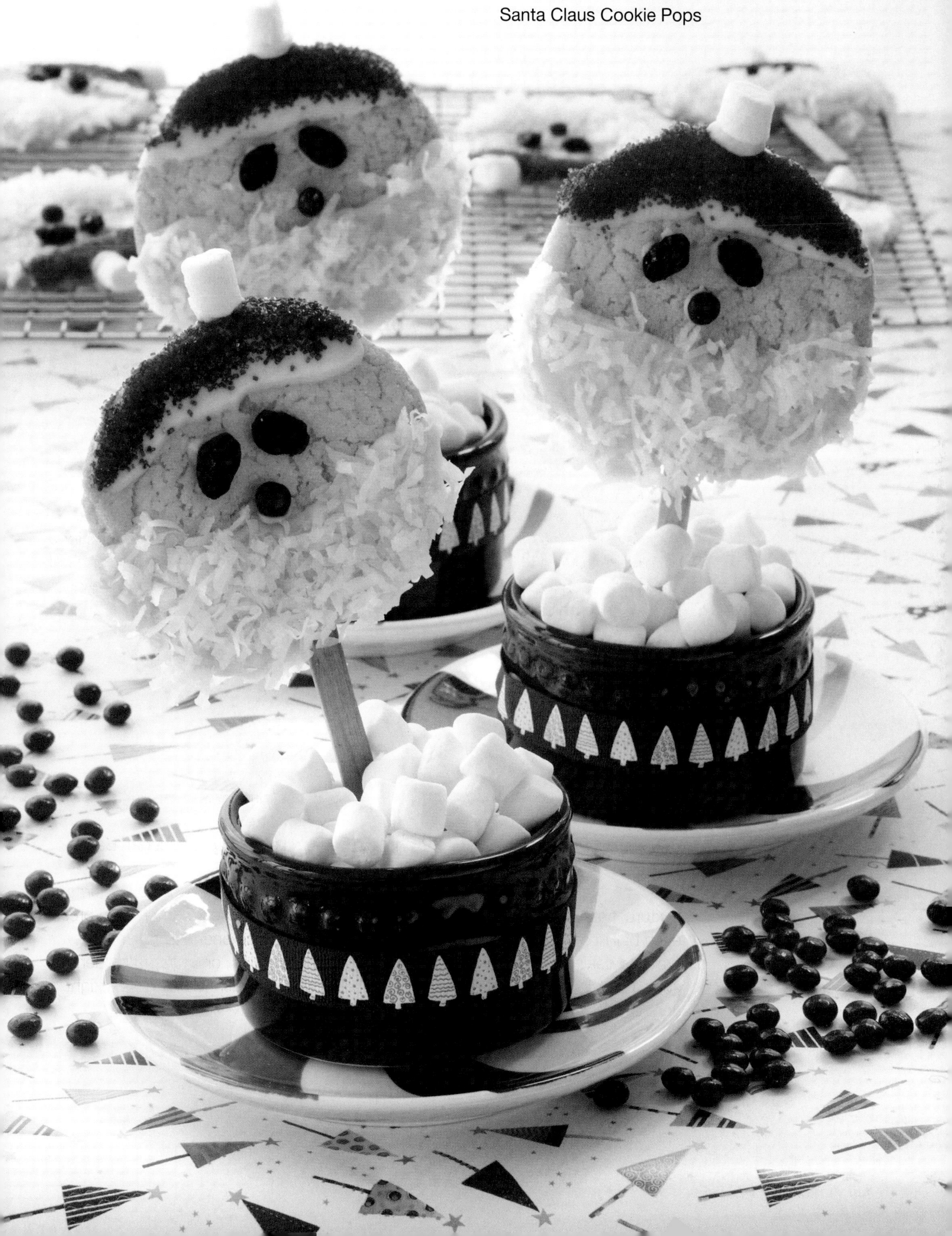

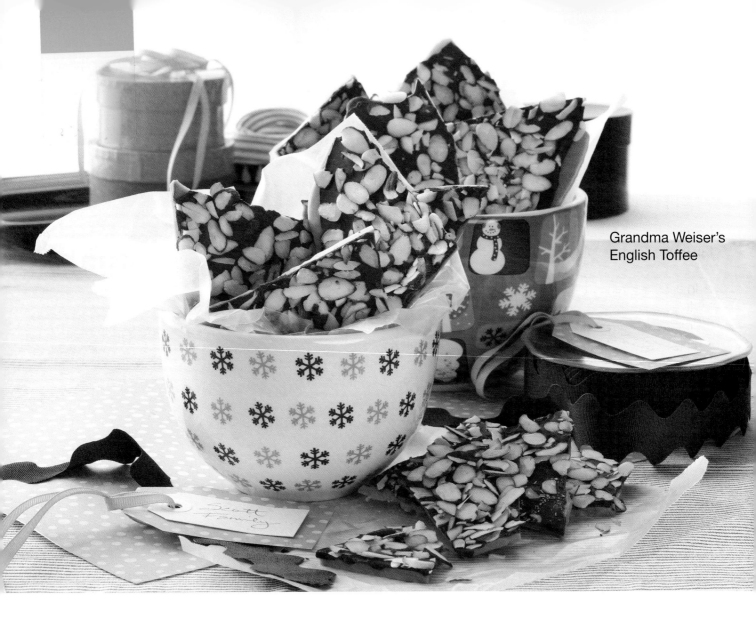

Grandma Weiser's
English Toffee

Grandma Weiser's English Toffee

Share this favorite
family recipe.

1 c. butter
1 c. sugar
1 T. light corn syrup

2 T. water
1 c. chocolate chips
1 c. almonds, sliced

In a heavy saucepan, combine all ingredients except chocolate chips and nuts. Stirring constantly, cook over medium heat until candy thermometer reads 300 degrees or until candy is thick and golden. Spread on a greased baking sheet, and then sprinkle with chocolate chips. Spread chips evenly until melted and top is completely covered. Sprinkle with almond pieces and refrigerate to set. Break into pieces before serving. Makes about one pound.

Crunchy Caramel Snack Mix

3 c. chocolate puffed corn cereal
3 c. bite-size square oat cereal
2 c. small pretzel twists
1 c. unsalted peanuts
1 c. brown sugar, packed

½ c. butter
¼ c. light corn syrup
¼ t. baking soda
¼ t. cream of tartar
½ t. vanilla extract

Sweet and crunchy…a wonderful combination!

In a lightly greased 13"x9" pan, combine cereals, pretzels and peanuts; set aside. In a saucepan, combine brown sugar, butter and corn syrup. Cook and stir over medium heat until butter melts and mixture comes to a boil. Cook without stirring for 4 minutes. Remove from heat; stir in baking soda and cream of tartar. Stir in vanilla. Pour over cereal mixture. Bake at 300 degrees for 30 minutes, stirring after 15 minutes. Transfer to large shallow pan. Cool. Store in an airtight container. Makes 10 cups.

Comet's White Chocolate Crunch

(pictured on page 140)

10-oz. pkg. mini pretzels
5 c. doughnut-shaped oat cereal
5 c. bite-size crispy corn cereal squares
2 c. peanuts

16-oz. pkg. candy-coated chocolates
2 (12-oz.) pkgs. white chocolate chips
3 T. oil

A favorite of children and reindeer everywhere!

Combine first 5 ingredients in a very large bowl; set aside. Melt chocolate chips with oil in a double boiler; stir until smooth. Pour over cereal mixture; mix well. Spread mixture equally onto 3 wax paper-lined baking sheets; allow to cool. Break into bite-size pieces; store in airtight containers. Makes 5 quarts.

~~~~~~

"MY BEST HOLIDAY MEMORY RELATES TO GIFT-GIVING. When my children were little, I didn't want them growing up to be self-centered. So I began a holiday tradition of choosing the name of a young child from the "angel tree" at church. With the understanding that there would be one less present for them, I would take the children shopping to buy gifts for our angel child. Watching the joy on their faces as they rushed around the store looking for presents touched me. They were so excited to know that they helped to make another child's Christmas brighter! In a world where people tend to put themselves first, my family is blessed by this tradition, which we've continued for more than 14 years."

Korbi Slocum
Johnstown, PA

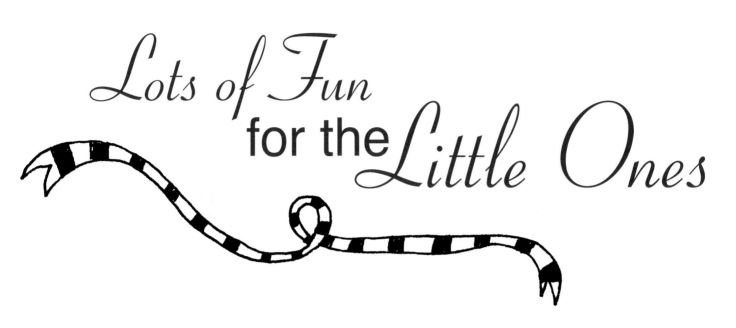

Lots of Fun for the Little Ones

Best-Ever Chocolate Finger Paint

For the budding artist in all of us, the tastiest finger paint of all! Try vanilla or butterscotch, too…

**4-oz. pkg. instant chocolate
    pudding mix
2 c. milk
white paper**

Prepare pudding mix according to package directions. Let the pudding set until thick. Paint on white paper with pudding. Let masterpieces dry for several hours.

Nutty Snowmen

Make a whole bowl-ful to hang on the tree!

**Unsalted peanuts-in-the-shell
White acrylic paint
Small paint brush
Fine-tip black permanent marker
Fine-tip red permanent marker
Red yarn
Safety scissors**

1. Pour peanuts out on a newspaper and let the kids paint 'em white. Let peanuts dry and eat a handful of unpainted ones while you wait!
2. Use your markers to draw on eyes, nose and mouth...add buttons on the front of the snow peanuts, too!
3. Cut a 5" piece of yarn and tie it around your snowman's neck. All done!

P.S. Thread a thin ribbon or fishing line through the back of the yarn to make a hanger.

Magic Reindeer Dust

Secret Ingredients:
Oats
Glitter
Pint-size canning jars with lids

Secret How-To Instructions:
1. Fill jars with oats, sprinkling a little glitter throughout.
2. Top jars with lids and attach a copy of "Magic Reindeer Dust" instructions (below). You might glue it on jar, if preferred.

Instructions:
Come December 24th, as Santa flies here from the North,
Here's what you do, it isn't hard
Just sprinkle this stuff in your yard…

The sparkles draw old Santa near
And oats attract his 8 reindeer…

Then you just wait, they're on their way.

P.S. Happy Holiday!

Santa Shakes

Make up a batch of this cool yogurt shake to refresh the kids after they finish making nutty snowmen!

2 c. chocolate milk
2 c. chocolate frozen yogurt, softened
2 c. crushed ice

½ c. chocolate syrup
Garnish: crushed peppermints,
candy canes or peppermint sticks

   In a blender, combine all ingredients except garnish. Process until well blended. Sprinkle with crushed peppermint and serve in tall glasses with a candy cane.

Nutty Cocoa

4 c. milk
½ c. chocolate-flavored drink mix
¼ c. creamy peanut butter
½ t. vanilla
mini marshmallows

In a saucepan, combine chocolate drink mix with ½ c. milk until well blended. Mix in peanut butter, and add remaining milk. Heat cocoa 'til almost boiling. Pour into mugs and top with marshmallows.

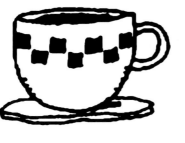

Chocolate Stirring Spoons

These are great for hot chocolate!

12-oz. pkg. semi-sweet chocolate chips
2 t. shortening
35 to 45 heavy plastic spoons

Line baking sheets with parchment paper. Place chocolate chips in a microwave-safe bowl; microwave on medium power for 2 minutes or until melted, stirring every 30 seconds. To thin chocolate, add shortening; gently stir. Dip each plastic spoon in chocolate mixture to cover the bowl of the spoon; place on parchment paper for chocolate to set. Cool thoroughly before wrapping. Makes 35 to 45 spoons.

Rainbow Toast

Is it more fun to make it or eat it?

Bread
Food coloring
Clean paintbrushes or cotton swabs

Place 4 drops of food coloring in each section of a muffin tin. Add 1 to 2 T. water to dilute colors. Dip paintbrush into food coloring and paint designs on bread. Place in toaster and toast. Butter & eat up!

Tortilla Treats

A perfect snack for your hungry young builders!

Flour tortillas
Peanut butter
Mini chocolate chips

Simply spread the peanut butter on the open tortilla. Sprinkle chocolate chips on the peanut butter, then roll up the tortilla. Scrumptious!

Mary Elizabeth's Super-Duper Play Dough

Great-smelling dough, perfect birthday party favors!

2½ c. all-purpose flour
½ c. salt
1 T. powdered alum
2 pkgs. unsweetened fruit-flavored
    drink mix

2 T. oil
2 c. boiling water

Mix together flour, salt, alum & drink mix in a large mixing bowl. Add oil. Pour boiling water over flour mixture; stir until well combined. Knead dough until smooth. Store in airtight plastic bag or covered container.

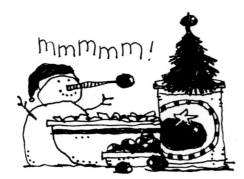

Pizza Cobbler

An easy and delicious snack!

Pizza sauce
1 can refrigerator biscuits
1⅓ c. shredded Mozzarella cheese

Grease an 8-inch square pan with vegetable oil spray. Place about ¼ of the pizza sauce in bottom of the pan. Cut each biscuit into 4 pieces. Roll biscuit pieces into balls and place in pan on top of sauce. Pour remaining sauce over biscuits. Sprinkle with Mozzarella cheese. Bake at 400 degrees for 15 to 20 minutes.

"Running Back" Popcorn 'N Peanuts

You'll go "running back" for more!

½ c. honey
¼ c. butter
6 c. popped popcorn
1 c. salted peanuts

Heat honey and butter until blended. Mix popcorn and peanuts in a large bowl, and stir in honey butter mixture. Spread mixture into 2 large pans. Bake at 350 degrees for 10 minutes.

Gift Giving & Packaging Ideas

Nifty Gifties

Those clear plastic bags that you use to pipe icing also make fun holders for holiday goodies! Fill them with…

- Red, green & yellow jelly beans (layered or all mixed up)
- Your favorite caramel corn
- Layers of different dried fruits
- Mixed nuts
- Snack mixes
- Red & green sugared jellied candies
- Chocolates

Finish your nifty gifties with rubber-stamped tags!

Giving Ideas

Give your gift tags & recipe direction cards a holiday sparkle…glue a sprinkle of glitter in the corner of tags & cards with easy-to-use spray adhesive. Clear crystal glitter is pretty, pretty, pretty.

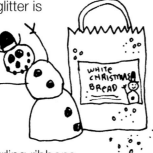

A white paper tote bag with a recipe card glued on the front will hold a merry mix…just add a piece of white tissue & a cascade of white curling ribbons… a wonderful white Christmas gift

Cookies

Here's a great way to package cookies for gift-giving…easy, elegant & keeps the cookies from crumbling!

- Find some clear glasses that are fairly tall (you know, the kind you sip those good, fruity, frosty drinks out of)…
- Now bake round cookies just a bit smaller than the glass in circumference…drop the cookies in carefully, stacking them inside the glass on top of each other 'til the glass is full.
- Finish it off with a wired ribbon tied around the glass vertically.
- Add a sticker on the glass, over the ribbon, for a last touch…you're ready to deliver!

Iced Jars

…so simple! Begin with a clean clear jar, any size. Just draw a design on the outside of the jar with fingernail polish…any color or clear. Now just sprinkle the wet polish with plain old table salt or glitter. Let dry, then use as a sparkling gift jar for a candle or any little favor…you are just too clever!

Mittens

Pack a small plastic bag full of treats and pop it inside a mitten or glove for a holiday gift. Shop after-season for on-sale mittens for next year! You can even personalize a mitten with a monogram in brightly colored yarn.

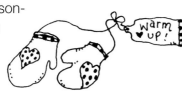

Handsome Holders...Cute Containers

No matter what you call them, don't forget that the presentation is half the fun of the present!

Jars can be easily recycled into terrific gift containers.

Cut a fabric circle and top a canning jar with it, securing it in place with ribbon, raffia, or even good old twine. You can fill it with homemade goodies, potpourri or store-bought candles.

A Fun Idea

Remember those old-time wire milk bottle carriers? Find enough old bottles or jars to fill it...and fill each bottle with a different colorful hard candy! Carry it off to your favorite friend with a sweet tooth.

Fun Things to Do with Santa's Hat

1. Fill it up with plastic zipping bags of homebaked goodies and deliver it to a neighbor...ring the doorbell, drop the hat and run!

2. Hang a row of Santa Hats on your mantel, just like stockings...personalize each one with a monogram, or tie on a name tag with a bright ribbon and a jingle bell.

3. Use a fuzzy red Santa hat under every plate at Christmas dinner... perfect placemats! And just for fun, tuck a personal letter from Santa into each hat, or a gift certificate!

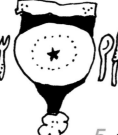

4. A Christmas bouquet of holly and greenery looks pretty in an upside-down Santa hat on a door or tacked on a gate.

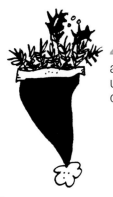

5. Make a very personal gift "basket" in a Santa hat:

- Fill with dog bones for a favorite pup.
- Balls of red & white yarn & knitting needles slip right inside a hat for Aunt Sue.
- Golf balls, tees and a glove are great hat-stuffers for a golf enthusiast!

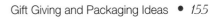

12 Days of Christmas Menus

1

Holiday Open House
SERVES 6 to 8

Caramelized Pecans
(page 10)*
Festive Cheese Ball
(page 12)
Barbeque Meatballs
(page 17)*
Artichoke-Parmesan
Squares *(page 16)*
Sonia's Holiday Sangria
(page 18)

2

Ladies' Luncheon
SERVES 8 to 10

Christmas Luncheon
Crabmeat Bisque *(page 79)**
Three Layer Ruby Red
Salad *(page 95)*
Savory Herb Biscuits
(page 105)

3

Kids' Classroom Christmas Party
SERVES 24 to 30

Santa Claus Cookie Pops
(page 146)*
Macadamia Cheesy Puffs
(page 16)
grapes and strawberries
hot chocolate, juice, or milk

7

Grab It and Go Breakfast
SERVES 12

Christmas Cranberry
Muffins *(page 99)* or Country
Morning Maple Muffins
(page 22)
Savory Brunch Bread
(page 25)
Chilled Vanilla Coffee
(page 19)**

8

Quick and Easy Lunch
SERVES 6 to 8

Penne Pasta with
Tomatoes *(page 38)*
Mandarin Orange Salad
(page 92)*
bread sticks

9

Make-Ahead Brunch
SERVES 6 to 8

Overnight Apple French
Toast *(page 22)* or Holiday
Quiche *(page 27)*
fresh fruit
coffee, milk, or juice
(see sunrise punch tip, page 26)

* *Double recipe*

** *Triple recipe*

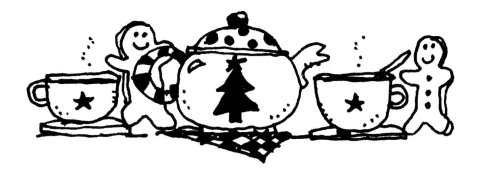

4

Desserts Mixer

SERVES 12

Pecan Pie Bars *(page 121)*
Marbled Pumpkin
Cheesecake *(page 136)*
Holiday Hot Fudge Dessert
(page 139)
Hot Spiced Wine Punch
(page 19)

5

Italian Night

SERVES 12

Spaghetti Casserole
(page 47)
green salad
Make-Ahead Dinner Rolls
(page 106)

6

Soup for Supper

SERVES 4 to 6

Burgundy Beef Stew
(page 81)
Sour Cream Cornbread
(page 106)
Holly's Chocolate Silk Pie
(page 133)

10

Christmas Eve Dinner

SERVES 4 to 6

Parmesan-Onion Soup
(page 73)
Slow-Cooker Turkey &
Dressing *(page 43)*
Green Beans Supreme
(page 59)
Orange-Maple Glazed
Carrots *(page 86)*
German Chocolate Cake
(page 126)
Old-Fashioned Eggnog
(page 66)

11

Santa Snacks

SERVES Santa Claus...and a
few reindeer, too!

Crunchy Caramel Snack
Mix *(page 149)*
Grandma Weiser's English
Toffee *(page 148)*
Gingerbread Babies
(page 113)
Don't forget the milk!

12

Christmas Day Meal

SERVES 8 to 10

Crunchy Granny Smith
Salad *(page 94)*
Pork Crown Roast with
Fruit Glaze *(page 56)*
Holiday Sweet Potatoes
(page 61)
Broccoli-Cheddar
Casserole *(page 84)*
Christmas Tree Pull-Apart
Rolls *(page 103)*
Maple-Spice Pecan Pie
(page 65)

Recipe Index

Our Story

Back in 1984, we were next-door neighbors raising our families in the little town of Delaware, Ohio. We were two moms with small children looking for a way to do what we loved and stay home with the kids too. We shared a love of home cooking and making memories with family & friends. After many a conversation over the backyard fence, **Gooseberry Patch** was born.

We put together the first catalog & cookbooks at our kitchen tables and packed boxes from the basement, enlisting the help of our loved ones wherever we could. From that little family, we've grown to include an amazing group of creative folks who love cooking, decorating and creating as much as we do.

Hard to believe it's been over 25 years since those kitchen-table days. Today, we're best known for our homestyle, family-friendly cookbooks. We love hand-picking the recipes and are tickled to share our inspiration, ideas and more with you! One thing's for sure, we couldn't have done it without our friends all across the country. Whether you've been along for the ride from the begining or are just discovering us, welcome to our family!

Your friends at Gooseberry Patch

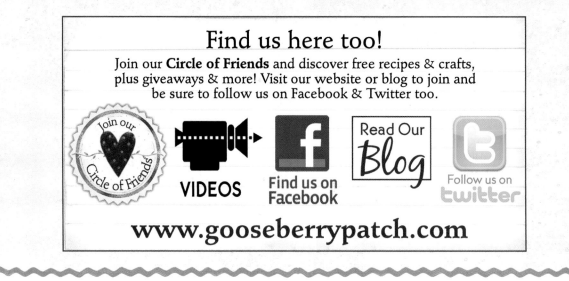

Find us here too!

Join our **Circle of Friends** and discover free recipes & crafts, plus giveaways & more! Visit our website or blog to join and be sure to follow us on Facebook & Twitter too.

Join our Circle of Friends

VIDEOS

Find us on Facebook

Read Our Blog

Follow us on twitter

www.gooseberrypatch.com